THE
BODY'S
KEEPERS

THE
BODY'S
KEEPERS

*A Social History of Kidney Failure
and Its Treatments*

PAUL L. KIMMEL, M.D.

MAYO CLINIC PRESS

MAYO CLINIC PRESS
200 First St. SW
Rochester, MN 55905
mcpress.mayoclinic.org

The information in this book is true and complete to the best of our knowledge. This book is intended as an informative guide for those wishing to learn more about health issues. It is not intended to replace, countermand or conflict with advice given to you by your own physician. The ultimate decision concerning your care should be made between you and your doctor. Information in this book is offered with no guarantees. The author and publisher disclaim all liability in connection with the use of this book.

The views expressed are the author's personal views, and do not necessarily reflect the policy or position of Mayo Clinic.

To stay informed about Mayo Clinic Press, please subscribe to our free e-newsletter at mcpress.mayoclinic.org or follow us on social media.

For bulk sales to employers, member groups and health-related companies, contact Mayo Clinic at SpecialSalesMayoBooks@mayo.edu.

Proceeds from the sale of every book benefit important medical research and education at Mayo Clinic.

Jacket design by Olya Kirilyuk. Front cover images: kidneys © Channarong Pherngjanda / shutterstock.com, background texture © Lana Veshta / shutterstock.com

Library of Congress Cataloging-in-Publication Data

Names: Kimmel, Paul L., author.
Title: The body's keepers : a social history of kidney failure and its
   treatments / Paul L. Kimmel, M.D.
Description: First edition. | Rochester, MN : Mayo Clinic Press, 2024. |
   Includes bibliographical references and index.
Identifiers: LCCN 2023028519 (print) | LCCN 2023028520 (ebook) | ISBN
   9798887700304 (hardcover) | ISBN 9798887701714 (epub)
Subjects: LCSH: Acute renal failure—United States—History—Popular works.
   | Acute renal failure—Treatment—United States—History—Popular works.
   | Hemodialysis—United States—History—Popular works. |
   Kidneys—Transplantation—United States—History—Popular works.
Classification: LCC RC918.R4 K56 2024 (print) | LCC RC918.R4 (ebook) |
   DDC 616.6/14—dc23/eng/20230706
LC record available at https://lccn.loc.gov/2023028519
LC ebook record available at https://lccn.loc.gov/2023028520

Printed in U.S.A.

First edition: 2024

This book is dedicated to my parents and sister, as well as my wife, without whom nothing would have been possible. The book also exists because of and for my teachers, students, and patients, who taught me more than I can ever know.

CONTENTS

Kidneys were in his mind as he moved about . . .

James Joyce, *Ulysses*

PROLOGUE

I was inspired to write this book because I have devoted most of my life to the study of a remarkable organ that almost nobody understands and to the care of patients affected by its poor workings. In contrast to the brain, the heart, and perhaps the guts, all we usually think about the kidneys is that they make urine—a bit of an inconvenience for older men and women, caretakers of the elderly, and travelers as well as for parents of infants and young children.

But when the kidneys don't work, whether we're old or young, we die unless we receive heroic treatment and therapies based on new, expensive technologies. These were not available until about seventy years ago and were then crude, experimental, and relatively scarce. Kidney disease affects a huge swath of the population—variably estimated in the United States to involve from 9 to 15% of adults, or up to 37 million people. For much of the world, kidney disease is the culmination of the endemic scourges of humankind—tuberculosis, malaria, schistosomiasis, HIV, and other parasitic as well as viral infections. These are often diseases of poverty and lack of public health interventions. But ultimately societal factors play dominant roles in determining health outcomes, including the consequences of kidney ailments. Many low-income countries do not have the resources to provide expensive life-sustaining treatments to their citizens who suffer from advanced kidney disease. And now we know that the new plague, COVID-19, causes kidney disease as well.

In the U.S., kidney disease is also often the result of indigence, poor sanitary conditions, and lack of access to adequate medical care. The two most common causes of chronic kidney disease (or, as doctors refer to it, CKD) nationally are hypertension and diabetes. Hypertension (or high blood pressure), although quite common, is often undetected and untreated, especially in underrepresented, underserved minority populations. An epidemic of obesity has fueled a striking increase in the number of people developing diabetes in the U.S. and globally, a byproduct of the economic success of the Western world that has provided easy access to food and diminished our reliance on physical labor. Both conditions markedly increase the risk of developing kidney disease in those who are already ill, magnifying personal losses as well as burdens, not to mention increasing health-care costs. In the U.S. end-stage renal disease (ESRD) program—which provides, at the cost of tens of billions of dollars, dialysis and kidney transplantation for those who have contributed to the Social Security system—African Americans are three times more likely to be enrolled than White patients. This inequality, however, is not the sole result of poverty or lack of access to care. Over the past decade, as a result of advances in the science of genetics, exemplified by the federally funded Human Genome Project, we have learned that people of African descent have inherited gene variants that magnify their risk of developing kidney disease by extraordinary levels. These adaptations, which may have protected people from parasitic diseases on the African continent, have become extremely maladaptive in Western societies, rendering those at risk susceptible to developing end-stage kidney disease (ESKD) as they age. Yet paradoxically, African Americans in the U.S. continue to have less access to kidney transplantation, the most desirable ESRD treatment, compared to patients of other race and ethnic groups.

The kidneys have been part of our collective consciousness since at least biblical times. The kidneys are mentioned eleven times in the Five Books of Moses, as both sacrificial items and the seat of some of humankind's most profound emotions. As biblical scholar Robert Alter opined, the kidney was the "organ of conscience."[1] That was long before classical, medieval, and Renaissance physicians and scientists identified the ureters as the connection between the kidneys and the bladder. These early investigators realized that the bladder was not the source of urine but merely its penultimate destination after its creation by the kidneys and subsequent transport through the ureters. The understanding of the excretory function of the kidney worked against its previous spiritual standing. The loftier aspects of emotional life were then assigned by the authors of the King James Version of the Bible to the "reins," after the Old French name for the kidneys. That ancient notion of the deep importance of the kidneys to an individual's personality persists in somewhat older bits of the English language. Shakespeare's 17th-century Falstaff is dismayed by the treatment he receives from the Windsor folk, treatment that "a man of my kidney" (in effect of his temperament, disposition, or standing) should never experience. In the 19th century, James Fenimore Cooper's and Benjamin Disraeli's use of the phrases "pretty much of the same kidney" and "but all of the right kidney," respectively, meaning the same sensibility or the right set of people, conveyed similar ideas. (We might now say, as the kidneys have lost their clout, that "she's a woman after my own heart.") Meanwhile, in Italy and England, investigators elucidated some of the less romantic inner workings of the organs.

Kidney disease, however, couldn't be easily or widely diagnosed until the latter half of the 19th century. Dr. Richard Bright, in Victorian London, linked anatomical disease of the kidneys with patients' symptoms, an important advance in medical science. Until then, how kidney disease manifested itself was unclear, really a conundrum of swelling and other complaints and maybe, if the doctor looked, or had the tools, abnormalities in the urine.

Since the diagnosis of kidney disease was difficult to make—and therefore its presence so obscure—we know little about pre–Victorian era people who had kidney disease. The legend of Mozart's death from uremia (or poisoning resulting in kidney failure) stands out in this regard. We do know Emily Dickinson died of kidney failure (because her death certificate so states), although how the diagnosis was made remains unknown. As kidney disease became better understood as a common affliction, however, the number of people who died with or from the illness has been astonishing. They include actresses Sarah Bernhardt, Jean Harlow, and Veronica Lake, showman Buffalo Bill Cody, playwright George Bernard Shaw, composer Cole Porter, pianist Art Tatum, and General Douglas MacArthur. For those who expired before 1973, the diagnosis of uremia was typically a death sentence. The ESRD program was enacted in the early 1970s through the joint efforts of Belding Scribner and other physicians in the new specialty of nephrology in coordination with patients who raised their voices in public, as well as through advocacy groups and specialty societies, with the help of politicians and considerable legislative legerdemain. The U.S. led the way for the entire world in providing therapy to patients with advanced chronic kidney disease. Since then, using differing implementation strategies and levels of commitment in different countries, therapies for ESRD have diffused across the globe, usefully allowing affected patients to live to a ripe old age.

More contemporary people who survived through ESRD care include Greta Garbo, Sandra Dee, Erma Bombeck, and Marion Barry, to name a few. Bobby Fischer and Bernie Madoff were among those who declined to start dialysis, resulting in their deaths. Howard Hughes, the seventy-year-old billionaire entrepreneur, aviator, and filmmaker, who endowed a medical foundation in his name that currently finances, among other endeavors, ongoing sophisticated research on the causes and treatment of kidney disease, paradoxically died in 1976 of kidney failure, with classic features of uremia, seemingly without taking advantage of contemporary strides in ESRD care. His kidney disease was attributed to the use of licit and illicit nephrotoxic drugs, including painkillers.

The death of the prolific and popular novelist James Michener in 1997, at the age of ninety, who voluntarily and of sound mind withdrew from dialysis after many years of successful treatment, brought to the attention of the public key considerations in the care of elderly ESRD patients, including the issues of participant quality of life and the high rates of discontinuation of therapy as a cause of death in the program.

Twentieth-century physiologists, such as Homer Smith, figured out the chemical measures of kidney function. Physicians found the appropriate laboratory tests and working with pathologists, using renal biopsies (where a doctor sticks a needle into the flank of a patient, engages some kidney tissue, pulls it out, and puts it on a slide for examination under the microscope) defined the various kinds of kidney diseases. Since the 1960s, the quest to establish diagnoses and define appropriate therapies has been in motion, as physicians and scientists have sought to determine the best treatment for the individual patient with a specific disease.

Many advances have subsequently been made over the last several decades. For instance, the HIV epidemic in the 1980s and 1990s shed much light on the ways in which kidneys may be injured, and these studies underpinned the understanding of genetic factors linked to kidney disease. Similarly, we learned from the coronavirus pandemic that the kidneys may become collateral damage of infection from that virus, in part because of a ubiquitous human protein that provides a portal for its introduction into the lungs while simultaneously playing a role in determining blood pressure levels and kidney functional changes. The pandemic has wreaked havoc on ESRD patients—halting kidney transplantation, delaying entry into dialysis programs, killing patients with advanced kidney disease, and magnifying the disparities in favorable outcomes between patients of different groups.

The Body's Keepers begins with the story of someone who developed kidney disease under extremely unlikely circumstances. His journey, however, includes considerations of almost every form of kidney disease and their treatments in existence today. The book ends with a perspective on the technologic advances made over the last seventy years that have revolutionized the quantity and quality of lives of patients with kidney disease today. However, big science functions in the context of government funding and regulations, big business imperatives, and corporate greed. An incredible technologic advance, the biosynthetic hormone and drug erythropoietin, truly a scientific tour de force, was marketed in a way that valued profits over patient survival. To right present and historic wrongs in the access to and outcomes of care for patients with advanced kidney disease from different socioeconomic, racial, and ethnic backgrounds, a concerted effort by health-care providers, policymakers, the pharmaceutical industry, patients, and the general public will have to emerge triumphantly.

The story is told, where possible, in the words of the protagonists. I have included the scientific writings of the investigators who performed critical studies and have highlighted the voices of patients who suffered from and surmounted the challenges of kidney disease. Science is a collaborative, competitive part of society, and in many cases, where the government is involved in funding programs or regulating the use of new medications, committees were formed to make decisions. Where committees have determined the outcomes that affect patients across the nation, I have listed the members and documented their deliberations, often in the notes, so the reader can decide if scientific and medical government reviews serve the populace. The funding sources for many of the scientific papers cited are also usually highlighted, since it is generally acknowledged that those who support research often anticipate financial gains from the resulting findings. When the funding comes from a corporate entity, potential conflicts of interest must be scrupulously evaluated by the reader.

The Body's Keepers focuses on acute kidney injury and the treatment of end-stage kidney disease by hemodialysis and kidney transplantation, primarily in the United States. Because of space limitations, much cannot be discussed, including polycystic kidney disease, diabetic kidney disease, glomerulonephritis, kidney stones, peritoneal dialysis, kidney biopsies, the kidney diseases of HIV infection, the chronic kidney disease of unknown etiology that has ravaged tropical agricultural communities, or 19th- and 20th-century pioneers who sought to understand the workings of the kidneys. The book is informed by the idea that race is a social construct rather than a biologic entity.

There are a lot of acronyms and abbreviations in medicine, so please avail yourself of the glossary at the end of the book, with many helpful definitions, including the abbreviations for medical journals, medical societies and advocacy groups, and federal agencies.

I hope you enjoy this history of the treatment of diseases of an unsung organ. If you are as fascinated as I am by the workings of this marvelous organ and the successes and challenges of current treatments for its diseases by the end of the book, I will have accomplished my goals as fully as when I led a group of young physicians through the hospital in the care of patients whose kidneys were damaged. As classic authors suggested, let's begin in medias res, in the late 1960s.

1

***

TWO ROOMMATES AND FOUR KIDNEYS

We met the first day of college. As Kevin's father drove him up to Phelps Gate in a battered yellowish 1963 VW Bug, I called out a noncommittal greeting. "Where are you from, Nu Yawk or Philadelphia?" Kevin replied. Our friendship was instantly sealed.

Kevin was interested in music, had an expensive Ampex reel-to-reel tape recorder, and forty or fifty tapes that he had carefully harvested from broadcasts and records. He had an AR turntable, a McIntosh amplifier, and powerful speakers. I was deeply envious. I had a clock radio.

We ended up in different rooms on different floors of the same entryway of Farnam Hall. Kevin's coursework included art history and music. I took Biology 10, Math 15, and Chem 14. We enrolled in the same English 29 seminar, "The Epic." The year was spent going to classes, writing papers, staying up late at our desks, falling asleep in club chairs in reading rooms, holing up in study carrels at Sterling Library, walking miles up snowy slopes to Science Hill, attending teas and seminars with visiting academic and cultural celebrities, driving to women's colleges, going to mixers where we hadn't known any of the visitors, playing bridge, and drinking alcohol of various colors in elegant and low places and at inappropriate times. By the beginning of sophomore year we were roommates.

By senior year, Kevin had developed a special interest in architecture, building ornamentation, and decoration. He wrote a paper on the architecture of the Pentagon and followed this with a senior thesis on the influence of governmental architecture in Washington, D.C., from the Civil War to World War II. Kevin set his sights on a career in public service and headed to Washington, D.C., to begin work with the U.S. government. Unable to balance the myriad requirements of coursework, eight hours of lab work a week, an embryonal social life, and a taste for extracurricular activities, including concert-going and cinema attendance, I switched from a biology to an English major. I did not look at it as a defeat. Rather, it was a reflection of differential interests and aptitudes. I inveigled my way into medical school in New York through an interview that focused on Fellini's filmography, Shaker furniture, and trends in contemporary art rather than on the details regarding my organic chemistry grades. I graduated from college—on time, by golly, by the skin of my teeth. My diploma featured the magic words *cum laude*.

Medical school was not easy for me, possibly because of my lack of scientific background comparable to my classmates' high level of preparation. Perhaps an inclination to spend time at the cinema, theater, and opera house rather than in the library had something to do with it. Nevertheless, those first two years were busy, focused on taking examinations, failing examinations, and having to remaster the material. This intensive and rather inefficient approach to education meant that real free time was limited. I did not have sufficient time or funds to visit Kevin in Washington, D.C. We did see each other about once a year if Kevin came to New York to listen to an opera at the Met.

I had wanted to be a psychiatrist. I envisioned myself in a Park Avenue office, in a tweed jacket with leather elbow patches, interpreting the nuances of speech that would explain my patients' conflicts and their inability to achieve love and success. I would use these found chunks of knowledge to repair my patients' battered egos, souls, and lives. Plan A was scotched when I took my first clinical rotation on the Bellevue Hospital psychiatric wards and encountered patients with schizophrenia who were either so highly tranquilized with gram doses of Thorazine that they appeared to be actors in a horror movie or violent enough to scale barriers and attack staff members in the small, cluttered nursing stations. I'd had enough academic training and clinical experience to understand that a rotation in psychiatry had made me profoundly depressed. In an unusual case of considering my feelings rather than my thoughts, I realized I would never be able to make it through a psychiatric internship. Forget about a residency.

Luckily, there was a plan B. In the first year of medical school, I attended physiology lectures, which began with the study of the heart and its functions. Physiology had great appeal. Unlike those of anatomy, histology, and biochemistry, physiologic concepts could be apprehended from first principles. With a knowledge of limited basic facts, approaching a complex system with logical inferences, one could predict the consequences. I thought physiology must be similar to mechanical or electrical engineering. But I was unprepared for the beauty of the kidneys.

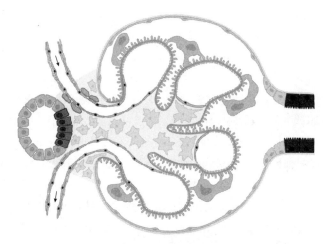

Figure 1a. The glomerulus is the filtering portion of the nephron. It is a modified, ramified set of blood vessels, in which plasma may cross the blood barrier to move into Bowman's space, where it becomes "glomerular filtrate." Bowman's space becomes the beginning of the tubular system of the nephron, starting with the proximal tubule. Glomeruli come off the afferent arteriole and re-emerge into the efferent arteriole, where blood will re-enter the renal and ultimately the general circulation. (The direction of blood flow is shown by arrows.) The glomeruli are composed of three types of cells—the endothelial (blood vessel), mesangial (multifunctional and support), and epithelial cells. Capillary loops, covered by podocytes (a specialized form of epithelial cell), are where filtration takes place. Image provided with permission of the Kidney Precision Medicine Project Consortium.

Each kidney serves as a filter of the blood, retaining important chemicals and proteins and removing the toxins and impurities that were consumed on a daily basis or that resulted from the breakdown of ingested foods. The kidneys also excrete the byproducts of the activities of the different cells of the body. If we are what we eat, the kidneys do an almost exact job of excreting the detritus of the daily diet. To do this, the kidneys filter the equivalent of up to two hundred quarts of fluid a day. The kidneys are able to separate the fluid portion of the blood into a compartment that ultimately forms the urine while relegating the red and white blood cells and all the important proteins circulating in the plasma to a pathway whereby these critical blood components are protected and retained by the body. The kidneys are so good at their work that normally almost no protein is found in the urine. I learned, fascinated, that the kidney tubules are able to transport bulk fluid in their early segments back into the blood after filtration without any change in their chemical composition. At the end of the tubules, which would eventually form a large conduit for urine to exit the kidney and enter the ureter, the kidney is able to separate ions like potassium, sodium, calcium, phosphate, and magnesium, so what is needed by the body is retained and what is excess ends up in the sewers. I thought it was an organ with a brain! And I was amazed at the elegance of the linkage between its structure and function. Before starting medical school, I had no interest in these obscure organs located in the middle of the body where low back pain plagues middle-aged office workers.

In the second year, I learned that there is a disease, primarily affecting children, in which the natural barrier that prevents the appearance of protein in the filtered fluid is abnormal. A simple clinical feature emerged. The suffering children had loads of protein in their urine. The consequences for the patient, however, were devastating. Parents were horrified to see their children swollen, with gallons of water sequestered in their faces, in their bellies, and in their ankles and feet. The level of the protective protein, albumin, in their blood was dangerously low. They had sky-high levels of cholesterol and might have abnormal blood clots, infections, or even heart attacks. The disease could appear out of the blue. One day the child would be perfectly normal. The next she might be a swollen, monstrous caricature of her former healthy self. Kidney tissue taken by the new technique of renal biopsy inspected under the

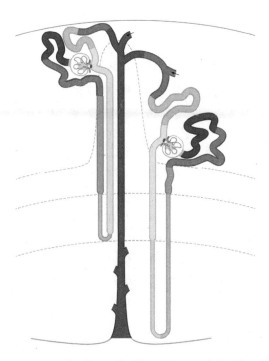

Figure 1b. The tubules process the glomerular filtrate, in normal situations, in response to the needs of the body. The tubules are aligned in sequential segments (such as the proximal tubule, loop of Henle, and collecting duct) composed of different cell types, which have different physical-chemical properties and unique responses to different hormones. Much of the energy of the tubular system, used to transport water, ions, and molecules across their membranes, is embedded in the tight anatomical relationship between the different segments. The tubules will ultimately drain into the papillae, which will join at the hilum to allow tubular fluid to enter the ureter. Image provided with permission of the Kidney Precision Medicine Project Consortium.

microscope could appear paradoxically completely normal. No one knew why the kidneys suddenly couldn't separate and retain protein. And no one knew how to treat the disease, although some studies had shown a salutary response to therapy with the newly available glucocorticoids, otherwise known as steroids.

I also learned that some people, with otherwise perfectly normal kidney function, might have subtle changes in a protein in the tubules that would prevent the kidneys from excreting acid in the usual manner. Acid production by the body is a feature of daily life, in part a consequence of the digestion and metabolism of the food we eat. It is the kidneys' charge to remove that daily acid load from our bodies. Some patients had a mild disease that did not progress but saddled them with very abnormal blood tests, which could prove a challenge for the primary practitioner as well as frightening to the patient. Other patients had a progressive disease, in which the level of acid in the blood gradually increased to life-threatening levels, and kidney function, as well as bone health, deteriorated perilously. Many of these disorders did not show up on routine physical examinations but caused panic when the laboratory analyses came back a day or two later. Curiously, although these rare abnormalities might be seen in children, suggesting that these were inherited disorders, the identical diseases appeared in adults, implying that they were also a result of degenerative processes or a consequence of other diseases of aging.

I was hooked. I discovered to my surprise that most clinicians and students did not find these ideas interesting or compelling. The math involved could be daunting, and my colleagues were content to skip these aspects regarding the more recondite processes of kidney function during their education or to invite a consultant to provide additional information on the disorder in a hospitalized patient rather than approaching the problems themselves. Abandoning the depressing field of psychiatry, I decided to become a member of the priesthood of nephrologists and solve physiologic puzzles that other physicians did not consider in their bailiwicks.

Internship and residency, following medical school, were hurdles to overcome before I could apply for a fellowship in kidney disease. Those efforts took time, and I could not easily reconnect with Kevin, 250 miles away in the nation's capital. After my residency, I spent four years in Philadelphia, learning the intricacies of kidney function in health and disease. I took care of patients with acute renal failure who would have died without emergency dialysis, which had become widely available in the U.S. only a decade or two previously. I cared for patients treated with chronic maintenance dialysis, available in the U.S. only since 1973 as a result of the efforts of physicians at Mount Sinai Hospital in New York City, the Peter Bent Brigham Hospital in Boston, and, perhaps most saliently, at the University of Washington (UW) in Seattle, where they demonstrated that dialysis would be feasible on a weekly basis to keep patients whose kidneys had failed completely alive for years. In testimony before Congress the UW group and National Kidney Foundation representatives supported the initiation of a government-financed dialysis program. Congress had also been influenced by the testimony of a patient who was treated with dialysis during a meeting in the House of Representatives. I had taken care of patients who had received a kidney transplant from someone who had had normal kidneys but had died, from the time the donated kidney was implanted into the recipient, through the period when high doses of drugs designed to impair the recipients' immune response were administered, while they developed the inevitable exotic and potentially deadly infections associated with immunosuppression. I continued to care for them as outpatients as their kidney function gradually improved and their quality of life soared, while they were in good health, and after their kidneys had been rejected. I also witnessed those patients on dialysis or nearing end-stage renal disease who were incredibly fortunate enough to have received a kidney from a parent, child, or perhaps a sibling who was a perfect match. In such cases the kidney could be removed from the donor by an extensive and laborious operation, in which a large incision from spine to umbilicus was made, through muscle and other tissue, to isolate a living kidney. Then the kidney and its artery, vein, and ureter were removed. Afterward the surgeon would reestablish the integrity of the blood vessels and prevent bleeding, and finally secure the incisions. The donated kidney, inserted into the groin of the patient, who might not have urinated for many months, sometimes began to work immediately, evidenced by urine gushing through the catheter into the bag at the bottom of the bed. In many cases, the newly invigorated, happy recipient might be up and about in a day, ready to leave the hospital after a short stay. In contrast, the donor might be laid up in a hospital bed for a week or two, receiving potent pain medications as the giant incision healed and the new patient learned how to walk again.

I decided to take an academic position in Washington, D.C., at a hospital I had never heard about during my training. I wanted to renew links with my old friend Kevin, from whom I had not heard in a while. I sent Kevin a letter, telling him I would be in Washington that fall. It said I would really like to get together and resume our friendship. Imagine my shock when I received a brief reply on a National Gallery notecard depicting a Japanese woodcut.

"Great that you are coming to D.C. I may not be able to meet you when you arrive. Will be having kidney transplant surgery. Regards. Kevin."

As a newly minted nephrologist, I was dumbfounded and crestfallen. How could my friend, Kevin, a healthy young man, have kidney disease to the extent that he would need transplantation? What kind of kidney disease could he have had? Kidney disease in the U.S. was mostly a disease associated with high blood pressure or diabetes and was a disease of the elderly rather than the young. Kevin had not had either of these problems. Kidney disease was encountered far more frequently in people of African descent in the U.S., than in White patients. In young people, the disease was often hereditary, and I did not know of anyone in Kevin's family who had had kidney disease. I knew that the lifespan of a kidney transplant recipient was not comparable to that of a person of the same sex, age, and ethnicity in the general population and that the burdens posed by complications were substantial.

I wrote a hasty letter to Kevin saying I would do everything I could to help, for him to please call on me and let me know the details, and that I wished him the best of everything. I did not get a response before I moved to D.C., by which time the operation had been performed.

When I called Kevin's house, I was pleased to hear a hearty voice answer the phone. The former roommates would meet for lunch in D.C. I would be able to hear the story in detail. I hung up—I couldn't wait to get together.

A robustly healthy Kevin strode into the West End Cafe.

"It's so nice to see you. Sit down. I've been anxious to see you. How are you?"

"Fine."

"Well, how are you doing? The drugs? What's your kidney function like?"

"Oh, they told me it's normal for the procedure. I'm not on any medications. They said I didn't need them."

"What? After a kidney transplant, a patient usually takes a myriad of drugs. I want to know how you're doing."

"I didn't have a kidney transplant. I was the donor! Would you like to see my scar?"

Kevin had donated his right kidney to his younger brother, who had had a long and complicated poorly characterized multisystem illness for years, culminating in kidney failure in the early 1980s. Kevin's brother had been treated with dialysis for a few months before receiving the transplant. Kevin's altruistic gift of a perfectly matched kidney allowed his brother to have a normal life in spite of the failure of his own kidneys. For forty years, Kevin's brother's kidney function (in fact the function of one of Kevin's kidneys) remained relatively stable. Kevin's brother had not needed any further dialysis and was able to pursue work and hobbies. Kevin, like most kidney donors, had had absolutely normal kidney function before his kidney was removed, an operation called nephrectomy. A curious aspect of kidney donation is the fact that, after removal of one kidney, the remaining kidney undergoes growth, so that it usually functions at a slightly higher level than one of the two kidneys in a normal person of the same sex, age, and ethnicity. The mechanisms underlying this phenomenon are still not completely understood, but the response allows kidney transplant donors to live normal lives. Actuarial data available since the late 1970s shows that patients who had had a nephrectomy—for kidney stones, bleeding in the kidney after trauma (such as after an automobile accident), urinary tract obstruction, or because of a tumor in one kidney—had survival rates comparable to those of the general population.

Kevin and I—and our wives—settled into a long-standing friendship in Washington, enjoying the opera together, as well as family events and vacations over the years. Kevin enjoyed the outdoors and went white-water canoeing and hiking in the area. He also continued his interest in culinary arts, hosting cooking classes in his kitchen, as well as enjoying occasional meals in 5-star restaurants.

After thirty-four years, the weakening of the abdominal wall where the incision healed (technically a "hernia") was causing Kevin some distress. Kevin spoke to his internist who suggested surgical consultation. The surgeon ordered a computed tomographic (CT) scan of the abdomen in preparation for surgery to repair the hernia.

Kevin called as we were preparing to go out to dinner with our wives. The CT had revealed the expected weakening of the abdominal wall but also that the remaining kidney was not normal. A mass had been detected in the kidney. I heard the news and surmised, thinking fast, that it was probably a kidney tumor, a renal cell carcinoma. Kevin would need a nephrectomy, which would establish the diagnosis, and probably result in a complete cure. As slow thinking kicked in, I reacted with horror and despair. Rather than being a relatively common and curative procedure, a second nephrectomy would result in Kevin immediately becoming an end-stage renal disease (ESRD) patient, who would require dialysis or transplantation. This was an extraordinarily ironic fate for a kidney transplant donor, but the possibility of needing dialysis in the near future was a clear consequence of that act of fraternal love thirty-four years before.

Dinner was a complex and eerie interplay of bonhomie, good will, love, friendship, anxiety, and the urgent need for the exchange of frank medical information. Yes, new medications, the checkpoint inhibitors, which had been approved recently by the Food and Drug Administration (FDA), had had spectacular success in treating renal cell carcinomas. Yes, new kidney tissue–sparing surgery had been employed successfully in patients recently. Where was the mass? What was its appearance? The friends left the restaurant, hugged, and got into their cars with their own individual thoughts, questions, feelings, and forebodings.

Most of the time, a mass in the kidney with a typical appearance is a renal cell carcinoma, or malignant kidney cancer. The cancer, if left untreated, can spread to the lungs, brain, and bones and lead in advanced cases to death. In rare instances, however, the typical appearance can be associated with an often-benign tumor called an oncocytoma, which can be treated relatively easily, with limited surgical approaches, and without the removal of much kidney tissue. I had momentarily forgotten about this escape hatch. Kevin was scheduled for a radiologic test, a Sestamibi scan, which in some cases has been successful in differentiating the two types of kidney masses. Upon consideration, I was convinced that the mass would be benign and shared my optimism with Kevin. Kevin had been healthy all his life, and he had no obvious risk factors for kidney cancer. At the same time, I let Kevin know I was a hopeless optimist and might lose objective medical judgment in the cases of those near and dear to me. Both Kevin and I, as well as our wives, were delighted to hear the scan suggested a benign mass. The surgeon, exercising the requisite caution, suggested the diagnosis should be confirmed by a renal biopsy. A procedure was scheduled and a radiologist, guided by scans, inserted a needle into Kevin's kidney to sample tissue from the mass. The patient, the nephrologist, and their wives were dismayed by the report, which determined the mass was indeed the more ominous of the two, a renal cell carcinoma.

Kevin was seen by an eminent urologist (a surgeon specializing in treatment of diseases of the kidneys and the genitourinary tract), Dr. Muhammad

Allaf, at Johns Hopkins University, who after an extensive evaluation considered the medical dilemma presented by his patient. The mass was in the center of Kevin's solitary kidney, a region called the hilum. In this area, at the heart of the kidney, the renal vein and artery, the renal nerves, and the ureter are intertwined in close conjunction of structure and function. Could an operation remove the tumor yet spare the most vital parts of the organ? Could a kidney be divided into three parts, the middle part excised, and the two remaining thirds be brought together, reestablishing all the intricate anatomy of the normal organ? Could a patient have enough kidney function remaining after the operation to sustain life without needing dialysis or kidney transplantation?

What were the long-term consequences even if the immediate prognosis was favorable? Would this single kidney be injured during surgery? How long would the patient be in the hospital? How big would the incision be? Would there be much pain? Could one drive after the operation? How would one exercise after surgery? What would Kevin's diet be like after the surgery? Kevin's wife had thoughtfully anticipated many of these questions, central to the patient's experience, over the days before the consultation.

Doctors are taught to never say never and never say always. We try to be truthful as well as hopeful in our encounters with patients. Often patients are anxious. Doctors know that trust is an elusive aspect of the patient/physician relationship but that it is a necessary concomitant of excellent care, especially when the stakes are high. Kevin was told that the operation could be performed. The surgeon told him he had the requisite experience, that the operation was risky, but the outcome could be good. There could be no guarantee about the ultimate level of kidney function, but Dr. Allaf was optimistic. Indeed, the kidney could be injured during surgery, but the doctor hoped this would not be the case. Kevin would be in the hospital for a week to ten days. The incision would be comparable to that on his other side. There would certainly be postoperative pain, but newer medications would be very helpful. The wounds would heal, and Kevin would certainly be able to drive. But first things had to come first, like walking and building up stamina after the surgery—all in good time. Kevin's diet might have to be restricted, but that would all depend on the level of kidney function. The level of postoperative kidney function could not be predicted preoperatively. Kevin and his family would probably have to consult a dietician experienced with patients with kidney disease. The operation would transform Kevin from a person in good health to a patient with chronic kidney disease, or CKD. Kevin would be treated before his operation, as an outpatient, with one of the new checkpoint inhibitors that had proved so effective recently. It was a good thing that Kevin, as a federal employee, had excellent health insurance. He would need it.

Many of the questions Kevin and his family raised could not be answered precisely, leaving them with a lingering sense of uncertainty. Kevin and his wife came away with the certainty that the operation was necessary, that the prognosis for treating the cancer was good, but that much was unclear about how his lone kidney would respond. They both were distressed that kidney failure and its treatment was a distinct possibility for which they must prepare.

Kevin and his wife appeared at the hospital before dawn for the surgery. Preoperative care was routine, and they were both optimistic. Kevin's was one of the earliest cases of the day, and his bed was wheeled into the Recovery Room in the late afternoon, after surgery was completed. Nurses rushed in and out of a space delineated by curtains hung from the ceiling on runners. The next patient was inches away. His wife was aghast at his appearance. Kevin's face was bloated, and his eyes were shut. He was responsive but sedated. As the anesthesia cleared, he gritted his teeth in pain. Opioid medications were administered intravenously intermittently in the Recovery Room, which alleviated the pain and resulted in a welcome return to sedation. His surgeon walked into the space, beaming, with a confident stride. Dr. Allaf told Kevin and his wife that the operation had gone very well and that he was pleased with the results. You could tell that the surgeon was quite proud of his handiwork. He told them he expected a rapid recovery. Kevin had no recollection of this conversation. After transfer to his room, Kevin remained alternately in pain or in a sedated state for the next day or so.

Kidney function was monitored daily by a blood test, which measures the serum creatinine concentration, or S[Cr]. The normal level is variably between approximately 0.6 and 1.3 milligram per deciliter (mg/dL) in different people. The higher the S[Cr] is, the worse the level of kidney function. After the surgery, Kevin's S[Cr] increased about 1.0 mg/dL a day, suggesting the kidney was not working at all. Was this a result of redistribution of body fluids during the surgery, so the kidney did not have enough substrate to act on? That situation would cause an increase in the S[Cr], although the kidney might be working normally. Alternatively, was the kidney injured and shedding vital cells into the urine?

Kevin was visited daily by the surgical team. They checked the wound, monitored the urine output and the S[Cr], and were in charge of all aspects of postoperative care. He was also followed each day by members of the nephrology team, who noted the S[Cr] and answered questions about the course and prognosis circumspectly. The surgeons gave Kevin large amounts of salt solution, through catheters connected to his large veins. His legs and abdomen swelled, but the S[Cr] continued to rise. I, essentially an interloper in a hospital in which I did not have privileges, went to the residents' laboratory with a specimen of Kevin's urine. I took a small volume of the urine, put it into a centrifuge tube, and set the dial that determined the number of revolutions per minute. After spinning the tube for five minutes, I removed and inspected it. A little red pellet remained at the bottom of the tube. "Not so good," I thought. I decanted the urine, and spread a bit of the pellet, reconstituted with a small amount of the urine, on a glass microscope slide. I put a thin cover slip on the fluid, trapping it between the two pieces of glass. I put the slide under the microscope and looked at it through the microscope. I saw the urine was not normal. Rather than being clear, field after field under the microscope showed debris and the remnants of tubules that had been sloughed by the kidney, called "muddy brown casts." It was a tour of a kidney battleground. I returned to Kevin's room.

"I looked at your urine. It was not normal—filled with casts and cellular debris. That suggests you have acute tubular necrosis—or ATN for short. That's a disease that we know a lot about since it was described in injuries during World War II and the London Blitz. It now often happens as a complication of surgery, especially if the patient is unstable. It doesn't mean the surgery was done incorrectly or badly. We're still unsure exactly why it occurs. We do say the kidney does not like to be insulted. I can sympathize.

"Anyway, this disease has a rather characteristic but highly variable course. The period of kidney dysfunction generally lasts up to two weeks.

Patients can have normal or high urine output, which we call a 'nonoliguric' state. Such patients have a relatively good prognosis, perhaps because the urine output provides a bit of a safety margin. Urine output allows excretion of potassium and sodium. You're making a fair amount of urine each day, so you're nonoliguric, which is great! Other patients may make less than 300 milliliters of urine a day, which we call 'oliguria.' It means there's relatively little urine. Polyuria means that there is a lot of urine. You have neither.

"Nonoliguric patients generally won't need dialysis. But your creatinine is going up about 1 mg/dL a day. That suggests that there is almost no kidney function. That's a bad sign. So the nephrologists will watch you each day to make a decision about your care. The indications for acute dialysis in this setting include developing congestive heart failure, a state where there is so much fluid in your body that the heart can't pump well enough to keep the fluid from backing up to your lungs, creating a state of extreme breathlessness. Another reason to start dialysis would be if the potassium concentration in your blood climbed too high, which could cause your heart to beat irregularly or even to stop. If the K+—that's what we call the potassium concentration— goes up too high, the nephrologists will recommend some medications to bring it down, with or without dialysis. If they recommend dialysis, I wouldn't refuse it.

"It's also possible that the acid level in your blood will increase to high levels. That could mean that you will need dialysis. If there's too much sodium in your body, like when the surgeons give you fluids hoping to make a sick kidney well without having a specific medication to treat ATN, you become edematous, as you are now.

"The indications for acute dialysis also include terrible things like inflammation of the pericardium, the sac that surrounds the heart, or the development of seizures, stupor, or coma. No good 21st-century nephrologist will let something like that occur.

"So you see, a normal kidney regulates all these factors: the sodium, acid, and potassium content of the body and their concentrations in the blood; other ions necessary for health, such as calcium, phosphate, magnesium, and zinc; and the production of red blood cells, as well as your vitamin D stores and bone responses. I love this organ. That's why I'm a nephrologist."

——— ✦ ———

The surgeons rounded every day, looking at the wound, assessing Kevin's pain, and bearing the news of the latest creatinine. Kevin had entered the hospital with a S[Cr] of 1.6 mg/dL. The day after surgery it was 2.2, as could be expected. On day 3 it was 2.8, and on day 4 it was 3.3. He gained twenty pounds. His legs were quite swollen and had to be elevated while he was in bed. The urology chief resident came into the room to speak to the family.

"We often see the creatinine go up after this type of surgery and want you not to be alarmed. But we have to maintain your safety. We've spoken to the nephrologists, and we think if the creatinine is not lower tomorrow that we will need to do dialysis."

"OK. What will that mean for me?"

"You'll need to have a catheter put in one of your large veins, probably in your chest or leg, to provide access to the bloodstream. We'll send you to the dialysis unit. You'll probably have dialysis three days in a row, and then we'll observe the creatinine to see if it starts to decrease. That will tell us that the kidney has started to recover."

"What are the side effects?"

"Oh, I think you should go into that with the nephrology team."

"And why are my legs so swollen?"

"The injured kidney and loss of renal mass have prevented the body from excreting all the sodium we gave you to try to 'open the kidney up.' The swelling will get better as the kidney recovers. If you need more details, I'm sure the nephrology team will be happy to discuss them with you. We're really glad you're doing so well from a surgical standpoint."

Kevin and his wife and daughter took in the news with a mixture of resignation and sadness. They had hoped that the kidney would have done better than this. Kevin was not ready to become an ESRD patient. Everyone had been so optimistic before the operation. He prepared for the worst but kept a smile on his face. He was glad the tumor had been successfully removed, and his pain had improved.

The next day the creatinine was 3.3, unchanged, which was a good sign. The chief resident said because Kevin was making "good urine," the surgical team could continue to observe him without his needing dialysis. The day after, the creatinine was 3.0, and general rejoicing echoed across the unit. Kevin and his family were elated, all because of a single number. He would not need dialysis! Dr. Allaf came in, congratulated him, and said they could make plans to return home the next day. The nephrology team on rounds said the kidney was recovering. They could not prognosticate regarding the exact course and timing of the recovery. Kevin would need to have his creatinine checked, probably twice a week as an outpatient. One of the possible complications of the diuretic phase of ATN (further discussed in chapter 3) is high urine flows for a week or two. Other clinical consequences of this complication include low blood pressure, weakness and dizziness from loss of sodium, and loss of potassium and magnesium, which can be as problematic as high levels of these ions. A little sobered, the family was still delighted that Kevin would be going home.

"What about his diet?" his wife asked.

"That's a good and important question," the nephrologist replied. "We'll have to limit your potassium and sodium intake, and you'll have to speak with the dietician. She'll give you information on what foods you can and can't eat."

"I'm not really eating anything. I don't have any appetite. I'm only on clear fluids."

"You'll be back on a normal diet soon." That was the last they heard about diet in the hospital.

Kevin was discharged the next day. Although it was painful for him to get in and out of the car, Kevin and his wife were thrilled that he was out of the hospital and that they were on their own, even if that meant frequent return trips to the hospital to see the surgeon as well as outpatient visits with the nephrologist and to the laboratory for the necessary tests. It was great to be home, but his new condition posed many challenges.

Kevin was an accomplished cook and had distinct preferences regarding meals. He had never considered the protein, sodium, and potassium content of specific foodstuffs and what happened to these during preparation. Kevin and his wife learned in the hospital that he'd be following a "renal diet." This consisted of restrictions to about 0.7 grams of protein per kilogram (2.2 pounds) of body weight per day, a 2 to 3 gram sodium restriction, and no more than 1 milliequivalent (mEq) of potassium per kilogram of body weight per day. This was a whole new medical and largely chemical vocabulary that needed to be understood to craft menus, stay on diets, and cook food. It really was a foreign language of medical cuisine. Where could they find out how much of this stuff was in each different product? They were directed to several websites but were disappointed to find that few gave exact amounts of the ions per weight of food. Even worse, many of the sites provided contradictory information. They learned that there were "bad" foods. Citrus fruits and tomatoes were full of potassium. No more tomato juice with breakfast! They were also saddened to learn that all the dishes they loved—often based on veal and fish—were rich in protein. Sauces and portions would have to be cut back. Luckily, they had a scale. They learned about an Italian diet that had been developed in the 1960s and 1970s. Carbohydrates were well-tolerated by people with kidney disease. This diet was based on pasta, bread, and butter, and patients had eked out several months before either needing dialysis (if it was available) or succumbing to the inevitable.

Pain was a constant but unwelcome companion. When would be the time for the next pill? Would he ever be weaned off these opioids? He learned common nonsteroidal anti-inflammatory drugs such as Aleve and Advil could worsen kidney function and, what's more, impede sodium and potassium excretion. Kevin was shocked to see that both his nephrologist and the surgeon preferred him to be on oxycodone rather than ibuprofen.

To help healing, Kevin set on a daily routine of walks, increasing his distances gradually to two miles a day. He gradually lost the weight he had gained in the hospital, and the swelling diminished and then disappeared. He visited the nephrologist twice a week over the next two months. The creatinine slowly dropped. From 2.8, to 2.5, to 2.1, it finally settled down to 2.0 over a period of a couple of weeks and his nephrologist told him it was "stable" and that his kidney function was "about a third of normal." The nephrologist told Kevin that he now had CKD, although all his physicians understood he had no disease in his tissue. Kevin had given away half his kidney function as a young man and now had lost one-third of the remaining function. (These procedures entailed the loss of about two-thirds of the mass of his original two kidneys. You do the math.) His surgeon and nephrologist were both rightfully thrilled with the present outcome. The surgery had eradicated the tumor and left Kevin with as much normally functioning kidney tissue as possible.

Over time, Kevin needed fewer and fewer pain pills, and he was eventually able to stop them altogether. He and his wife weighed portions, avoided particular vegetables, consulted apps, and monitored his potassium with the nephrologist. They bought a home blood pressure cuff. He weighed himself daily and checked for swelling around his ankles. Kevin and his family learned what it was like to have CKD, even if he had never had diabetes and didn't come from a disadvantaged background that impeded access to medical care. After two months, Kevin went back to work.

Kevin's case touches on almost all aspects of kidney disease in industrialized societies at present. While his story may seem unusual, it is not uncommon to encounter patients with disease in the solitary kidney after altruistic donation. Currently, chronic kidney disease in the U.S. is, in many cases, an illness of poverty, neglect, lack of access to care, and racial discrimination. Powerful genetic susceptibilities in a particular population lead to inequities in the burden of those who must undergo treatment for ESRD in the U.S. The treatment of ESRD is relatively new—in reality only about fifty years old—and is based on innovative technologies developed during and shortly after World War II. New dialysis and transplantation technologies have allowed the quality and quantity of patients' lives to improve. But a therapy supported by tax dollars in the U.S. and in various ways in other high-, mid-, and low-income nations is, in reality, a business. Although the therapy is lifesaving, the quality of life of patients treated with dialysis is severely compromised. Approximately 800,000 people in the U.S. have ESRD. This number represents only the tip of the iceberg for a condition, CKD, that has been estimated to affect approximately 37 million people nationwide. Recent estimates for Medicare costs for hemodialysis for the U.S. population are approximately $28.5 billion a year. Medicare's yearly costs for CKD patients are approximately $85.4 billion. Roughly one-fifth of the Medicare budget goes to the care of CKD and ESRD patients. A large proportion of ESRD patients who want a kidney transplant must languish on waiting lists, hoping for a kidney that may never arrive. Many patients will die awaiting their transplant. Each year, more than 100,000 patients remain on kidney transplant waiting lists. Living donors may provide recipients with the gift of life, but the long-term consequences for some of the donors are unknown. Until recently, living donors did not receive financial reimbursements, but recent administrative changes have allowed more benefits to accrue to donors, a collection of policies that are proving to be a game changer. Living donors, however, do not receive benefits, such as insurance or long-term medical care, in exchange for their altruism. Erythropoietin—whose production by the biotech industry represented a major medical advance, one based on the revolution in molecular medicine that started in the 1960s and 1970s and was fueled by tax dollars designated for biomedical research—has improved the quality of life of thousands of CKD and ESRD patients with anemia. Nevertheless, therapy with erythropoiesis-stimulating agents, which is the major source of revenue of several giant international biotechnology corporations, can be associated with mortality when too much drug is given to reach inappropriate laboratory value–based goals. The most recent history of the kidneys involves incredible scientific advances, with limited translation to patient care, in a social landscape where genetics, geographic heritage, racism, poverty, and corporate greed interact in a complex and often unhealthy manner.

Kevin's individual case is extremely rare, affecting approximately 1 of 2,500 donors.[1] The vast majority of living donors do well after their surgery, but Kevin's course illustrates the current state of the art of treatment for common kidney disease. This book explores these thorny issues. We'll start with a brief review of how the kidneys work, learn about acute renal failure (ARF, now termed acute kidney injury, or AKI), the problem that affected Kevin's life after his surgery, and progress to consider the birth and maturity of hemodialysis and transplantation, mostly in the U.S.

2

———— ✦ ————

WHAT THE KIDNEYS DO AND
WHEN THEY DON'T

Why do we have kidneys? Homer Smith, the New York University physiologist of the early and mid-20th-century who became the father of modern nephrology, suggested that evolutionary changes in kidney structure and function were the key factors that allowed vertebrates to move from the nurturing environment of the sea and survive in the harsh terrestrial landscape, eventually becoming humans roaming the savannahs and building huge cities.

People know they have kidneys but don't know why—or much about them. We know we need to urinate several times a day, and as we grow older, perhaps a few times after we go to sleep. The workings of the kidney are thought to be obscure—even to medical students and some seasoned practitioners, who often avoid the esoterica and leave the screening, diagnosis, and management of kidney ailments to superspecialists, the nephrologists. The intricate mechanisms underlying the work of the kidneys regulate our most basic physiologic processes.

What Do the Kidneys Do?

The kidneys, however, are also the amazing accountants of the body—the body's keepers. When they work normally, they literally balance the books of body chemistry. The kidneys match all the nonnutritional components of the foods we eat with equivalent losses in the urine and tightly regulate the composition of the blood, which feeds every organ in the body. Evolution has provided a fantastically dense array of tubules to put the blood through labyrinthine manipulations—a beautiful system, indeed, that allows exactly the right amount and type of waste products created in the body to be removed on a daily basis. The kidneys are also intrinsically involved in the integrated response to mortal threats to our integrity, as in people who experience rapid blood loss. The function of the kidneys is dependent on precise relationships in tiny spaces.

When the system doesn't work, you die—often a lingering death with terrible breathlessness and delirious states followed by coma and cardiac arrest. This was the fate of most people with kidney failure in the United States and around the world until 1973, when Congress changed our national therapeutic agenda by establishing an entitlement for people with end-stage renal disease that provides dialysis and kidney transplantation to practically every American, regardless of financial status, through the Medicare and Social Security programs.

This chapter will introduce the functions of the kidney in the body and provide some examples of how the kidneys work under normal circumstances as well as under stressful or emergency conditions. We'll start with an investigation of the kidneys' functions related to increasingly magnified views of the kidneys' microanatomy, and we'll end with an attempted murder.

The Body Fluid Spaces, Sodium Distribution and Homeostasis

The kidneys maintain the balance and amount of salt and water in our bodies. They don't do the work alone, but they are essential to this task. Physicians have known the body is composed mostly of water for many years. About two-thirds of us is water. A human weighing 220 pounds (100 kilograms) is composed of about seventeen and a half gallons of water. The body water is divided into two parts. First, there is the larger compartment: the fluid within cells, called the intracellular fluid, which makes up about two-thirds of the total volume of the body's water. The second component, which bathes the cells and includes the plasma water, is termed the extracellular fluid (ECF). The plasma component of the blood is relatively small, making up about 5 to 7% of the total body water (and about 20 to 25% of the extracellular fluid).

The sodium concentration of the extracellular fluid, and therefore the blood, is strikingly similar to that of sea water. The critical importance of the ECF is implicit in the poetic term that has been used to describe it: "the sea within us." This environment, often termed the internal milieu, is remarkably constant in healthy people. This concept of constancy and the necessity to reset conditions to their baseline status when physiologic changes occur is called homeostasis. Homeostasis was conceived of by the great 19th-century French physiologist Claude Bernard, and the term is still in use today. Illness often poses a threat to the stability of the internal milieu, its homeostasis. Kidney disease frequently results in abnormalities of the volume and chemical composition of the extracellular fluid, specifically affecting the plasma component of the blood, our internal surroundings.

Maintaining that internal environment—the liquid portion of the blood that has the same concentration of salt as the ocean—prevents us from either having high blood pressure and swelling (if there is too much fluid) or experiencing severe fatigue or fainting from low blood pressure if there is too little fluid in our bodies. Paradoxically, the kidneys perform the function of maintaining the fluid volume mostly by managing the salt economy of the body rather than directly regulating water metabolism.

The Kidneys, Salt, and Water

The amount of fluid in the body—particularly the extracellular fluid, including the plasma volume—is determined by its sodium content. One of the key tasks performed by the kidneys is maintaining the balance between retaining and excreting sodium chloride (common table salt). The size and the composition of the sea within us is regulated by the kidneys. That's why Smith suggested the move of fish from the sea to freshwater was an essential step in kidney evolution, since marine vertebrates have a much simpler job of regulating salt and fluids, and hence simpler kidneys, than terrestrial verte-brates, including humans. The internal and external milieu of marine fish is almost identical. This is manifestly not the situation in humans.

The kidneys, however, are also the preeminent managers of the amount of water in our bodies. Some people drink only a little bit of water a day. They don't like to be bothered with going to the bathroom while they're traveling, at their desks, or in meetings. Other people like to drink relatively large amounts of water, to "flush out the kidneys" or to maintain their skin in what they sup-pose is its best condition.

How do the kidneys maintain an internal environment where the concen-tration of all the elements in the plasma is stable over days, weeks, months, and years in someone who drinks a quart of water a day and in others who might drink two gallons of liquid, on a whim, on a particular day? How do the kid-neys deal with a body that drinks three quarts one day and only three pints the next? The answer may seem fairly obvious. Some people void relatively small amounts of urine, with a deep color. Others excrete much larger amounts of pale urine, several times a day. Just how is this accomplished?

The answer lies in the microscopic structure of the kidneys—their blood vessels, glomeruli, and tubules (with distinct protein composition in different segments)—and the ability of the different tubular segments to respond to hor-monal signals of changing conditions. Although the endocrinologists may be jealous of this wonderful organ not usually included in their specialty, they must acknowledge the kidneys are a primary source of production of several hormones critical to life and well-being. This puts the kidney in a class with the thyroid gland and the pancreas. The kidneys produce renin, an important hormone that is ultimately involved in the regulation of blood pressure and the control of sodium excretion, in response to a decrease in blood pressure or because of low blood flow to the kidneys. Renin acts at the beginning of a cas-cade that ultimately produces angiotensin II, which controls blood pressure and acts to enhance the reclamation of sodium by the kidneys. Angiotensin II also stimulates the adrenal gland to produce aldosterone, another hormone that acts in tandem with angiotensin II to defend the body from sodium loss. In general, the more renin, the higher the blood pressure.

Other Functions of the Kidneys

The kidneys also perform other functions that are vital to life and well-being. For instance, the kidneys are critical in regulating the level of red blood cells in the body, preventing anemia. The kidneys respond to anemia by releasing a hormone, called erythropoietin, when they sense that the oxygen-carrying capacity of the blood is diminished.

The kidneys promote bone health and strength by facilitating the final step in the body's manufacture of the active form of vitamin D from vitamin D precursors ingested with food or activated in the skin by sunlight. One can think of kidney vitamin D, or 1,25 dihydroxycholecalciferol (its scientific moniker), as a hormone. This vitamin is critical in supporting gut calcium absorption and bone structure and integrity. (By the way, 1,25—as it's known at home—is also a mediator of good immune function.)

The metabolism of ingested food, and the everyday work of the body's systems, generates about 1 mEq per kilogram of body weight of hydrogen ions on a daily basis. For a 176-pound person, that would be 80 mEq of hydrogen ions produced a day. If not handled carefully, such a large acid load might damage delicate tissues or change the reactivity of chemical processes within the various cells of the body. The kidneys excrete these hydrogen ions not as strong acids (such as hydrochloric or sulfuric acid) but harmlessly neutralized in the urine each day. This occurs as the kidneys combine the acids with ammonia, which they synthesize. The urine never gets so acidic that it can injure kidney or other tissues. This process ensures the safety of the urinary tract, keeps the fluid surrounding and within the cells at an optimal state to allow catalysis of biochemical reactions, and maintains the blood pH at a relatively constant 7.4, year in and year out. We don't get too acidic or overly alkaline if we eat certain foodstuffs, thanks to the kidneys.

The kidneys are responsible for managing the balance of potassium, calcium, phosphate, zinc, copper, and other trace elements in our bodies and their concentration in the bloodstream on a daily basis.

What Happens When the Kidneys Don't Work?

Patients with extremely poor kidney function have a constellation of problems and symptoms. This syndrome is called uremia, coming from the notion of abnormal urinary wastes in the blood. The kidneys are critical in maintaining our ability to think and respond to the world around us by supporting brain and hematologic (or red and white blood cellular) function. In extreme cases, when decreased kidney function is close to no longer being able to sustain life, as it is in a uremic patient, neurological changes occur. Patients in late stages of kidney disease often develop lassitude, depression, lack of awareness of their surroundings, and excessive and irresistible sleepiness. Patients at the end of life from lack of kidney function often develop seizures, lapse into coma, and die if they are not appropriately treated. Providing appropriate therapy is usually within the purview of nephrologists. If the condition is chronic or irremediable, the treatment is usually either a form of dialysis or kidney transplantation.

Another key function of the kidneys is metabolism of drugs. This is important primarily with toxic substances such as poisons, which can be excluded rapidly from the body through the urine if the kidneys are working optimally.

When the uremic syndrome develops, either quickly or slowly and insidiously, all the functions of the kidneys are impaired, resulting in abnormalities in many of the body's physiologic systems. Patients experience multiple systemic consequences of the failure of the kidneys that physicians will diagnose and attempt to treat, with variable success unless the kidneys recover or the patient undergoes dialysis or transplantation.

Kidney Physiology 101

To appreciate better how these functions of the kidney come into play and work in concert in healthy people without kidney disease, let's consider some typical cases, just as medical students do in Clinical Physiology 101.

Let's suppose that the three most important organs in the body are the brain, the heart, and the kidneys, in no particular order, although nephrologists are prejudiced in this regard.

We can't live without a functioning brain. The experience of death, in the Intensive Care Unit, in a person maintained on artificial life support, is often determined by monitoring brain activity. If there is no activity, patients can be declared "brain dead," the equivalent of dead, and their organs can be used to save the life or improve the quality of life of other patients through organ donation.

The heart is a great pump, circulating the blood, which is responsible for providing oxygen and nutrients to all the cells in the body, no matter how far removed they are from its center. The brain is dependent on blood flow, and the oxygen and sugar the bloodstream supplies to its cells maintain its integrity as well as its life. The brain receives about one-fifth of the cardiac output.

The heart pumps an amazing 5 liters (about 1.3 gallons) of blood a minute to all the cells of the body. The kidneys also receive about a quarter of the cardiac output. Therefore, renal blood flow is about 1.25 liters per minute, or approximately an astonishing 1,800 liters (475 gallons) a day. Blood is composed normally of about 40% red cells. Plasma, with its dissolved proteins, constitutes the remaining 60%. Therefore the renal plasma flow is about 750 milliliters (about 0.8 quarts) a minute. The task of the kidneys is to filter the vast amount of blood they receive each minute without losing the plasma proteins and reclaiming (or, as physiologists call the appropriate function, reabsorbing) the vital sodium ions and trace elements.

The kidneys also need to eliminate the precise amount of water necessary to keep the concentration of molecules in the plasma stable, as well as the waste products accumulated by the ingestion and metabolism of food. The water eliminated usually matches the volume consumed each day. As the blood courses through the renal arteries, a portion of it is filtered. This fraction is about 20%, or up to about 150 milliliters per minute (ml/minute) (about a third of a pint a minute), in this example. (Any plasma not filtered will be on the next go-rounds.) The rest of the renal blood flow bathes and feeds the cells making up the tissues of the kidney. That filtered 150 ml/minute adds up to about 220 liters of fluid a day, or about 58 gallons. If the typical output of urine is about a quart a day, we see the kidneys reabsorb more than 99% of the filtered fluid.

To grasp these concepts better, we must review the anatomy of the kidney and consider its functional unit, the nephron. To do so, we start at eye level and then delve deeper and deeper into the kidneys' microscopic anatomy to elucidate their structure and function.

One can see (with the naked eye) the renal artery, which provides the inflow of blood into the organ. The renal vein allows blood to exit the kidney after it makes its way through the network of smaller, microscopic blood vessels, which we next consider. The ureter acts as the conduit for the urine, the product of the tubular system, to leave the kidney, enter the bladder, and then exit the body. This was the level that physicians and scientists could evaluate kidney anatomy before the invention of the microscope by Antonie van Leeuwenhoek in the latter part of the 17th century. Even so, many of the outstandingly prescient observations of the 19th-century father of kidney disease, Dr. Richard Bright, were made by visual inspection of cut kidney tissue.

The smaller blood vessels as well as the anatomic organization of the working components of the kidney can only be appreciated at a microscopic level. Pride of place is given to the relationship between the blood vessels, the glomerulus, and the tubular system. These associations were delineated by the 17th- and 19th-century anatomists Marcello Malpighi of Italy and William Bowman of England, as well others (like the 19th-century German anatomist Friedrich Henle), who benefited from the advances in microscopy and optics over the years since Leeuwenhoek's initial inventions and discoveries.

The kidneys are composed of a vast, ramifying vascular system, leading to the glomeruli, the tubules, and the interstitial cells that support the structure of the kidney. Nerve fibers branching from the central renal nerve surround each tubule. The functioning unit of the kidney, the nephron, is composed of a glomerulus (its filtering portion) and a tubule that emanates from the glomerulus in its intricate circuitry surrounded by the vasculature. Malpighi first described the glomeruli (labeled renal corpuscles) and the tubular system of the kidneys.

There are approximately 500,000 to 1 million nephrons in each kidney, which filter and treat the tiny volumes of plasma presented to each of them. Each glomerulus, the filtering unit of the nephron, is surrounded by Bowman's capsule, which opens at its far end into the beginning of the tubular system (the proximal tubule). Bowman first described the relationship between the renal corpuscles and the tubules, opening up the field of kidney physiology into consideration of functions such as filtration, reabsorption, and secretion. The entire tubule is a long and winding system that descends, ascends, and descends again on itself in a complicated, snake-like trackway designed to harness the energy of anatomy. Along its looping, serpentine course the tubule is composed of distinctly different parts that have contrasting biological structures and physiological functions.

The glomerulus fits into Bowman's capsule, the beginning of the tubular system, like a doorknob fits into a hand. (See Figures 1a and 1b in the preceding chapter.) The tubular system is composed of many individually different segments (by some counts ten or more) and perhaps twenty or more different cell types arrayed throughout these segments. Some components of the tubule include the proximal convoluted tubule (composed of three parts), the descending limb of Henle, its hairpin loop, the thin ascending limb of Henle, the thick ascending limb of Henle, the connecting tubule, the diluting site, and the collecting ducts, which converge into one of the papillae. Fluid draining from the papillae enters into the ureter, which exits the kidney and joins the bladder below.

Blood courses to the kidneys from the aorta, the largest blood vessel in the body, which first emerges from the heart, and subsequently enters the renal arteries. Each renal artery usually splits into branches at its entry point in the central part of the kidney, the hilum. These branches extend to the kidney periphery, or cortex, further dividing into the interlobar arteries, and finally the arcuate arteries. At the end of this series, the afferent (going in) arteriole is seen, which will connect to the glomerulus. Blood moves out of the glomerulus through the efferent (going out) arteriole, ultimately to travel into the vasa recta and then the renal vein. From there the blood drains into the vena cava, the largest vein in the venous system, which will complete the circuit by conveying blood back to the heart.

The work of the kidneys begins at the tiniest microscopic level. The plasma presented to the glomeruli undergoes a process by which some of it is filtered, the rest flowing through the efferent arterioles and ultimately back into the systemic circulation. This fraction is dependent on a normally beating heart, normal blood flow to the kidneys, and finally the balance of the pressures and the resistances between the afferent and efferent arterioles and the beginning of the proximal tubule, at Bowman's capsule. (That's a lot to take in and is not critical to understanding the major points of kidney functions, so you can relax.)

The fate of the fluid entering the beginning of the tubular system is to ultimately become urine, if it is not reabsorbed by the tubules. The fluid filtered by the glomeruli entering the beginning of the tubules may total from 150 to 180 liters a day (about 40 to 48 gallons) in a young healthy person. Since people generally void 1 to 2 liters (about one to 2.1 quarts) of urine a day, it is clear that the tubular system acts to reabsorb more than 99% of the fluid presented to it, as we previously calculated. If the glomerular filtration rate (GFR) is 150 to 180 liters a day, and the kidneys have up to 2 million nephrons, each microscopic nephron is responsible for processing the infinitesimal volume of about one-tenth of a milliliter of fluid a day. Therefore, the number of nephrons is important—or really essential—for the existence of good kidney function.

This fluid treatment system is all put together as the tubules course through their passage from proximal tubule, down to the thin descending limb, then up through the thin and thick ascending limbs, to the diluting site and cortical collecting ducts and papillae. The papillae coalesce to form the beginning of the ureter. Each individual nephron contributes to the outflow of the tubular fluid from the kidney as it exits as urine through the ureter into the bladder. Each segment of the tubule has different permeabilities, and capacities for reabsorbing sodium, water, potassium, and calcium, as well as other ions, proteins, and protons (hydrogen ions).

Why would such an elaborate system be necessary?

The task of filtering the blood also involves retaining the red blood cells as well as the vital plasma proteins in the body. In addition, ions, such as sodium and potassium, have to be treated differently from the water, according to variations in dietary intake and the daily needs of the body. A complex, multi-looped and coiled system exists to perform these functions. The energy for differential transport of water, sodium, potassium, and other ions is provided by the intricate architecture of the kidney tubules, creating a countercurrent system, similar to that in residential heating systems but much tinier. The different protein composition of the cell membranes in every segment of the tubule—primarily composed of submicroscopic protein pumps, each with different physiologic and physicochemical characteristics—allows each segment to transport different substances in different places within the kidney.

For instance, the main transporter in the thick ascending limb of Henle, involved in creating sodium and concentration gradients that facilitate the concentration of the urine, is the sodium potassium 2 chloride channel, known affectionately to renal physiologists as NKCC2. A key transporter in the distal convoluted tubule is involved in regulation of the urinary calcium excretion, which determines, in part, the total body calcium content, critical for preventing bone diseases, such as osteoporosis. These different proteins, with different ion and water transport capabilities, placed at different segments of the tubule, enable the kidney to achieve the goal of differential management of water and ions at different anatomic sites, allowing for wide-varying changes in the volume and composition of the urine. Energy in the form of anatomical complexity and consistency, as well as the spatial representation of different proteins along the length of the tubules, allows the kidney to accurately separate the metaphoric wheat from the chaff or, rather, to retain the nutrients and ions that are needed while excreting precisely the amount of waste necessary.

What Happens When We Don't Have Access to Water?

Let's see how this system works in a typical case where the patient, as well as the kidney, is subjected to mild stress. The kidneys have two main functions. They handle the volume of water ingested each day by regulating urine flow and concentration and also balance sodium outflow to match the intake as well as the needs of the body. We all know people who have been advised to drink three or four quarts of water a day because it's "good for the kidneys." To understand this situation, it is perhaps more instructive to first see how this system works in the case of a person who has been deprived of water for twelve to twenty-four hours. Let's start simply, by considering the challenge of fasting without drinking any water for a day or more.

We already know that about two-thirds of our bodies are made up of water. The kidneys, working in tandem with the organs of a normal body, are exquisitely good at maintaining the balance of water needed to keep all the organs, including the blood, working at optimal levels. But they and the body are not perfect. We lose about 600 to 700 milliliters (about 1.25 to 1.5 pints) of water a day through exhalation (the breath is humidified by the lungs) and through the skin as sweat. Water loss through these routes increases as metabolic demand increases—when we exercise, sweat excessively, or hyperventilate, and when it's hot. So we must drink a certain amount of water—say, at least a liter each day—in order to stay in water balance and to survive. Marathoners must drink more.

If we don't drink enough water, the levels of salt and other minerals in our blood increases, perhaps at first very slightly. If the plasma sodium concentration (P[Na]) rises slightly in a person who is fasting and not drinking water, vasopressin (also known as antidiuretic hormone, or more familiarly, ADH) is swiftly released from the posterior portion of the pituitary gland, nestled in the brain, into the bloodstream. ADH works to increase the permeability of the distal portion of the nephron (the collecting ducts) to water, increasing water reabsorption. Most of the water filtered by the kidney will be reabsorbed by the collecting ducts under the influence of ADH. The urine flow will be low, it will have a high concentration of filtered substances, such as sodium and urea, and the person voiding it will note that it is deeply hued. The concentration of the urine will be high, but the plasma mineral levels will remain relatively stable. The net result is that the plasma concentration of minerals, a quality of the internal milieu, or the sea within us, is tightly regulated and maintained. Homeostasis is preserved. Constancy is achieved as the characteristics of the urine change dramatically. Of course, this system can be overwhelmed if the insensible water losses are not replaced after a day or two. Without access to water, this water-deprived person will die, albeit with a very concentrated, physiologically appropriate low volume of urine—renal success but failure to survive.

What Happens If We Drink a Lot of Water?

What about when we drink too much water? (Is this possible?) If the P[Na] decreases more than 2 or 3%, consistent with excessive water ingestion or water intoxication, ADH release from the pituitary gland is suppressed, and the hormone will be absent from the bloodstream and, therefore, unable to affect kidney tubular function. In this example, the collecting ducts will be impermeable to the water delivered to them, and all the water presented to that part of the tubule will be excreted as urine, so long as the rest of the body systems are normal. If a normal person drinks enough water to dilute the plasma, say a gallon or so, it will all be excreted in the urine. There will be a brisk flow of urine, the urine will be clear, and it will have a low concentration. The person is peeing water to get rid of the extra water ingested, a quite normal event. Once again the net result is that the plasma mineral concentrations, that internal milieu, is tightly regulated within the normal range.

But just how much water can a person drink without overloading the system? That would result in dilution of the plasma, a medical state called hyponatremia. Hyponatremia can occur in a normal person from drinking too much water, but it takes a lot of water ingestion to achieve this state.

The kidneys of normal people filter about 150 to more than 180 liters of plasma a day. Let's use 180 liters (about 48 gallons) as our example, since it's a number divisible by so many other numbers. If the proximal tubules reabsorb about two-thirds of the filtered load, that leaves 60 liters (16 gallons) for the rest of the nephron to process. The descending limb of Henle has the special property of being highly permeable to water but impenetrable to dissolved salts whether we are water deprived or overloaded, a result of the protein composition of its distinctive cells. By the time the fluid reaches the hairpin loop, up to 40 more liters (about 10 to 11 gallons) of tubular fluid will be reabsorbed. The ascending thin and thick limbs of Henle primarily reabsorb sodium in a relatively fixed manner, processing about 15 to 20% of the entering load. Water follows the sodium transport passively in the thick ascending limb. Therefore, this section of the kidneys removes up to about 3 liters (about 0.8 gallons) of the filtered fluid in a day. That leaves about 17 liters (about 4.5 gallons) to be processed. The collecting ducts are unique in that they reabsorb water when ADH circulates in the bloodstream. When ADH is absent from the blood, as is the case in a person who quickly ingests a gallon of water, the collecting ducts do not reabsorb any of the water coursing through. Practically all of the water presented to the collecting ducts will be excreted as dilute urine. So, a healthy person would have to drink more than 17 liters of water a day to overwhelm the body's defense against overhydration, resulting in the development of a dilute plasma, the medical condition called hyponatremia.

Such cases of hyponatremia do exist, typically in patients with mental illness. The medical diagnosis describing this state is psychogenic polydipsia. Studies suggest, however, that even in those cases, patients are not drinking more than seventeen liters a day. (That's almost three-quarters of a quart an hour—ingested day in and day out. It's hard to imagine someone keeping up that pace throughout the day. We do have to sleep, after all.) In most instances of hyponatremia, the patients' kidneys are not normal, reducing their water excretory capacity, or the patient is taking a medication that limits the ability of the kidneys to efficiently excrete the water. (Such common drugs include antidepressant medications, nonsteroidal anti-inflammatory drugs, and, perhaps counter-intuitively, thiazide diuretics, among many others.) We see that the kidneys, by easily excreting water, are extremely efficient at defending the body against overhydration. So we can keep our skin supple, wrinkle-free, and smooth. And new findings indicate that the better we are hydrated, the better are our chances of long life.

What Happens When We Lose Sodium?

Let's consider a more dramatic example, one where the kidney is involved in defending the body from a potentially fatal assault on blood volume. Consider a person stabbed on a city street during a robbery.

A knife wound to the heart or a tear in the aorta usually results in immediate loss of blood from the circulatory system. While bleeding continues unimpeded, the heart pumps blood less efficiently with each contraction, and blood flow to the brain, the kidneys, and the heart itself becomes markedly diminished. Blood pressure drops precipitously. This response to stress involves multiple organs, rallied together to save the organism. Stress hormones, notably epinephrine, norepinephrine, and cortisol, are released from the adrenal glands in the well-known fight-or-flight response. The master gland, the pituitary, located in the folds of the brain, rapidly releases the ancient hormone vasopressin into the blood stream.

Vasopressin (also known as ADH) has two main effects. It increases blood pressure by squeezing (or, in medical terms, vasoconstricting) the blood vessels. Simultaneously, vasopressin causes a dramatic increase in the reabsorption of the water presented to the final portions of the tubule. Even though the heart rate increases to compensate for the diminution in its stroke volume, the kidneys immediately sense the reduction in blood flow.

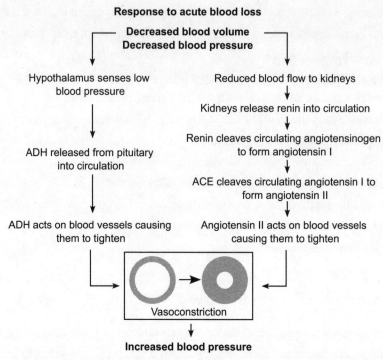

Figure 2. Flow chart depicting the integrated systemic and kidney responses to blood loss. Image courtesy of Erik Koritzinski.

As a result of decreased delivery of fluid to the tubular system, a highly choreographed set of physiologic events occurs in rapid sequence to defend the blood volume. The executive organ responding to hormonal commands will be the kidney. A specialized part of the glomerulus, the juxtaglomerular apparatus, releases renin, which acts as an enzyme, into the bloodstream. Renin converts angiotensinogen, produced by the liver, quickly into angiotensin I, which circulates through the bloodstream. The inactive precursor angiotensin I is rapidly metabolized to angiotensin II by the angiotensin-converting enzyme (ACE), produced by the lungs. Angiotensin II is a powerful vasoconstrictor like vasopressin. In other words, angiotensin II also squeezes the blood vessels, decreasing their caliber, which causes blood pressure to increase. (This happens literally in seconds.) Again, like vasopressin, angiotensin II affects specific portions of the kidney.

In particular, the small artery, or efferent arteriole, leaving the glomerulus is clamped tightly shut under the influence of angiotensin II, resulting in a shunt of blood flow away from the rest of the kidney, specifically into the glomerular circuit to maximize filtration by the kidneys. The GFR is maintained in this situation.

Angiotensin II also stimulates the adrenal glands to produce the hormone aldosterone, which has a dramatic effect to increase the reabsorption of sodium by the kidneys at the collecting ducts, similarly defending the body fluid volume. (Luckily, there will not be a quiz.)

The diminished volume of plasma that is filtered by the glomeruli is largely reabsorbed in the proximal tubules as a result of changes in the concentration of the proteins in the small arteries surrounding the tubule and the newly resultant pressure ratio between the tubule and the surrounding blood vessels. Instead of the typical proportion of about two-thirds of the fluid being reabsorbed at this early level of the tubular system, an increase in tubular fluid reabsorption of up to 90% may be seen because of the integrated response to the patient's vascular collapse. Reabsorption of salt and water continues in Henle's descending and thin and thick ascending limbs. The collecting duct, which usually fine tunes the reabsorption of salt at the end of the course of the fluid through the tubules, receives almost no fluid. Under the influence of vasopressin, the little water that is presented to the collecting ducts is reabsorbed into the bloodstream. Sodium will soon be reabsorbed in the collecting ducts as well, through the action of aldosterone, the production of which has been stimulated by angiotensin II. The result is a marked decrease in the loss of fluid and salt from the body. This intricate interplay of maneuvers between hormones, blood vessels, and end organs acts to defend the blood volume, all working in concert to try to maintain blood pressure in the face of massive blood loss.

The surgical intern on call won't care at all about angiotensin, vasopressin, or aldosterone when confronted with a patient brought into the emergency room. She will see a person with marked pallor of the linings of the eyelids who is minimally responsive or unresponsive, with a very rapid pulse that can barely be felt and a very low blood pressure. The intern will call for help to put in intravenous lines in all available large vessels. The staff will quickly instill a great deal of salty fluid into the patient and will type and cross the blood so that a transfusion of red blood cells may take place as soon as possible. The patient will be hooked up to an electrocardiographic monitor, which will beep in tandem with the rapid heartbeats. A catheter will be inserted into the urethra to monitor any changes in urine flow, which will provide another practical way to monitor how the patient's vascular system is responding, through the work of the kidneys. (See how important the kidneys are?) At the beginning of the procedure, there may be no urine at all in the drainage bag, or the urine may be highly concentrated, deeply yellow in color, and low in volume. When it is sent to the laboratory for analysis, the urine will have almost no sodium. That will indicate a normal response of the entire body—lungs, liver, adrenals and kidneys, all working together to maintain the blood volume, and life.

The patient will be transported to the operating room, and after induction of anesthesia and successful repair of the laceration, the anesthesiologist will note, among many other details, the urine flow. The patient will be brought to the recovery room, and as saline solutions and transfusions are administered, the hemoglobin concentration of the blood will rise toward normal. The intern will be gratified on rounds the next morning to tell the attending surgeon that the urine flow is now brisk, that the urine is not concentrated, and that the urinary sodium concentration is more than 70 milliequivalents per liter. Those tests show the kidneys are no longer retaining salt and water, since the heart is functioning normally and the blood volume has been restored. If they were measured, the epinephrine, norepinephrine, cortisol, vasopressin, renin, angiotensin II, and aldosterone levels all would now be normal. The hormones have done their job, and their glands can now relax. The patient will recover.

I have summarized a great deal of physiology and pathophysiology here and have provided contemporary and classic references for those who are interested in further readings on the subject.[1] You can see that the highly complex, intricate system of glomeruli and tubules superbly responds to physiologic stresses and hormonal signals to adjust to minor and major changes in access to water as well as emergency losses of sodium or blood. The kidneys are truly the guardians of our homeostasis—our body's keepers.

3

---- ✲ ----

ACUTE RENAL FAILURE—WORLD WAR II, THE BLITZ, AND DRS. KOLFF AND MERRILL

It is one of the most devastating diagnoses a patient can receive. It is one of the most clinically inauspicious events that can happen during a patient's hospitalization. It can happen immediately, often when a patient is already gravely ill, and instantaneously changes patients' lives and their chances for survival. Acute renal failure (ARF), currently known as acute kidney injury, or AKI, significantly increases the risk of death in hospitalized patients. A 2006 paper in the *Journal of the American Society of Nephrology* (*JASN*) titled "Incidence and Mortality of Acute Renal Failure in Medicare Beneficiaries, 1992 to 2001" showed, in a study of hospitalized patients, that a diagnosis of acute renal failure, although representing only about 2.4% of the total number of cases, was associated with a 3.3- to 7.1-fold increase in the patient's risk of death compared to the rest of the patients without acute renal failure.[1] Older people, men, and Black patients were more likely to have a diagnosis of ARF. Acute renal failure, now a defunct diagnosis (killed by committee in 2007), itself did not exist until the latter part of the first half of the 20th century, although the disorder had obviously been present as a medical entity for thousands of years. Prior to then, physicians didn't have the names to classify the illness or the tools to identify ARF when it occurred.

The Discovery of Acute Renal Failure

Captains Davies and Weldon of the British Royal Army Medical Corps reported cases of "war nephritis" in the *Lancet* in 1917.[2] On autopsy, the microscopic kidney pathology showed disease affected primarily the tubules but spared the glomeruli. The authors stated granular casts were invariably found in the urine of such patients when it was examined. Because of the short length of the report, it is difficult to ascertain the clinical course of the patients described or the cause of the kidney disease in these cases. Davies and Weldon suggested the development of kidney disease was relatively common as a result of military injuries and that its occurrence was associated with a high mortality rate. The study was not quoted in the key papers on the subject emanating from World War II. The first cases of crush injuries resulting in kidney failure (in three World War I soldiers) were reported in Japan by Seigo Minami in *Virchows Archives of Pathologic Anatomy* (now the *European Journal of Pathology*) in 1923.[3] The article seems to have gone largely unnoticed, perhaps because of its publication during peacetime. (Dr. Garabed Eknoyan has provided a nice review of the history of acute renal failure before World War II.)[4]

The diagnosis of acute renal failure entered the consciousness of the public and, perhaps more importantly, hospital physicians as a result of the Blitz—the German bombing of London in the 1940s. But it was not yet called kidney failure. During the bombing of Britain by the Nazis, buildings became the tombs of people trapped within their collapsed shells. Patients might have survived the injuries to their muscles and limbs, often sustaining amputations, but they frequently later died of kidney failure, despite recovering from their surgical procedures. In the beginning, acute renal failure was a wartime diagnosis. The reasons underlying the development of the kidney disease were unknown at the time. The English, as a result of widespread, extensive casualties, led the academic field in studies of acute renal failure in the 1940s. Leadership in the field would move to the Netherlands and then to the U.S. as the century unfolded.

Drs. D. Beall, Eric G. L. Bywaters, and colleagues reported a case of crush injury with renal failure in the *British Medical Journal* (*BMJ*) in March 1941:

When a bomb demolished a hostel . . . a young male leatherworker of 20 . . . was buried beneath the debris . . . his left leg was crushed against the side of an iron bedstead by a heavy metal girder. When he was first seen at 1:30 PM the left leg was still trapped, his mental condition was apathetic, the extremities were cold, and no pulse was palpable. . . . He was finally released at 2:15 p.m., 10 hours and 15 minutes after the accident.

On admission. . . . He was pale and lethargic but not cyanosed, and complained of no pain. The left leg was swollen and tense. . . . There was no external wound of the limb. . . . Physical examination revealed no further injuries.[5]

On the third hospital day, the patient's urine output became frighteningly decreased, to about 200 milliliters (less than half a pint) over twenty-four hours. His urine was brown, and microscopic examination showed a large dark brown sediment with "blood pigment casts." Laboratory evaluation showed increased levels of urea, potassium, and phosphate in the patient's blood. On days four to six, the patient's clinical condition worsened. However, on day six, the patient appeared improved. His urine output had increased. Urinary microscopic findings were almost normal. However, despite some further limited clinical improvement on day seven, the patient later suddenly exhibited low blood pressure and an irregular heartbeat and soon thereafter died.

An autopsy was performed. The most important findings were those of the microscopic examination of the kidneys.

Other cases of the syndrome of crush injuries accompanied by acute renal failure were published in the same issue of the *BMJ*. R. Mayon-White and O. M. Solandt reported another heartbreaking case:

A girl aged 11 was pinned under bomb debris for about three hours. . . . In this position she was compressed, though not actually crushed, by the dead bodies of her parents; a heavy beam lay upon her left thigh. On admission to hospital she was conscious and rational. . . . Though rather pale and complaining of pain in both legs, she seemed comparatively unhurt. Full examination revealed no evidence of injury save some swelling of the left thigh. . . . During the early morning she passed 4 oz. of smoky red urine which was . . . positive . . . for blood. . . .

　　She presented a typical picture of uraemia. She was drowsy and irritable, her skin was dry. . . . Her mouth was dry, the tongue covered with brown fur, and the lips cracked. The left thigh was very much swollen, pitting oedema extending from the hip to the toes. The greatest swelling was in the thigh. . . . The left arm was also oedematous. During the next five days the whole body below the level of the nipples showed pitting on pressure. . . . The bladder was never palpable. There was complete anuria save for a few cubic centimetres passed incontinently. . . . Attempts to collect a specimen of urine by catheterization proved the bladder to be empty. Her condition progressively deteriorated. She was conscious, though increasingly stuporous, until an hour before her death. She died at 4.30 p.m. a week after admission. At no time was the patient jaundiced, nor was there an icteric tinge to the plasma.[6]

Treatment was not effective. An autopsy was performed and the failed kidneys were examined under the microscope:

Most of the tubules contained a granular debris that stained a brickred colour. . . . This material could be found in all parts of the tubule. . . . Proximally it was small in amount . . . but in the collecting tubules the granules were tightly packed, forming a solid cast of the lumen . . . some of these granules seemed to be red blood corpuscles . . . it was evident that the tubular contents were frankly granular, though "ghosts" of broken cells could be seen in some places . . . the tubular contents were the golden-red colour of unstained red cells. The tubular epithelium in some places showed evidence of degeneration. Some of the cells had lost their outline. There were some pyknotic nuclei. This degeneration seemed to bear no constant relation to the amount of material in the tubule. The glomeruli were normal; the capsular space was not dilated.

The authors emphasized the patient had not had a blood transfusion, as occurred in other cases reported in the same issue. The newly named "crush syndrome" seemed to produce some factor that injured the proximal tubules of the kidney enough to destroy the function of the entire organ and result in the inexorable death of the patient because of the impairment.

Beall and Bywaters, in a major article in the same issue of the *BMJ* in 1941, "Crush Injuries with Impairment of Renal Function,"[7] reported four cases of kidney failure associated with the crush syndrome and established it as a new clinical entity. The case reports were accompanied by extensive anatomic and microscopic descriptions of the injured kidneys of three of the patients, which all resembled each other. The authors suggested the renal pathologic features consisted of "degenerative changes in the proximal convoluted tubules and pigment casts in the more distal part of the nephron" and noted the glomeruli were not affected. They reported that the urine suggested severe injury was sustained by the kidney tubules. The authors emphasized the similarity of the kidney pathologic changes to those seen in transfusion reactions. They also remarked that the patients' histories and physical examinations were not consistent with typical transfusion reactions. Bywaters and Beall suggested that muscle injury and subsequent leak of intracellular ions and proteins might affect heart and kidney function, respectively. The Bywaters and Beall paper recalls those of Bright, linking a clinical syndrome with uniform pathologic characteristics, a set of aberrant laboratory findings and abnormal urinalyses, and has become a classic.

In August 1941 a case report in the *BMJ* by Ronald G. Henderson, a surgical resident, offered a glimmer of hope for patients with crush syndrome and the physicians caring for them:

A man aged 32 was admitted to hospital as an air-raid casualty . . . May 7, 1941. From about 1 to 9 a.m. on May 6 he had been pinned down by heavy debris across his left shoulder and upper arm; he had suffered no other serious injury. He had received first-aid treatment in the neighbourhood of the air raid and had been in bed in a damaged hospital for about thirty-two hours before being transferred. No transfusions had been given. On admission his general condition was very satisfactory. The left arm was grossly swollen and reddened. . . . The circulation was intact and the radial pulse palpable. . . . Despite a liberal intake of fluids the output of urine for the preceding twenty-four hours had been only 30 oz. The blood urea was 390 mg. per 100 c.cm. Active treatment was begun immediately, 40 c.cm. of 25% glucose being given intravenously, followed by 540 c.cm. of isotonic sodium sulphate solution.... During May 12–16 ... the patient was restless and rather childish, though otherwise rational. On the 17th his local and general condition began to improve and thereafter continued to do so. At the beginning of June ... some hyaline and a few granular casts were present in the urine. (At the beginning of the illness there were very numerous granular casts, no hyaline casts, a few red blood cells, but no blood casts . . .) The patient had never suffered from nephritis or any disease likely to predispose to it.[8]

Henderson differentiated his case from the other crush injuries previously reported, emphasizing that his patient had not had a transfusion, and had experienced spontaneous recovery. The urea levels in the blood declined, and urine urea excretion increased while the patient's urine output simultaneously increased.

Acute Renal Failure, Lower Nephron Nephrosis, and Acute Tubular Necrosis

Dr. Maurice Strauss, a faculty member at Harvard Medical School whose clinical position was medical director of the Cushing Veterans Administration Hospital in Framingham, provided a comprehensive description of what we would now call acute tubular necrosis, including its clinical course and pathologic anatomy in a paper in 1948 in the *New England Journal of Medicine* (*NEJM*), perhaps infelicitously titled "Acute Renal Insufficiency Due to Lower Nephron Nephrosis."[9] The term lower nephron nephrosis (LNN) had been coined by Colonel Balduin Lucké in 1946 in an article in *Military Surgeon* entitled "Lower Nephron Nephrosis: The Renal Lesions of the Crush Syndrome, of Burns, Transfusions, and Other Conditions Affecting the Lower Segments of the Nephrons."[10] The moniker LNN was used in many articles between 1946 and 1950. In 1950, for the first time, the term acute tubular necrosis (ATN) appeared in the title of a paper in *Clinical Science* by G. M. Bull, A. M. Joekes, and K. G. Lowe.[11] The same authors also wrote several other papers using this latter nomenclature. The term ATN was evidently well enough understood for Lowe to publish a paper in the *Lancet* in 1952 titled "The Late Prognosis in Acute Tubular Necrosis: An Interim Follow-Up Report on 14 Patients."[12] The designation of lower nephron nephrosis subsequently descended into oblivion, putting the legacy of Strauss's report into jeopardy.

Strauss described a diverse set of clinical situations in which acute renal failure could occur, including transfusion reactions and heat stroke, after abortions, infections and surgery, from "non-traumatic muscle ischemia," complicating burns, and as medication reactions as well as "from various poisonings of diverse origin, including the most common offender, carbon tetrachloride." Strauss briefly described the characteristic clinical phases of loss and recovery of kidney function in patients and outlined the consequences of a prolonged injury phase. In a beautiful turn of phrase, Strauss presciently noted the "magnitude and severity of the general manifestations frequently so divert attention from what at the moment seems a minor matter that it is often difficult to determine just when the urine volume declined or became nil." He cataloged the pathology that had been reported in previous cases and diligently quoted Lucké's paper. Strauss described the dismal survival statistics of the patients and presented electrocardiographic evidence of severe abnormalities in the concentration of salts dissolved in the bloodstream of patients with LNN. Strauss proposed general principles of treatment that are still in practice today, grounded in sound physiologic observations and well-informed theory, including restriction of sodium, paying careful attention to the balance between the input and output of fluids, and provision of the right amounts and kinds of nutrients, including oral and intravenous routes of delivery for patients who suddenly were put at risk of death because impaired kidney function limited the excretion of fluid and potentially dangerous mineral ions from the body. Strauss reviewed an impressive list of therapies that had been employed in the treatment of lower nephron nephrosis that had largely been found ineffective. Some of these included spinal anesthesia, "splanchnic block," diathermy or irradiation to the region of the kidneys using X-rays, irrigation of the renal pelvis, surgical removal of the capsule of the kidney, transfusion of compatible blood or plasma, intravenous administration of sodium sulfate or hypertonic fluids (such as glucose, sodium chloride, or lactate solutions), and flushing the abdominal cavity with fluid delivered by catheters. At the end of this long list, Strauss added "use of an artificial kidney." Strauss mentioned that the "artificial kidneys developed by Kolff and Alwall offer considerable promise for the future," but opined that conservative management would be much more widely used, even if these technical advances became a reality. (Strauss quoted three papers by Nils Alwall published in the Scandinavian literature and in the *Lancet* in 1947 and 1948 and one by Willem J. Kolff, published in the *Journal of the Mount Sinai Hospital* in 1947.)[13] Seven illustrative cases were presented by Strauss in great detail in the paper, to acquaint clinicians with the clinical aspects and disparate presentations and complications of the syndrome. The paper was a tour de force, now probably forgotten because of its unfortunate title.

Strauss, a distinguished student of the kidney before there were nephrologists, went on to become the coeditor of one of the first modern comprehensive textbooks on kidney disease—Strauss and Welt's *Diseases of the Kidney*.

These first reports established the clinicopathologic syndrome of acute renal failure, associated with the kidney tissue diagnosis of acute tubular necrosis. The patient would experience a period of dramatically decreased urine flow (termed oliguria) or diminished urination, lasting a few days to two or three weeks, followed by an increase in urine flow, which could be very sudden or gradual over days or weeks (the diuretic phase). Occasionally the urine flow could become very high, termed polyuria, or "much urine." During the period of decreased renal function (the oliguric phase), the S[Cr] (first described as a marker of renal function in 1926, by Poul Brandt Rehberg, of the University of Copenhagen)[14] increased, and then, hopefully during the diuretic phase, the S[Cr] would progressively diminish, perhaps to normal levels, reflecting recovery of the kidneys. The rise in S[Cr] was potentially associated with dramatic increases in circulating levels of blood potassium, phosphate, and acidity, all of which could result in fatal derangements of heart function. The patient might exhibit fluid overload, resulting in heart failure and congestion of the lungs. Neurologic symptoms, such as irritability and drowsiness, could and often did progress to somnolence or coma. Abnormalities of blood chemistry jeopardized heart function—potentially causing disturbances in its rhythm that might result in cessation of the heartbeat and death. The characteristics of the syndrome described in the 1940s remain relatively unchanged to the present time. No therapies have been developed yet to improve or "cure" this type of AKI. Physicians at the time had few clinical tools to ameliorate the patient's condition. Their task was to provide support through the period of acute renal failure and hope the kidneys would recover before the patients died of the biochemical or cardiovascular complications of the failed kidneys. Acute renal failure became an accepted name for the syndrome after about 1951, in part because of its use in a chapter heading in Homer Smith's *The Kidney* and in a long article published in the *Journal of Clinical Investigation (JCI)* by Dr. Jean Oliver and colleagues.[15]

Acute renal failure, or acute tubular necrosis, resulting from crush injuries or infections, however, might have remained a death sentence with occasional reprieves but for the work of a young Dutch physician during the Nazi occupation of the Netherlands in World War II.

Dr. Kolff and the Genesis of Hemodialysis

Willem Johan Kolff was born in 1911 in Leiden, the eldest of five sons of a physician. Kolff received his M.D. degree from Leiden University and afterward trained in internal medicine at the University of Groningen. In 1938, the care of a patient with advanced kidney disease due to nephritis inspired Kolff to search for a treatment for a disease that had stubbornly defied therapy. Kolff told his story in the *Annals of Internal Medicine (AIM)* in 1965,[16] as well as elsewhere, including several of his books and during prize presentations. Kolff hoped that if he could remove relatively small amounts of urea from the patient, perhaps on a daily basis, some of the symptoms of uremia (the clinical constellation of signs and symptoms constituting kidney failure) could be ameliorated. A professor of biochemistry at Groningen, Dr. Robert Brinkman, introduced the young physician to some of the biophysical properties of cellophane, a semipermeable membrane. Kolff also became acquainted with the work of John Abel and colleagues Leonard Rowntree and Bernard Turner published in two papers in the *Journal of Pharmacology and Experimental Therapeutics* and another in the *Transactions of the American Association of Physicians*, that first described dialysis in 1913 and 1914.[17] The Nazis invaded Holland in May 1940. While the Germans and sympathizers took charge in Groningen, in 1941 Kolff moved to the town of Kampen, where he became the lead internist in the hospital. The hospital supported his research efforts, and Kolff continued his investigations on the possibility of treating uremia in humans with dialysis. Kolff noted in the *AIM*:

> Earlier attempts to make artificial kidneys had failed for lack of reliable anticoagulant, lack of good dialyzing membranes, and insufficient capacity of dialyzing equipment. Since I had both heparin and cellophane, all that remained to do was to build a dialyzer of sufficient capacity to make the application clinically worthwhile.[18]

Kolff obtained the requisite calculations from simple in vitro experiments he performed. With the assistance of Mr. Berk, a director of an enamel factory in Kampen who donated the efforts of his company, Kolff built crude dialysis machines, using enamel bathtubs and cellophane that would have otherwise been made into sausage casings. The cellophane tubing was wrapped around an aluminum drum. The patient's blood, circulating through the tubing as the drum turned, was exposed to a large amount of fluid containing no urea to facilitate its diffusion into the wastewater. The rotation of Kolff's apparatus was facilitated by components used by Henry Ford in the rotating joints in his automobiles, supplied by a local Ford dealer. Eventually wooden drums were used as aluminum in wartime became scarce. Berk subsequently was an author on one of the first papers Kolff wrote on dialysis in humans.

The first dialysis treatment of a patient with an artificial kidney was performed on March 17, 1943, in Kampen. The patient was a twenty-nine-year-old woman who worked as a housemaid. She had

> malignant hypertension and contracted kidneys, who upon admission not only had uremia but also cardiac insufficiency. She soon developed pericarditis, parotitis, and otitis media. Her blood pressure at the time of admission was 245/150 mm Hg. . . . During the following days we dialyzed consecutively 1, 1.5, 3.5, 4.5, and 5.5 liters/day. Serious reactions

were not observed, and from then on we began to dialyze continuously, which meant that blood was let into the artificial kidney at one end and after having run through it was immediately returned to the patient.

The patient died despite treatment. From March 17, 1943, until July 27, 1944, Kolff dialyzed fifteen patients.

Of those 15 patients only 1 survived. . . . The artificial kidney reduced his blood urea from 222 to 104 mg/100 ml . . . the next day one ureter was unblocked by retrograde catheterization, and he had a diuresis. I have never thought nor said that this man's life was saved by the artificial kidney . . . he might not have needed the artificial kidney had we done the cystoscopy first. At that time I felt that the patient's general condition, cardiac failure, atrial fibrillation, pneumonia, continued hiccuping, and vomiting, justified the sequence that we chose. . . . I sometimes wonder what would have happened to this project if I had done it not in the Netherlands but in some location in the United States and if having treated 15 patients in 1½ years I could not have claimed a single therapeutic triumph. However, many things were established about clinical dialysis during those war years in Kampen. It was established beyond doubt that urea, creatinine, uric acid, and phosphates were removed by dialysis. . . . It was proven that sodium and chloride were increased if they were too low and decreased if they were too high before dialysis . . . we did show that potassium high before dialysis was still low a few days later. . . . The observation that dark venous blood became bright red in the cellophane indicated that oxygenation through the membrane took place and formed the basis for the later development of membrane oxygenators.

Although Kolff's first fifteen patients died, he was able to observe improvement in their symptoms of uremia, such as the recovery of visual and cognitive abilities in some of the patients, as well as the amelioration of their nausea and vomiting during treatment. A few of the patients who had been unarousable or drowsy woke up and were able to interact with medical staff and their family members. In addition, technical aspects of the dialysis procedure worked.

Successful treatment of a patient with uremia by dialysis came after the liberation of the Netherlands. As Kolff recalled,

> after the liberation we finally received one patient who probably owed her life to treatment with the artificial kidney. This was Patient 17, treated on September 11, 1945. She was 67 years old and had cholecystitis with pericholecystitis and icterus, and probably acute glomerulonephritis. She was treated with sulfathiazole and her fever decreased, but she remained anuric. Her blood urea rose to 396 mg/100 ml, the potassium to 55 mg/100 ml. The clinical condition of the patient deteriorated to the point where she snored all day. Cystoscopy and retrograde catheterization of the ureters showed a normal pyelogram on the right side, and the next day, while anuria persisted, the patient was treated with the artificial kidney. Eighty liters of blood flowed through the artificial kidney in 11½ hours. Sixty grams of urea were removed, and the blood urea fell from 396 to 121 mg/ml. The potassium decreased from 55 to 19 mg/ml. The patient's clinical condition improved dramatically, and she spoke much and easily. The first understandable words she spoke that I remember were that she was going to divorce her husband, which indeed in time she did. Further recovery was uneventful. It is significant that this 67-year-old patient, at least in our eyes at that time, was not considered to be a very useful member of society. As a matter of fact, she was admitted to the Kampen Hospital from a prison in which my politically unreliable—that is national socialist—countrymen were at that time detained. Many of our fellow citizens would have accepted her death without regret. May those who decide whether a certain patient should be admitted to a dialysis center in the year 1965 remember that the physician's primary responsibility is towards the patient.

After the war, Kolff sent dialyzers to several Dutch cities as well as to Hammersmith Hospital in London, Mount Sinai Hospital in New York City, and the Royal Victoria Hospital in Montreal. Drs. Bywaters, A. P. Fishman, and N. K. M.

de Leeuw, and colleagues all published accounts of successful treatment of patients with kidney failure using the Kolff machines.

Kolff emigrated to the U.S. in 1950 and accepted a position at the Cleveland Clinic. His early work there included the development of smaller dialyzers that were more portable, and disposable, allowing the treatment of patients with acute renal failure with hemodialysis to become more generally available. Kolff's initial published studies established him, without question, as the father of dialysis as a treatment for kidney disease in humans. His technique revolutionized the care of people with acute renal failure.

Dialysis Spreads from Europe to the United States

Although other reports of dialysis devices and treatments in humans and animals were soon published—by Gordon Murray of Toronto and colleagues in 1947, 1948, and 1949, by Leonard T. Skeggs Jr., Jack R. Leonards, and colleagues of the School of Medicine of Western Reserve University in 1948, 1949, and 1950, and by Nils Alwall and colleagues in 1947, 1948, 1949, and 1950—Kolff established his primacy in the field by quoting his 1946 thesis, *Die Kunstmatigie Nier* (The Artificial Kidney), describing the development and use of the dialysis apparatus.[19] (The thesis was accepted by the University of Groningen, with a rating of summa cum laude.) Kolff also quoted his papers published in the Dutch literature in 1943 and 1946, in *Acta Medica Scandinavica* in 1944, and in the U.S. in 1947, as well as a 112-page book published in London in 1947, *New Ways of Treating Uraemia*.[20] Kolff jealously but truthfully guarded his priority in the field as others joined it. As he pointed out in the *Annals* paper in 1965, "Alwall's paper on his artificial kidney was published in the *Acta Medica Scandinavica* in 1947, Murray's in 1947, and Skeggs and Leonard's was published in 1948. Ours had been published in Dutch in 1943 (3) and in English in 1944 (4)."

In 1945, an unsigned editorial entitled "Artificial Kidney" appeared in the *Journal of the American Medical Association* (*JAMA*).[21] The editorial reviewed the work of Abel, Rowntree, and Turner from 1914 as well as that of the American physician Dr. William Thalhimer (1884–1961) and colleagues. Thalhimer had been Abel's student at Johns Hopkins and went on to become a hematologist. The editorial noted his studies, including "exchange transfusions" and use of dialysis techniques in normal dogs and dogs that had undergone surgical removal of their kidneys, rendering them uremic. (One of Thalhimer's coauthors was Dr. Charles H. Best, the codiscoverer, with Dr. Frederick G. Banting, of insulin.) The editorial also cited Kolff's work in Kampen and described his dialysis apparatus and techniques in detail. The editorial referenced the paper by Kolff and Berk in *Acta Medica Scandinavica* published in 1944[22]—its title translated into English was "The Artificial Kidney: A Dialyzer with a Great Area." The editorial concluded,

> From the experiences of these authors the artificial kidney of the future apparently would not find its greatest usefulness in patients with chronic nephritis and uremia; these lesions are irreversible. As originally suggested by Thalhimer, dialysis of the blood may find its application in instances in which an individual with previously competent kidneys suddenly develops loss of renal function, as after a severe burn, in a prostatic patient who develops anuria after relief of intravesicular pressure, and in anuria after operative procedures. Conceivably if the renal secretion is temporarily taken over by the artificial kidney the patient's kidneys may return to their previous competence.

It remained for others to adapt this therapy for the care of patients with chronic kidney disease.

First Dialyses in the United States

I first met A. P. Fishman when I was a second-year research fellow in the Renal-Electrolyte Section of the Department of Medicine at the Hospital of the University of Pennsylvania (HUP) in 1980. At that time, Fishman was the William Maul Measey Professor of Medicine at the University of Pennsylvania. He was a large distinguished-looking fellow, with a bright smile, a shining pate, close-cropped gray-white hair, and a colorful bowtie anchoring a splendid, starched white shirt. He looked the patrician, with a somewhat forbidding demeanor in spite of his smile. Fishman was the world-renowned head of the Cardiovascular Pulmonary Division at HUP and was deeply involved in research in the physiology of the lungs, the care of patients with pulmonary disease, medical administrative affairs, and national and international academic committee work. I respected him and was a little afraid of him, although he always had a kindly word for lowly renal fellows if they collided with him at the copying machine located in the corridor between the two sections. Perhaps the pulmonary fellows did not enjoy the same relationship with their chief. Little did I know that Fishman had started his career as one of the pioneering nephrologists before that specialty had a name and before he became one of the world's leading pulmonologists.

Fishman was born in Brooklyn, New York, the son of Lithuanian immigrants. He achieved his M.D. degree in 1943, from the University of Louisville, after he completed undergraduate and graduate work at the University of Michigan. He did military service with the Army Medical Corps between 1944 and 1946 and then started postgraduate training in pathology and medicine at Mount Sinai Hospital in New York City, all before he was thirty.

Kolff had given one of his dialysis machines to Mount Sinai Hospital, in part because its chairman of medicine, Dr. Isidore Snapper, was his friend. Shortly after the publication of the unsigned editorial on the artificial kidney, Snapper introduced Kolff's work to the U.S. medical community in a letter written to *JAMA* in 1946 entitled "Treatment of Uremia" in which he, too, described the dialysis apparatus and the necessary technical procedures in detail.[23] Kolff visited Mount Sinai Hospital in March 1947, as described by Fishman, Irving Kroop, H. Evans Leiter, and Abraham Hyman in an article published in the *American Journal of Medicine* (*AJM*) in 1949.[24] They acknowledged the previous work of Abel, Rowntree, and Turner and that of Kolff as well as that of Alwall and the Canadian surgeon Gordon Murray. In addition, Fishman and colleagues cited the work of the relatively obscure Georg Haas (1935) (1886–1971), and Heinrich Necheles (1923) (1897–1979) (who performed dialysis in dogs whose kidneys had been surgically removed) in the German literature, and the American William Thalhimer, who reported use of an "artificial kidney to treat complications" of transfusion reactions in 1938.

As described in a 1994 reminiscence by Fishman in *The Pulmonary Circulation and Gas Exchange*,[25] he had just completed his chief residency in medicine at Mount Sinai Hospital and was assigned to use the artificial kidney machine in the care of patients with acute renal failure. A team composed of urologists, a cardiologist, and others was assigned to the task as well. Fishman remembered that physicians from the Peter Bent Brigham Hospital in Boston came to New York to observe how the apparatus worked. In the *AJM*, Fishman and colleagues described six uremic patients who were treated with the Kolff apparatus by the Mount Sinai team between 1947 and 1948. Although the authors realized that the duration of acute renal failure could be limited, they noted that the first four patients described in the paper were "dying of uremia." Fishman attributed the success of the technique to cellulose, which supplied the semipermeable membrane that allowed diffusion to occur (resulting in dialysis), and to heparin, which allowed anticoagulation of the blood. Their first case was a "Puerto Rican woman twenty-five years of age" who had inserted five sublimate of mercury tablets intravaginally in order to induce abortion after she had been raped earlier in the month. "All observers agreed that the patient was virtually moribund." Her dialysis treatments started on the day of her transfer to Mount Sinai from another hospital, January 26, 1948, using the Kolff apparatus. The patient was described at the time as being "semi-comatose." "There was a precipitous drop in blood non-protein nitrogen, urea nitrogen, phosphorus, creatinine and uric acid. . . . On the eighth day after use of the artificial kidney she appeared more rational, with only occasional disorientation and periods of delusion and paranoia. She responded well to questioning and appeared to be convalescing well." After dialysis treatments she was able to eat and drink, and her nausea and vomiting subsided. Her urine output and urinary urea excretion gradually increased, as her kidneys recovered and her clinical condition improved. Fishman and colleagues described the favorable outcome of the procedure in the patient.

> During treatment with the artificial kidney all were impressed by the apparent innocuousness of the procedure and the clinical as well as chemical improvement manifested by the patient. It is believed that the artificial kidney may have provided additional time for spontaneous improvement to occur. A report from the Rockland State Hospital, Orangeburg, N. Y., indicated that analyses made on March 5th showed the following: urea nitrogen, 13 mg. per cent; creatinine, 1.4 mg. per

cent; uric acid, 2 mg. per cent; non-protein nitrogen, 30 mg. per cent. The specific gravity of the urine was 1.013.

These values were taken by the physicians at Mount Sinai to demonstrate recovery of renal function, but nephrologists today would suggest that the S[Cr] indicated that the patient may have made a transition from acute to chronic renal failure. The case of the woman could be reported with very little change in 2024.

Although the patient's medical condition improved, her psychiatric status deteriorated, and she was transferred to another hospital for care of her mental illness.

A second patient, a thirty-year-old man who had been exposed to carbon tetrachloride fumes, was transferred to Mount Sinai Hospital in April 1948 with acute renal failure, as well as acute liver disease. He was first dialyzed on April

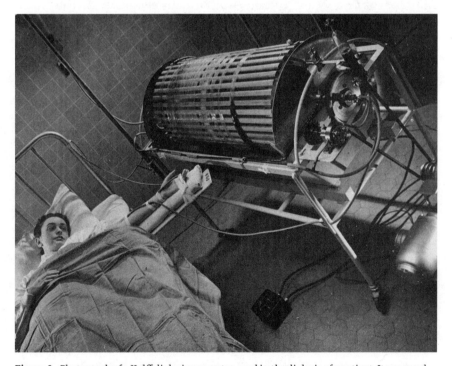

Figure 3. Photograph of a Kolff dialysis apparatus used in the dialysis of a patient. It appeared in the April 28, 1947, issue of *Life* magazine. The article did not provide details regarding the patient or physicians involved, but mentioned that the device built by Kolff was used at Mount Sinai Hospital in New York. Image used under license from Shutterstock.com.

10, and after a second treatment, his kidney function began to improve. The authors wrote, "Recovery of normal tubular function evolved slowly. It is believed that in this instance the artificial kidney served as a temporizing measure which potentiated spontaneous restoration of kidney structure and function." A third patient, a sixty-three-year-old man, was transferred to Mount Sinai on May 7, 1947, with diagnoses of prostate disease, infection, and acute renal failure. (This was actually the first patient treated by the team with the artificial kidney.) "However, the patient continued to deteriorate. Coma and uremic frost appeared on May 11th. All other available measures having been exhausted, on May 11th treatment with the artificial kidney was started and continued for four hours." The patient died shortly after dialysis, and an autopsy was performed.

A fourth patient, a thirty-three-year-old woman, was transferred to Mount Sinai Hospital on July 18, 1947, with an infection after an attempted abortion using potassium permanganate, with extremely elevated levels of BUN and S[Cr]. She was described as "comatose and virtually moribund." Although dialysis was started, the treatment could not be completed because of the patient's low blood pressure, presumably a concomitant of infection. An autopsy revealed evidence of "lower nephron nephrosis." The fifth case was a fifty-six-year-old man who had an operation for adenocarcinoma of the rectum in July 1947. "On July 16th he could not be roused. . . . The lungs were full of coarse, moist rales. All observers agreed that the patient was in extremis. It was thought that all other available measures had been exhausted and that the artificial kidney could certainly do no harm." The patient underwent dialysis the same day and regained some neurologic function but became "semicomatose" thereafter. The patient died three days after treatment. An autopsy revealed changes in the kidney consistent with a transfusion reaction. The authors speculated that dialysis treatment should have been started earlier and noted that the amount of heparin administered might have been excessive. The last patient was a man who had acute renal failure after his gallbladder surgery was complicated by severe infection. He was not making any urine. The patient had one dialysis treatment at Mount Sinai. His dialysis was complicated by oozing from his surgical wounds after being exposed to the anticoagulant heparin. He died shortly thereafter. An autopsy showed cortical necrosis of the kidneys, presumably from shock associated with the infection.

The cases were not presented in chronological order—presumably because the first four patients died. In light of current events, it is important to note in both of the women (a third of the cases), acute renal failure was the result of attempted abortions. In all cases, dialysis resulted in the desired intermediate outcomes—the high level of waste products circulating in the blood decreased after the procedure. The patients' chances of survival depended in large part on whether they had previously been healthy, if the underlying disease had improved, and if the kidneys were recovering. The patients who recovered had been poisoned and did not have other underlying acute or chronic illnesses. To this day, even with provision of dialysis to patients with AKI requiring treatment, the syndrome is characterized by high mortality. It is said nowadays that "patients do not die of AKI, but with AKI." Fishman's article detailed some of the theoretical chemical and physiologic principles underlying dialysis, demonstrated its technical feasibility in patient care, and listed complications of the procedure. The authors concluded,

> It is obvious that this treatment is not curative but can aid in prolonging the patient's life until spontaneous regeneration of the damaged renal tissue may occur. By the same token it is obvious that the artificial kidney should be reserved for those cases in which restoration of renal function can be anticipated rather than for cases of chronic progressive renal disease.

The paper also included a photograph of Kolff's dialyzer. You can see the machine, presented startingly at an angle, as well as, if you look closely, part of a person's arm that is extended on a board with blood-filled tubing connecting it to the Dutch physician's marvelous apparatus. A story about the Mount Sinai dialyzer was also reported in the popular press, with photographs, in *Life* magazine, in April 1947.

Fishman later obtained a fellowship to work in Homer Smith's laboratory at NYU for six months before beginning his illustrious career studying the pulmonary circulation with Dr. André Cournand and Dr. Dickinson W. Richards Jr. at Bellevue Hospital. (What could he have done if he had remained a nephrologist?) Cournand and Dickinson (with Werner Forssmann) went on to win the Nobel Prize in Physiology or Medicine for their "discoveries concerning heart catheterization and pathological changes in the circulatory system" in 1956. Mount Sinai Hospital has gone on to become a medical school and medical center with a large kidney transplant program and a distinguished record of treating patients with acute and chronic kidney disease.

Dr. Merrill and the Brigham: Dialysis as a Common Clinical Tool for Treatment of Acute Renal Failure

Next, we turn to considering the impact of acute renal failure on a major U.S. teaching hospital—the Peter Bent Brigham Hospital in Boston, under the medical leadership of Dr. George Thorn—as the locus of excellence in dialysis technique moved east. John Putnam Merrill's second paper was published in 1949 in the *Transactions of the American Clinical and Climatological Association*.[26] Merrill had had a bird's-eye view of the development of dialysis for humans, citing the work of Abel, Rowntree, and Turner, Nils Alwall in Sweden, and Gordon Murray in Toronto. But pride of place in the article was reserved for Willem Kolff, who had also been invited to visit the Peter Bent Brigham Hospital in Boston, Massachusetts, in 1947, as a visiting professor, when its physician in chief, Dr. Thorn, decided that the hospital should shift its attention to the care of patients with advanced kidney disease. Thorn also decided that young Dr. Merrill would lead the clinical and research efforts related to patients with kidney disease, creating one of the first patriarchs of modern clinical nephrology. Kolff shared blueprints of his dialysis machine with his hosts, Drs. Thorn and Merrill, who recruited Dr. Carl Walter, who then built the Peter Bent Brigham version of the rotating kidney with the help of the machinist and engineer Edward R. Olson. Kolff, in his 1965 article in the *Annals*, claimed that "the Harvard group with John P. Merrill probably did more for the further propagation of dialysis than any other group."

Merrill's short article dealt with chemical composition of the dialysis bath and changes that needed to be made to adjust to the concentration of salts and sugars in the blood of individual patients and described the evolution and culmination of Kolff's technique in Europe in detail. Merrill also reported sixty dialysis "experiments" in forty-eight patients the Brigham team had treated over the previous year and a half. The paper described modifications made to the original Kolff design, which Merrill suggested had decreased complications, such as clotting in the dialysis system. The authors stated the first indication for dialysis treatment was anuria (no urine output) in a patient with a "reversible renal lesion." The treatment would remove harmful waste metabolites and correct the chemical derangements in the blood of people with acute renal failure, such as high levels of blood potassium concentration, or hyperkalemia. Dialysis could also help patients with anuria and fluid retention because of congestive heart failure. The authors further recommended treatment with the artificial kidney for patients with decreased kidney function who had nausea or vomiting or had lost the desire or ability to eat (anorexia). The article outlined the contemporary indications for dialysis in patients with acute renal failure more than seventy years ago. This short early benchmarking paper established Merrill and the Brigham group as the international leaders in dialysis for acute renal failure.

Merrill did not waste time building on this reputation. He followed this report with numerous papers on the artificial kidney, acute renal failure, dialysis treatments, and other topics over the next almost four decades. In April 1950, Merrill published two papers, with several distinguished coauthors, in the prestigious *JCI* on the technique and clinical applications of the artificial kidney.[27] The introduction suggested

> our results seem to indicate: (1) that the use of an artificial kidney is a feasible method for the removal of specific diffusible substances from the circulating blood; (2) that it can be accomplished without excess hazard to the patient; (3) that it can be repeated if necessary; (4) that its use should not be postponed so that it is offered to the patient as a last resort because other methods of treatment have failed; and (5) that in addition to nitrogen metabolites it is possible to remove other diffusible substances which may be toxic in high concentrations, such as the barbiturates and sulfonamides. It is also possible selectively to remove sodium, potassium, calcium, and water. In patients with specific mineral depletion these substances may be restored without the addition of other electrolyte or water. In anuric, sodium-depleted patients this last function may be extremely valuable.

The clinical paper presented summaries of each of the forty-three patients treated and outlined the responses to and complications of therapy. The authors also presented a range of clinical conditions where hemodialysis might be effective. This paper was almost immediately followed by a publication summarizing a talk Merrill had given at the preceding American College of Physicians meeting.[28] Merrill was the only author. In this paper, really a set of clinical aphorisms as well as vignettes of individual cases, Merrill reviewed the salutary consequences of dialysis for patients with acute renal failure and hinted that dialysis for patients with "chronic uremia" could improve their course as they faced clinical challenges, such as the need for emergent surgery. This was followed by several clinical papers on aspects of dialytic treatment, including "potassium intoxication," culminating in the single-author publication of "The Artificial Kidney" in the *NEJM* in 1952—in case you had missed any of his previous papers.[29] "The Artificial Kidney" was a beautiful paper summarizing the basic science underlying dialysis techniques, including the physiochemistry of cellophane, and clinical information about the new procedure that could be appreciated by generalists. Merrill described the different types of dialyzers commercially available at the time and traced their lineages to such pioneers as Kolff, Alwall, Murray, and Skeggs and Leonards. This period of Merrill's life culminated with groundbreaking reports in a slightly different field of nephrology in 1955.

Dr. Murray Epstein, a former Brigham Renal fellow who worked under Merrill's supervision, published a deeply felt reminiscence of Merrill, in the *Clinical Journal of the American Society of Nephrology (CJASN)* in 2009, twenty-five years after his death in 1984.[30] Epstein, a distinguished nephrologist at the University of Miami, was interested in the interactions between kidney and liver disease and had worked on the roles adrenal hormones played in mediating abnormal renal responses (a central theme of the work of Dr. George Thorn). Merrill was born in Hartford, Connecticut, in 1917. He received an undergraduate education at Dartmouth and graduated Phi Beta Kappa in 1938. Merrill graduated from Harvard Medical School in 1942. Merrill interned at the Peter Bent Brigham Hospital and then fulfilled military service in the air force. He served as the flight surgeon on the *Enola Gay* mission, which included the release of a nuclear bomb over Hiroshima in 1945. In 1947, Merrill returned to the Brigham to complete his training in internal medicine, under Thorn's tutelage, just in time for Kolff's visit to the institution, at the behest of the senior physician.

The first dialysis at the Brigham, on June 11, 1948, has been described several times over the years by different authors in varying narratives. George Thorn referred to it in a brief memoir. Merrill wrote about Kolff (who survived him) in one of his last articles. In "The Legacy of 'Pim' Kolff," published posthumously in *Nephron*, an international kidney journal, in 1986, Merrill recalled:

> In 1948, there took place the first dialysis in the United States with a machine built in this country. Present at the dialysis were: Dr. Thorn, Dr. Carl Walter, myself and a fourth-year student who had spent 2 months of elective time working with me on the artificial kidney. His name was Lloyd "Holly" Smith and he is now Chairman of the Department of Medicine at the University of California at San Francisco. Our first experience with dialysis was a minor disaster. The tubing was polyethylene which, when autoclaved, flowed so that the joints became loose. All four of us in the room held the joints together by hand and we finally achieved a 3-hour dialysis in a patient who was chronically uremic and who had been comatose and convulsing for several days. On the following day, a Saturday, when I saw the patient in the morning he certainly was no better and his convulsions continued. We were bitterly disappointed. However, 2 days after dialysis, I walked in to see him sitting up in bed, reading the comic strip and eating breakfast.[31]

Note that Merrill stipulates that this was the first hemodialysis in the U.S. using a machine manufactured "here," undercutting the glory of Fishman and Mount Sinai Hospital (shades of Red Sox versus Yankees!). Ironically the first hemodialysis at the Brigham was in a patient with CKD, rather than AKI. (Merrill also didn't mention Dr. Jarvik, Kolff's protégé, in his discussion of Kolff's subsequent work on the development of the artificial heart.) He signed himself director emeritus of the Renal Division, Brigham and Women's Hospital. Merrill would be hesitant regarding the possibility of the widespread use of dialysis for the long-term treatment of patients with chronic uremia, now known as

CKD, for quite some time. Another physician from another city on the opposite side of the country would lead that battle, after he heard a lecture by Merrill on the possibilities of the Kolff-Brigham apparatus.

The diffusion of dialysis from the Netherlands to other parts of Europe occurred in part because of mediation through the Boston channel. Dr. Gabriel Richet ([1916–2014], who later became an editor of *Kidney International*), from Dr. Jean Hamburger's group in Paris, visited the Brigham and was able to establish the use of Kolff-Brigham dialysis machines at Necker Hospital and subsequently throughout Europe. Necker Hospital became one of the great world-class centers of kidney disease research. Industry took the lead in manufacturing more portable dialysis components, and companies such as Travenol and Drake-Willock created machines that could be more quickly and easily set up at patients' bedsides. Dialysis technology spread across the U.S. as well as internationally for the treatment of patients with acute renal failure beginning in the 1950s.

Acute Kidney Injury Today

As the syndrome of acute renal failure became more appreciated by hospital clinicians, who called on nephrologists to dialyze their sick patients, by the late 1950s nonclinical laboratory scientists began to establish the relationship between the release of myoglobin, a key protein constituent of muscles, into the circulation and the subsequent development of acute renal failure in patients. Such studies continued to be published over the next several decades, establishing myoglobin release into the blood stream as a toxic exposure to the kidneys. By the early 1970s, acute renal failure from the muscle protein myoglobin released during trauma or surgery or in nontraumatic settings had become a commonly appreciated clinical syndrome, as well as an accepted cause of acute renal failure.[32]

Clinicians had refined the syndrome of acute renal failure to include three broad categories. The approach to diagnosis centered on the presence of azotemia. Patients could have azotemia (high nitrogen in the blood stream, assessed by the blood urea nitrogen [BUN] test) because of the kidneys' response to the stresses of other diseases, such as heart failure or liver disease, or the loss of blood, dehydration, or other causes. In this case, the kidneys functioned well, but blood tests, such as BUN and S[Cr], were abnormally elevated. An astute clinician could assess the responses of the patients' kidneys using simple chemical tests, and the abnormalities would be corrected if the underlying cause could be treated successfully. This situation was termed prerenal azotemia. Secondly, urinary tract obstruction from prostatic disease or genitourinary or reproductive organ tumors could result in azotemia that might be corrected and thereby enable the return of normal renal function. The obstructive form of acute renal failure is often referred to as post-renal azotemia.

If prerenal azotemia and urinary tract obstruction were excluded, the clinician could conclude that a third diagnostic category, an "intrinsic renal disease," was present. Analyses would identify the locus of disease anatomically: in the arteries leading to the kidneys, the smaller vessels, the glomeruli, the tubules and their surrounding supporting interstitium, or perhaps the renal veins. In this manner, a tenable clinical diagnosis could be established to help the physician approach the cure of the patient's malady. This approach is still used today to diagnose patients with AKI. Although the diagnosis of a course consistent with ATN is usually clear, occasionally, to establish a diagnosis in a patient with an unusual case of ARF, performance of a kidney biopsy may be necessary.

Kolff went on to lead the Institute for Biomedical Engineering at the University of Utah. He pioneered work on the artificial heart, with another one of his illustrious trainees, Dr. Robert K. Jarvik. Kolff led studies in the development of extra-corporeal membrane oxygenation, or ECMO, which enabled the growth of open heart and lung surgery, and encouraged work on the development of artificial eyes and ears. His techniques allowed surgery to develop for pediatric patients who needed support for their heart and vascular systems. Kolff received the prestigious Lasker Prize in 2002 for work that enabled the care and survival of large numbers of patients with ESRD to become a reality. The person honored with him at the time was Dr. Belding Scribner.

———— ✢ ————

The mortality associated with an episode of AKI has not improved substantially over the last sixty years. Patients with AKI now, however, are older and sicker than patients who had the syndrome in the past. AKI, rather than affect-ing the kidneys alone, nowadays often presents in debilitated patients with severe infections or cancer after receiving toxic chemotherapies or in surgical patients after operative misadventures. The dialytic techniques developed by Fishman, Merrill, and other pioneers, based on the primitive Kolff apparatus, are similar conceptually to contemporary treatments, although the design of the equipment has changed radically. Dialyzers have become compact plastic boxes enclosing thousands of cellophane tubes or sheets of other semiperme-able membranes. The old, giant baths have been replaced by pump systems that remove water from municipal supplies and reconstitute its chemical composi-tion into fluids suitable for use in dialysis. Setup times have decreased from hours decades ago to minutes today, as equipment has become smaller, modu-lar, and digitized. Nephrologists, however, still sit by their patients' bedsides during acute dialysis treatments when their blood pressures are perilously low. Dialysis, although a lifesaving procedure, is often a harbinger of death for many of the patients undergoing treatment. Nephrologists still administer dialysis treatments to deathly ill patients with ATN, while waiting for the nat-ural reparative systems of the body to result in the recovery of kidney function.

Does AKI Cause CKD?

Although some early papers suggested the kidneys completely recovered after an episode of acute renal failure, close scrutiny of the reports, using the always available retrospectoscope, shows some patients never regained normal renal function. This is currently a substantial area of research, as basic and clinical scientists search for the factors associated with recovery, in addition to trying to delineate the causes of progressive damage. The field is now termed the AKI to CKD Transition.

Papers by K. G. Lowe in the *Lancet* in 1952 and Merrill and John T. Finken-staedt in the *NEJM* in 1956 describe the long-term course of patients who sur-vived an episode of ATN.[33] The papers emphasized the survivors regained enough kidney function to sustain life but were misinterpreted and taught to subsequent generations of renal fellows as implying that renal function in the patients returned to normal. Close examination of these data from the 1950s in the 21st century shows that a substantial proportion of the patients who survived an episode of ATN had moderate deficits in kidney function compared to what would be expected in age-matched people without kidney disease.

Members of the Division of Renal Diseases and Hypertension in the Department of Medicine at George Washington University (GW) became interested in the long-term course of patients with ATN at the beginning of the 21st century. They wished to evaluate the course of patients with ATN for longer periods than studied in the work of Lowe or Merrill and Finkenstaedt. One evening in the late 1990s, while I was in the hospital laboratory with medical students, housestaff, and fellows looking under the microscope at the urine of a patient with ATN, which was filled with muddy brown casts, I related the oft-told fable of ATN. "If the patient survives the oliguric phase, a diuretic phase will ultimately ensue, and the patient's renal function will eventually return to normal." As soon as these words left my mouth, I realized I was participating in the medical version of an old wives' tale, handed down from attending physician to fellow ad infinitum, across the generations of medical trainees. How did we know "renal function would return to normal?" Where was the evidence? Had anyone done the appropriate studies designed to accept or refute this idea? If so, did the old findings hold up in a new era of AKI typified by elderly patients with multisystem illnesses (often with underlying kidney and heart disease or cancer) that were treated with nephrotoxic drugs?

I collaborated with epidemiologists at the National Institute of Diabetes and Digestive and Kidney Diseases (NIDDK) and the United States Renal Data System (USRDS), to show, in an article in *JASN* in 2009, that patients in the Medicare system who had a diagnosis of acute renal failure were far more likely to enter the ESRD program than those without the diagnosis.[34] The risk of becoming an ESRD patient rose even more steeply if the patient had a diagnosis of both ARF and CKD. GW investigators, led by Dr. Lakhmir (Mink) Chawla, a young nephrologist and critical care physician, followed up in *JASN* in 2009 with a paper from the Veterans Administration system showing a subset of VA patients (mostly men) with a diagnosis of ATN but without evidence of preexisting kidney disease developed, over time, loss of renal function consistent with a diagnosis of chronic kidney disease.[35] Chawla and colleagues, including me, published two provocative reviews suggesting AKI and CKD were indeed one interconnected syndrome (a bit of heresy at the time) in *Kidney International* in 2012 and in the *NEJM* in 2014.[36] Investigators, including Chirag Parikh and colleagues at Yale and Matthew James and colleagues in Canada, as well as others, explored these issues using other databases and patient cohorts, coming to similar conclusions. It is difficult, however, to use such administrative data to establish causal relationships. A prospective study that followed patients after an episode of AKI would be necessary to confirm that AKI resulted in CKD.

The Assessment, Serial Evaluation, and Subsequent Sequelae in Acute Kidney Injury (ASSESS AKI) consortium was convened by the NIDDK in 2008, the brainchild of Dr. Robert A. Star, now the director of the institute's Division of Kidney Urologic and Hematologic Diseases. The NIDDK project officer for the initiative was Dr. Paul W. Eggers, an eminent epidemiologist of kidney disease who had previously focused on studies of the ESRD program. Eggers was assisted by me in the federal oversight of the project. The consortium, determined after a review of competitive applications by a team of physicians and scientists without conflicts of interest, was headed by Drs. Vernon Chinchilli of Hershey Medical Center at Pennsylvania State University, T. Alp Ikizler of Vanderbilt University, Chirag Parikh, then of Yale University, Alan Go of Kaiser Permanente and Jonathan Himmelfarb of the University of Washington. The group was assisted by many investigators with an interest in the long-term course of AKI. The consortium was charged, in part, with determining whether the long-term outcome of patients who had previously had normal kidney function but had sustained an episode of AKI would go on to develop chronic kidney disease. Thirteen years later, after a heroic effort of recruiting more than 1,500 patients, with and without AKI, and following them for an average of four and a half years, the investigators published their seminal paper in *Kidney International* in 2021.[37] The authors concluded patients with previously normal kidney function who had had an episode of AKI during hospitalization had a higher risk of developing CKD than patients who did not have AKI. Patients with preexisting CKD who had had an episode of AKI had a higher risk of progression of their kidney dysfunction, often to ESKD, than patients who did not have AKI. It is now widely recognized that a possibly substantial proportion of patients with CKD and with ESRD had an episode of AKI as their initial illness.

Technical Advances in Hemodialysis

Advances in dialytic techniques over the approximately thirty years after the use of the first crude dialysis machines were predominantly incremental. Dr. Juan P. Bosch, as a young faculty member at Mount Sinai Medical Center in the Renal Division of the Department of Medicine, built on the work of the German Peter Kramer (first reported in 1977)[38] and the American Emil Paganini (of the Cleveland Clinic) to improve the dialysis of critically ill people with acute renal failure and very low blood pressure. This technical advance, continuous arteriovenous hemofiltration (CAVH), built on the physiology of the normal kidney using the patient's blood pressure (even if very low) to drive the filtration outside the patient's body. The arterial circulation of the patient was directed into a dialyzer that could remove fluid and waste chemicals, slowly, over a period of hours or several days. It was a relatively low flow system. The technique had the advantage of being used over time to avoid rapid changes in blood volume and ease the work of the heart while providing large clearances of urea and other waste products of metabolism. Slow, continuous therapy could achieve so much fluid loss over time that it allowed the administration of nutrients intravenously to patients, even if they were not making urine. The loss of fluid often improved the tenuous condition of a patient with combined severe heart and kidney failure. Bosch and collaborators published their landmark paper in the *AIM* in 1983, adding to the nephrologists' armamentarium of hemodialysis and peritoneal dialysis for the very ill.[39] Bosch subsequently moved to George Washington University, where he pushed the research interests of the Division of Renal Diseases and Hypertension to include studies of acute renal failure and its treatment as well as spearheading programs in improving the efficiency of hemodialysis. Others, including Drs. Ravindra Mehta at the University of California, San Diego, and Claudio Ronco and colleagues in Vicenza, Italy, have advanced the field to include mechanical assistance pumps that facilitate and control the treatment, allowing the transformation of the procedure to involve only the patients' venous circulation, as continuous venovenous hemofiltration (CVVH). These procedures are now used commonly in critically ill patients in U.S. intensive care units and across the globe and are encompassed by the terms continuous renal replacement therapies, or CRRTs.

A paper in *Critical Care* in 2007 signaled the death knell for the diagnosis of acute renal failure, substituting acute kidney injury as the approved nomenclature. The authors of the paper comprised a distinguished group of international nephrologists (and a critical care physician)[40] writing for the Acute Kidney Injury Network, which hoped definitions and standard naming conventions would aid epidemiologic studies of the syndrome. (The group had originally met in Vicenza, Italy, in 2004, and Amsterdam, Netherlands, in 2005. The authors stated that the American Society of Nephrology, the International Society of Nephrology, the National Kidney Foundation, and the European Society of Intensive Care Medicine had provided input into the proceedings.) The abstract of the article stated, "The term AKI is proposed to represent the entire spectrum of acute renal failure. Diagnostic criteria for AKI are proposed based on acute alterations in serum creatinine or urine output. A staging system for AKI which reflects quantitative changes in serum creatinine and urine output has been developed." Although there was some grumbling from old-timers, the new moniker has held up over time.

Prospects for a Cure for AKI

Research performed in the 1990s and the first decade of the 21st century attempted to use drugs that had showed some success in ameliorating the long-term and inexorable decline of kidney function seen in animal models of AKI. Therapeutic trials in randomized studies of humans with ARF included administration of hormones and growth factors, which had been shown to improve acute renal failure in animals. None of these trials in patients was successful. In truth, the animal models do not reproduce the complex physiology and compensations that occur in humans after an episode of AKI. Two main avenues of research currently address these thorny scientific and clinical issues.

The NIDDK established the Kidney Precision Medicine Project (KPMP) in 2017. Meeting in the Washington, D.C., area, NIDDK scientists and academic scientists from around the country and the world agreed that animal models of AKI did not reproduce with fidelity the clinical characteristics of the human disease. A key aspect of this workshop was the participation of patients who had experienced an episode of AKI. Their stories galvanized the scientists attending the meeting by giving individual human faces to the suffering experienced during the episode and afterward. In addition, the patient participants validated the approach to evaluating the clinical problem using kidney biopsy material from human volunteers, affirming that the research could be conducted ethically and safely. The best way forward, members of the conference thought, was to obtain human tissue from patients with kidney disease to delineate the pathways involved in kidney injury as well as kidney repair in patients with AKI—only after first providing information about the risks and benefits of the study and obtaining informed, voluntary consent from the participants. These precious tissues would be analyzed by modern high-tech procedures (now often called 'omics studies), using up-to-the-minute, state-of-the-art methodologies. Some of these include evaluating the expression of specific genes in specific cell types in kidney disease or evaluating the presence of individual proteins or chemicals in tiny samples of the kidney tissue. All the cutting-edge tools of modern biology would be brought to bear to address the conundrum of the pathogenesis and cure of AKI. Patients with AKI attributed to the common syndrome of acute tubular necrosis only rarely are evaluated using the relatively invasive procedure of kidney biopsy because the clinical course of the disease entity is so well delineated. Clinicians watch for the oliguric phase, wait for the onset of the diuretic phase, and hope that the kidney will ultimately repair itself, just as Maurice Strauss described in 1948. The KPMP is predicated on the altruistic participation of patients with AKI who undergo the risk of a renal biopsy to provide a precious piece of tissue from their bodies to move science forward. In many cases, there may be no benefit to the patient from this gift. The participants in the study have been accounted as heroes. The biopsies performed under the aegis of the KPMP are done under the strictest ethical and safety provisions. An independent Data and Safety Monitoring Board (DSMB) reviews the study at frequent intervals. A patient representative, as well as ethicists, are included on the DSMB to maintain the high standards of the study. Over the next five to ten years, information from the KPMP may help resolve the thorny problem of a cure for the long-standing, well-known clinical problem of ATN.[41]

Marla Levy was a happily married forty-one-year-old woman in November 2013. She had one- and three-year-old daughters, a loving husband, and a satisfying job providing medical products to acute care units in Northern California hospitals. Levy had always been interested in medicine and felt she was serving the community through her work. True, she had had some medical problems. As a child, she knew she couldn't run or exert herself as much as other children, or she might pass out. This seemingly slight limitation didn't disturb Levy. "It didn't affect me at all." However, at the age of twenty-one, her college classmates became alarmed at her frequent fainting with exertion. She underwent tests, including an echocardiogram. She received a diagnosis of supravalvular aortic stenosis (a disorder involving one of the principal valves of the heart). Thereafter, she underwent cardiac catheterization. The diagnosis was confirmed, but Levy was told that she didn't need further interventions at the time. All was well until Levy was twenty-seven. At that time, when her clinical condition worsened, she underwent open-heart surgery, and a valve homograft was provided. Levy did well for fourteen years. In November 2013, however, she became gravely ill.

Because of the deterioration of the homograft, Levy needed to have an aortic graft replacement. During her open-heart operation, which unexpectedly required coronary artery bypass procedures as well, Levy's heart stopped and couldn't be restarted. She underwent the equivalent of a "code" for six hours. While her chest was open, Levy was treated with the extracorporeal membrane oxygenation device conceived of by Kolff more than a lifetime previously, in order to support the function of her heart and lungs. (Levy was delighted to learn of this connection between the originator of dialysis and the ECMO procedure.) Because of her severely weakened heart, her blood pressure was very low, a condition called cardiogenic shock. Levy's kidneys "shut down." She had no renal function. Levy was supported by continuous renal replacement therapy and hemodialysis for almost a month. At the end of her hospital stay, Levy was discharged to an outpatient dialysis unit. Her treatment there was characterized by a series of hospital readmissions and discharges with seemingly little coordination among the dialysis unit, hospital physicians, and outpatient physicians and staff.

Levy was horrified by her care after her discharge from the hospital:

It was such a shock. I went from being a completely healthy person to being tethered to a CRRT machine. I was very scared, and I thought I was dying. Nobody told me there was any chance of survival. I thought I had received a death sentence. My new outpatient dialysis unit treated me without any records. No one ever listened to me or treated me as an individual. They had their "policies and procedures." In several days I was in congestive heart failure with massive fluid overload. I wasn't breathing. I couldn't open my eyes. When I came home to see my children, I couldn't communicate with them, or hug them, I was so fluid overloaded. I could only communicate by blinking my eyes. My condition was so severe, I couldn't believe I was able to survive to get to the hospital. I was readmitted to UCSF. In the hospital they dialyzed me for five days in a row.

Afterward, they discharged me back to the dialysis unit. I was never scheduled as an outpatient to see a nephrologist who knew my history. I was sent back to UCSF to see surgeons to create a permanent vascular access. I was in a referral merry-go-round. Somebody sent me to Dr. Chi-Yuan Hsu, a nephrologist at UCSF. After reading my old records and examining me, Dr. Hsu told me "I want to take you off dialysis." I said, "Are you kidding me?" He told me "I truly believe dialysis is doing you a disservice." In the spring of 2014, I was hospitalized at UCSF for eight days, under close medical observation. Over that time, my creatinine spontaneously, progressively decreased, without dialysis. My recovery was slow. A physical therapist was sent to my home to help me walk. I was told I was too weak to profit from therapy and I never saw the therapist again. My husband helped me walk, slowly but over a period of weeks, from my living room to the kitchen. One day I was strong enough to walk from the living room to the kitchen by myself. That was quite a milestone for me! By 2016, I finally felt like I was back to my old self. But I had undergone an incredible ordeal.

Levy's story illustrates the fragmented care patients receive after an episode of AKI. Inexplicably, but reflecting the current status of care, she wasn't immediately referred to a nephrologist at discharge from the hospital. She faced problems reestablishing her place in her marriage and family, as she was desperately trying to regain her health and strength. Luckily, things turned out well for Levy as well as for her family. Her story can be viewed online.[42]

Realizing that a cure for AKI might still be a decade or so in the future, scientists at NIDDK proposed an alternative way of improving outcomes for patients who develop AKI during a hospitalization. Shockingly, as Levy's case illustrates, even in the best medical settings, it became apparent that very few patients who had sustained an episode of AKI were followed, by any physician, let alone nephrologists, after discharge from the hospital. After a workshop held in January 2019, NIDDK scientists proposed a study of radical changes in the follow-up of patients who had sustained an episode of AKI in the hospital.[43] Current plans for this randomized study include close follow-up of patients with AKI after hospital discharge, the use of nurses acting as "navigators" to help facilitate interactions within a complex, fragmented medical system, and frequent checks of the medications ordered for such patients. The work is being led by Dr. Ivonne Schulman at NIDDK with Dr. Kaleab Abebe from the University of Pittsburgh and Drs. Emilio Poggio of the Cleveland Clinic, Edward Siew of Vanderbilt University, Orlando Gutiérrez and Javier Neyra of the University of Alabama, and Chirag Parikh, now of Johns Hopkins University. Hopefully, information from the Caring for Outpatients after AKI (COPE-AKI) study will be available in several years to help clinicians guide the care of patients with AKI after their hospitalization, to improve outcomes. Ms. Marla Levy served as an active, highly regarded participant in the NIDDK workshop that led to the conception of the COPE-AKI study, and was a coauthor of its report. Levy is currently a consultant to the Scientific Data and Research Center of the study.

Looking Back and Forward

The Nobel Prize laureate Dr. Joseph Goldstein praised Dr. Willem Kolff as he won the 2002 Lasker Award for his work enabling the successful treatment of patients with end-stage renal disease. In his address, Goldstein reviewed Kolff's reasons for developing dialysis, his scientific forebears, the scientific underpinnings of the procedure and outlined Kolff's numerous initial failures and final success treating patients with acute renal failure with a contraption he built, that worked, during the Nazi occupation. Goldstein described the bathtub apparatus operationalized for clinical care. Goldstein retold the story of Kolff's patient who awoke from coma to divorce her husband. He described how dialysis machines had been sent by Kolff to hospitals in London, Poland, The Hague, Montreal, and New York City, jump-starting the field. He recounted Kolff's visit to the Brigham with blueprints of his device. Goldstein mentioned how this visit had been critical for the development of dialysis and transplantation in the U.S. and across the globe. He noted the inventor's other engineering achievements in heart surgery and lauded him shortly before Kolff's ninety-second birthday.

A steel Kolff-Brigham artificial kidney machine currently is owned by but "not on view" at the Smithsonian's Museum of American History. Kolff died on February 11, 2009, eight days before his ninety-eighth birthday. He was awarded the Harvey Prize in 1972 from the Technion Institute in Israel, "in recognition of his contribution to human health through his invention of the artificial kidney." In addition to the Amory Prize, among his many accolades he also received the Cameron Prize for Therapeutics from the University of Edinburgh in 1964, the Gairdner Foundation International Award in 1966, the Wilhelm Exner Medal in 1980, and the Japan Prize in 1986. The person who shared the Lasker Award with Kolff was Dr. Belding H. Scribner.

John Merrill began his fellowship at the Brigham under Dr. George Thorn in 1948, roughly thirty years before I began my training in kidney disease at the University of Pennsylvania. Merrill's copious, wide-ranging work in nephrology also included a call for the establishment of a national program that would support the care of ESRD patients. Merrill died suddenly in 1984 at the age of sixty-seven in a boating accident in the Bahamas while on vacation.

In 2004, there were almost 900,000 hospitalizations in the U.S. with a diagnosis of acute renal failure. The number of patients who experience AKI in the U.S. is undoubtedly greater today. A cure for AKI still seems to be off in the future. Dialysis for patients terribly ill with acute renal failure, however, was literally invented by a set of three pioneering thirty-somethings, from diverse backgrounds in Europe, New York, and Boston more than seventy years ago. In 1979, six years after the inception of the ESRD program, I did not even have a glimmer of how much my own work, and indeed the broadening field of treatment of acute as well as chronic kidney disease, was dependent on the work that Kolff did in Europe, Cleveland, and Salt Lake City and Merrill did at the Brigham over their long and illustrious careers.

4

---- ❧ ----

THE BIRTH OF THE ESRD PROGRAM

If you developed a rapidly progressive kidney disease, such as malignant hypertension, which also affected the heart, eyes, and brain, in the U.S. in the 1950s, and your kidneys failed, no option was available except death.

In 1960, if you became ill with uremia, you might have survived if you lived in Seattle, Washington, although the odds would be against you. You might have had a better chance at life if you were a White man, had a job, and were young.

By 1974, however, if you lived anywhere in the U.S. and had worked long enough to contribute some payments to the Social Security system and your kidneys failed, your life could be saved by treatment with dialysis for the newly designated illness end-stage renal disease (ESRD). (Although, if you were older than sixty-five or had diabetes, there was some concern that the program might not be for you, and your participation might be discouraged.) You even had a chance to receive a kidney transplant, paid for by the U.S. ESRD program. Your chances of receiving a kidney were higher if you were young and you were White.

The birth of the U.S. ESRD program is the story of many people. The tale involves life and death decisions, pathbreaking medical advances and experiments, ethical issues, political considerations, economic concerns, and legislative horse trading. The effort had a complex genesis and an intricate set of actors from different backgrounds who did not always work together but ultimately shared common goals. The establishment of the program involved patients, members of a new subspecialty called nephrologists, surgeons, engineers, nurses, social workers, psychologists and psychiatrists, philanthropists, journalists, politicians, and patients. The work required first and foremost patients and lastly and most importantly patients.

Since this medical crusade began more than a half century ago, most of the people involved in this story have died. But their efforts have had tremendous ramifications for the hundreds of thousands of people whose lives have been saved by the ESRD program and the more than 800,000 patients currently treated with dialysis or who have received a kidney transplant, according to the most recent statistics.[1] Dr. Richard Rettig pointed out that at least four leaders should be highlighted in recounting the history of federal coverage of the treatment of people with uremia: Drs. Willem Kolff, John Merrill, Belding Scribner, and George Schreiner.[2] Let's start somewhat out of order with the person who made the successful, ongoing treatment of patients with a chronic, previously fatal disease a reality.

By 1960, Dr. Belding Scribner had thought for many years about how to keep patients alive with chronic kidney disease whose illness had reached a crisis point—where the function of the kidneys could no longer support life. Scribner himself was standing on the shoulders of giants, whose work had progressed by fits and starts over the previous century, which culminated in the provision of dialysis to those with advanced kidney disease.

Early Experience with Dialysis

The Scottish chemist Thomas Graham (1805–1869) coined the term *dialysis* in 1861 to describe the movement of colloids and crystalloids across a semipermeable membrane. Abel, Rowntree, and Turner in Baltimore about a half century later reported in the *Transactions of the Association of American Physicians* (1913) and the *Journal of Pharmacology* (1914)[3] on the use of these techniques, including the application of hirudin, a substance that prevented blood clotting in live dogs, to demonstrate the feasibility of dialysis in living animals. To be useful to treat uremia in humans, the condition where retained toxins circulating in the bloodstream would eventually cause death, the procedure required (1) access to a patient's bloodstream, (2) a safe and effective anticoagulant (or blood thinner, as it is called colloquially), (3) a safe and efficient dialysis semipermeable membrane to allow wastes to flow out of the blood and be discarded, and (4) a pump to facilitate blood flow through the circuit. For patients with acute but reversible losses of kidney function, the system might be used for a week or two. For patients with chronic irreversible kidney disease, the system would have to last a lifetime.

Dr. Georg Haas (1886–1971) first treated humans with uremia with dialysis in 1924 in Germany, using the newly available anticoagulant drug heparin. However, faced with challenges and disappointing results, he gave up his work in 1928. It was left to Dr. Willem Kolff to move the field forward, amid warfare, through 1945. During World War II in the Netherlands, Kolff developed a rotating drum device, really a large container, using a cellophane membrane (made from the material used to create sausage casings) and a solution termed dialysate that would facilitate the diffusion of toxins and waste products from the patient's bloodstream into the device for disposal according to the principles laid out by Graham. After many attempts that culminated in the deaths of many patients, one of his patients, an elderly woman with kidney failure in the face of an overwhelming infection, recovered from acute renal failure after dialysis using Kolff's device. Kolff, still in his early thirties, reported his work and the survival of his first patient in 1944. Although many of the patients he had treated before this successful attempt had died, this single instance of survival was taken as proof that dialysis was a lifesaving procedure for patients with acute renal failure. The challenge remained to translate this heroic advance into clinical practice and build a system that could be used in day-to-day patient care in hospitals across the globe.

Kolff's dialysis machine design was modified and used to treat patients with acute renal failure by American physicians before and during the Korean War. A Kolff device was given to Mount Sinai Hospital in New York and used in the care of patients with acute renal failure. Physicians at the Peter Bent Brigham Hospital in Boston also adapted the Kolff design from blueprints Kolff provided to its physician in chief Dr. George Thorn. The new, modified machine was known as the Kolff-Brigham artificial kidney. The Kolff-Brigham artificial kidney was made available to other hospitals between 1954 and 1962.

Dr. Nils Alwall, a Swedish physician, as early as the late 1940s became interested in the treatment of uremia by dialysis. In 1947, he described a "dialyzer" that could perform the twin functions of removing waste and excess fluid from patients, more efficiently than Kolff's rotating drum.[4] This dialyzer placed cellophane membranes in a more compact device that could accommodate a blood pump.

Scribner and the Start of Chronic Dialysis in Seattle

Belding Hibbard Scribner was born in 1921 in Chicago. Scribner graduated from the University of California, Berkeley, in 1941 and received his medical degree from Stanford in 1945. One of his teachers there was Thomas Addis, a nephrologist who pioneered in the treatment of kidney disease with diet and had an interest in quantifying metabolism in chronic glomerular diseases of the kidney. Scribner pursued postgraduate studies at the Mayo Clinic and obtained a master's degree from the University of Minnesota in 1951. He started on the faculty of the University of Washington (UW) School of Medicine in 1951 and by 1958 was the chief of kidney diseases at UW, a position he retained until 1982.

Scribner became interested in dialysis after listening to a lecture by Dr. John Merrill of Harvard's Peter Bent Brigham Hospital given at the Mayo Clinic in 1950. Merrill, an early expert in acute renal failure and the new dialysis therapy, described the use of the Kolff-Brigham artificial kidney in the care of patients with kidney failure. Scribner understood that the overwhelming obstacle in delivering dialysis to patients with the more common, chronic form of kidney disease over a long period of time was obtaining repeated access to the circulation. Typically, the cannulation of blood vessels quickly scarred them, preventing their further use for dialysis, rendering ongoing care impossible. The treatment of the patient over an extended period of time, therefore, was a clinical improbability. Pondering this seemingly insoluble issue for weeks, he woke from sleep in the middle of the night with the answer to the problem.

Scribner conceived of a plastic cannula that could be connected and disconnected and accessed by tubing linked to a dialysis machine that would be surgically implanted between an artery and a vein, remaining on the outside of the body when not in use. Scribner consulted with Loren Winterschied, a surgeon at UW, as they met by chance on the stairs. Winterschied suggested the use of Teflon, which had been newly developed, as a material for the tubing. Teflon had already been shown in other studies to resist the propensity to blood clotting. Working with the engineer Wayne Quinton, in 1961, they devised a Teflon tube that formed an arteriovenous shunt, connecting the radial artery in the wrist to a vein in the forearm.[5]

On March 9, 1960, Clyde Shields, a patient of Scribner's, became the first person to have a shunt surgically created for use to enable chronic dialysis. Shields was thirty-nine years old, was employed, and had chronic glomerulonephritis, a disease resulting from the inflammation and subsequent destruction of the filtering portions of the kidneys. In advanced stages, the disease was uniformly fatal. Dr. David Dillard performed the operation. Shields became the first patient to be treated in what would become Seattle's Artificial Kidney Center. His ongoing survival could be taken either as a miracle or a revolution in medical technology and care.

Scribner did not have time to submit an abstract of this work for presentation at the meeting of the American Society for Artificial Internal Organs (ASAIO) in April 1960, but he attended the conference with Mr. Shields.

The meeting was conducted under the direction of Dr. George Schreiner of Georgetown University. The conference attendees heard a dramatic presentation on the advances that had taken place in Seattle. Scribner prepared two papers, both published by the society in its transactions, in which he recounted his progress in treating patients with uremia. One paper reported on the creation of the shunt, and the other outlined the development of a program to treat patients with chronic renal failure with maintenance hemodialysis. The papers, though published in a seemingly obscure technology journal, of course went on to be among the most highly cited in the medical literature.[6]

A National News Story about the Seattle Artificial Kidney Center

A little less than two years later, in November 1962, Shana Alexander wrote about the Seattle dialysis program in the popular weekly *Life* magazine.[7] She reported the case of John Myers, who had known he had kidney disease since his army discharge in 1945 but didn't have symptoms until 1960. At that time, working as a businessman, he began to notice headaches, with increased blood pressure. At age thirty-seven, he could barely go to work. In December 1961, he became acutely ill with a severe headache, cough, nausea, and swelling of his legs. His kidney disease had progressed to the stage of uremia. He was accepted as a patient at the Seattle dialysis program. Twice a week, Myers traveled the forty miles from Bremerton by ferryboat across Puget Sound to Seattle. He was dialyzed in the evening in an annex of Swedish Hospital. Alexander wrote that there was a "small, U-shaped plastic tube sutured into the blood vessels of his left forearm."

Alexander, somewhat dismissively, called the kidney "relatively simple in function," really only a "filter." To a nephrologist, this characterization is infuriating. How manifold are the functions of the normal organ is made clear as the author went on to describe the machine and procedures designed to attempt to replace the performance of the human kidney.

The article portrayed the dialysis apparatus as a "washing machine." Alexander depicted the procedure, including the connection of the shunt to the machine tubing, the flow of blood from the artificial shunt, through the tubing, into the dialysis machine, and then back into Myers's arm. Myers's dialysis treatment took ten to twelve hours a session. The procedure was reported to be "painless."

Alexander explained that, at that time, approximately 100,000 patients a year developed uremia and died of kidney disease in the U.S. She noted there were five patients cared for at Swedish Hospital with end-stage renal disease. The other patients were "a car salesman, a physicist, an engineer, and an aircraft worker." One of those patients was Clyde Shields. At that time, the program was scheduled to scale up to ten patients a year. The cost of dialysis in the program was, according to her sources, about $15,000 a year per patient. (The median family income in the U.S. in 1962 was about $6,000 a year.)

Alexander went on to recount the hard choices that had to be made at the start of this experimental medical program. Only one patient out of the fifty who needed treatment could be accommodated by the Seattle program. Alexander emphasized that Myers had not been chosen to receive the treatment by chance or by physicians but by a committee. She outlined the procedures of the Admissions and Policies Committee of the Seattle Artificial Kidney Center at Swedish Hospital, which consisted of seven people. They had been appointed by the King County Medical Society and had served anonymously and without pay. Alexander called the seven members a "Life or Death Committee." The committee met for the first time in the summer of 1961. Members included "a lawyer, a minister, a banker, a housewife, an official of state government, a labor leader, and a surgeon."

Physicians who briefed committee members suggested that patients over age forty-five and children should not be accepted because their treatment might be fraught with obstacles. It was thought that their care would be simply too difficult. Committee members decided to keep their identities anonymous. They also requested keeping the names of the potential treatment candidates unknown. Committee members created a list of factors they would use in making decisions. Some of these items included patients' age and sex, their marital status and number of dependents, their income and net worth, their emotional status, educational background, and "future potential." The committee also thought that references for the candidates from friends, acquaintances, and associates could be useful to inform choices. They agreed to limit candidacy for dialysis therapy to residents of the state of Washington. A key rationale was that the shunt had been developed at the UW School of Medicine and its university hospital using state tax revenues. A principle, however, was established. In life and death decisions, where medical resources were limited, nonmedical personnel should play crucial roles in their ethical allocation. Currently opinions from nonphysicians are sought by institutional review boards and, more recently, regarding the conduct of some clinical studies supported by the federal government.

Alexander presented a typical set of deliberations undertaken by the committee and also provided a brief interview with each of the committee members, focusing on their backgrounds, perspectives, and the way each viewed the choices he or she made. She related that at a meeting, five candidates were considered for two places newly available for dialysis treatment in the Center. The Kidney Center at that time contained only three beds to accommodate all the patients with uremia from the state of Washington. Alexander did not report interviews with people who had not been accepted by the program.

Alexander described Scribner's original conception of the shunt. She outlined the development of the shunt, starting in 1960, from Scribner's early morning epiphany, to its realization as a medical device two weeks later. The first patient who had a shunt inserted was described as suffering from "Bright's disease." That patient, Clyde Shields, a forty-two-year-old machinist, was alive two years later, when Alexander wrote the article. Patients underwent many shunt insertions during the course of more than two years as they wore out, clotted, or became infected.

Scribner's experimental program, including the selection committee, was funded by a $250,000 research grant from the John Hartford Foundation. Start-up funds were also supplied by the University of Washington.

Alexander ended the article by reviewing the ethical issues faced by the committee. "Who really is the more suitable patient under the present committee rules—the man who, if he is permitted to continue living, can make the greatest contribution to society; or the man who by dying would leave behind the greatest burden on society?" Alexander did not comment on the possible dialysis of women.

The article in essence set forth the ethical choices involved in the clash of incremental, practical responses with the development of a new, expensive lifesaving technology for a uniformly fatal disease when resources were scarce, not solely because of the lack of funds. The agonized emotions of the members of the committee, who were making existential choices, can be understood by anyone who had served on a jury or who had had to make a difficult decision that might affect someone's life. The story, however, served to place kidney disease and its treatment front and center in the national consciousness. A decade later, the ethical conundrum would be faced by the country's leadership as it considered patients who might be poor, unmarried, childless, unemployed, or of minority status. These choices involved, unwittingly, those who may not have made great contributions to society (subjectively determined) but who wanted to live. In 1962, a seed had been planted.

Technical Advances and Advocacy Efforts

The challenge now was to enable this therapy to disseminate throughout the nation. Physicians came to Seattle to learn how to create shunts as well as how to dialyze uremic patients to keep them alive, but often, returning to their own hospitals, they found that no structure existed to treat the sick. As the new subspecialty of nephrology came into being, there were no machines to cleanse uremic patients' blood. And if there were machines, who would pay for treatment that was deemed "experimental"? Insurance only covered traditional therapies. Dialysis would be expensive. The Seattle group estimated their costs at $15,000 per patient per year and speculated that 100,000 people across the U.S. needed and could benefit from the treatment. (If all those patients were to be treated, costs would be $1.5 billion a year.) Yet starting a unit might be daunting. The machines took up space, and treatment was delivered by technicians and supervised by nurses. Both nurses and technicians needed specialized skills and training. Social workers' and psychologists' assistance and expertise were critical to surviving an onerous but lifesaving treatment. Rents needed to be paid, and sources of salaries for doctors, nurses, technicians, and administrators had to be identified. Access to space, water, and electricity were essential. Units had to be cleaned regularly. The clinical status of the treated patients had to be monitored frequently with routine and special laboratory tests, and the tests had to be paid for. Rents, utilities, salaries, and laboratory evaluations all posed hurdles to diffusion of this new technology. In the absence of financial support from a charitable foundation, it appeared that no dialysis treatments could occur, even if they could save lives.

Dr. James Cimino, head of the Renal Unit, and Dr. Michael Brescia, a medical chief resident at the Bronx Veterans Administration Hospital in New York, with Reuben Aboody, reported in the *NEJM* in 1962 that simple, repeated puncture of veins could be used to support the dialysis of patients with chronic kidney failure.[8] In 1966, Brescia, by this time an attending physician, and Cimino (head of the Hospital Dialysis Unit)—working with Kenneth Appel, a surgeon, and

Baruch Hurwich, a physician on the Renal Service at the VA Hospital—reported in the *NEJM* on the creation of an arteriovenous fistula for hemodialysis.[9] The fistula, a connection between an artery and vein created surgically, had the ability to support the blood flows needed for dialysis and could be used repeatedly. The investigators had feared creation of a fistula could cause or exacerbate heart failure in patients. As the fistulas matured, increasing in size and permitting greater blood flows, such problems had not been detected in the thirteen patients who had undergone surgery, whose course was reported in the paper. Three of the patients in the series had been treated this way for over a year. The technique diffused across the nation (and around the world), changing clinical practice dramatically. The Brescia-Cimino fistula obviated or ameliorated some of the problems encountered with the Scribner shunt and was safer and more convenient for patients as well as dialysis staff. Over six years, physicians had learned how to dialyze patients. This innovation in vascular access could potentially enable the rapid growth of programs designed to treat patients whose kidneys had failed. Was that growth a possibility, practically and financially, in 1967?

The National Nephrosis Foundation developed as a result of parents wishing to find a cure for their children with nephrotic syndrome. The foundation was active through the late 1950s and early 1960s, with a focus on patients with kidney disease and their families. The organization responded to the recent advances in dialysis techniques and the new technology of kidney transplantation. The National Nephrosis Foundation became the National Kidney Foundation (NKF) in 1964. The NKF developed a unique organizational structure, linking physicians with patients and families, setting up regional centers with a coordinating national office. The NKF focused on patient welfare and the search for treatments and cures, while emphasizing patient well-being, patient education, and professional growth through educational and research meetings. The foundation engaged in efforts to secure federal funding to treat and cure kidney disease. Under the NKF's auspices, training centers for professionals engaged in the treatment of kidney disease, and public education became key missions. In addition, the NKF supported research by young and established physicians and pushed for the development, dissemination, and coverage of dialysis techniques. Dr. George Schreiner of Georgetown University in Washington, D.C., became active in the foundation.

Federal Responses

Richard Rettig has carefully documented, in several publications, the federal response to the burgeoning appreciation by patients, physicians, and policy makers of the clinical conundrum that a large proportion of the U.S. population had advanced kidney disease. Although a treatment for the malady existed, its cost was great, and it was largely inaccessible to those in need.[10] By 1963, the Veterans Administration decided to establish dialysis centers in some of its hospitals across the nation. The National Institute of Allergy and Infectious Diseases (NIAID) of the National Institutes of Health (NIH) established a program in 1964 to foster research in the immunology of organ transplantation to provide support for enhancing the initial favorable clinical results reported nationwide, hoping to provide a cheaper, more desirable alternative to dialysis. A sister institute at NIH, the National Institute of Arthritis and Metabolic Diseases (a forerunner of the NIDDK) started an artificial kidney and chronic uremia program in response to the advances emanating from Seattle in 1965 to encourage research in this new field. The U.S. Public Health Service started a program in 1965 to facilitate the development of dialysis centers across the nation, followed by issuing contracts to spur development of programs that would allow patients to perform dialysis in their homes the next year.

President Lyndon Johnson played a key role in the congressional enactment of Medicare in 1965, part of his Great Society program, to ensure the health of elderly people in the U.S. who could not afford medical care. Medicaid was enacted to provide access to care to the poor on a state-by-state basis.

As pressure increased from patient groups and physicians, and as the realization grew among the public and their legislative representatives that there were many people around the country who could live if given access to dialysis but who would die without receiving this treatment, the government realized there was a need to evaluate therapy both from policy and fiscal perspectives. Dr. James Kimmey, chief of the Public Health Service's Renal Disease Activity Branch in the Division of Chronic Disease, had advocated for a national dialysis program, but the costs remained uncertain.

Perhaps considering the costs of these clinical and research advances, the Bureau of the Budget, working with the White House Office of Science and

Technology Policy, convened a group of experts to assess end-stage renal disease, evaluate whether new treatments for the illness were effective and could be added to the clinical armamentarium, and suggest fiscally responsible and medically reasonable and ethical responses the federal government might undertake and support.

The committee needed to be multidisciplinary. Policy, economic, ethical, and medical issues would have to be simultaneously considered. The committee would address key scientific and societal questions. Was dialysis therapy feasible in the widespread clinical community? Was dialysis still "experimental"? Would chronic, ongoing dialysis treatment indeed make a meaningful clinical difference in patients' lives? How much would dialysis cost, how many patients would it affect, and would the cost be reasonable for the nation?

Members of the committee convened by the Bureau of the Budget included distinguished nephrologists, pioneers in kidney transplant surgery and immunology, a psychiatrist, economists, a lawyer, and others.[11] The government chose Dr. Carl Gottschalk to head the Committee on Chronic Kidney Disease. Gottschalk had an important role in selecting the medical scientists and ethicists on the committee.

Gottschalk was born in 1922 in Salem, Virginia. After graduation from Roanoke College, he matriculated at the University of Virginia and received a medical degree in 1945. He interned at Massachusetts General Hospital in Boston and subsequently, from 1946 to 1948, performed research while in the U.S. Army Medical Corps on the effects of cold climates and exposure on military personnel. He returned to Boston and, from 1948 to 1950, worked at Harvard Medical School, where he became interested in the kidneys. Thereafter, he served on the faculty of the University of North Carolina (UNC) until his retirement in 1992. Gottschalk's initial interest was in lepidoptery, and he identified a new species of butterfly as a teenager. At UNC, Gottschalk developed into one of the world's greatest renal physiologists. Mastering the vagaries of renal micropuncture, a laborious technique that required great manual dexterity and an ability to interpret limited information to formulate far-reaching conclusions about the workings of the kidney, Gottschalk investigated the ways in which the kidney concentrated and diluted the urine in response to water ingestion and dehydration and advanced understanding of its responses to disease. Gottschalk edited several editions of the original Strauss and Welt textbook *Diseases of the Kidney*, with eminent nephrologists such as Drs. Laurence Earley and Robert Schrier. By 1966, Gottschalk was widely renowned as one of the most important nephrologists in the country as well as internationally.

The distinguished, multidisciplinary Gottschalk Committee was well prepared to address the scope of advanced chronic kidney disease in the U.S., including the number of patients affected, the utility of the treatments, and their ability to be disseminated through routine medical care, across the country. Their work was informed by the need to show tangible results from the recent increased federal funding of medical science, through the NIH and other venues, as well as the newly established Medicare and Medicaid programs, which enhanced access to medical care for the elderly and the poor. In addition, it was evident, especially considering the inclusion of economists trained in cost benefit analyses and knowledgeable regarding allocation of scarce resources, including health care, that decision-making about the expense and coverage of these new treatments had to be confronted. Were dialysis and transplantation "experimental" therapies, therefore not covered by employee health insurance plans, or had they become routine parts of health care for the ravages of chronic illness? Irving Lewis of the Bureau of the Budget lamented that although several government agencies such as the NIH, the Veterans Administration, and the Public Health Service had become interested in these therapies, there was no "national approach." The committee had to come up with a well-founded federal response to the ethical, medical, economic, and policy problems presented by patients with this newly named end-stage renal disease.

The committee met seven times between July 1966 and May 1967. Its report was submitted to Charles Schultze, the director of the Bureau of the Budget, in September 1967. The report affirmed that treatment of end-stage renal disease with dialysis and kidney transplantation was not experimental. Dialysis and transplantation were life-saving procedures that should be available to all who needed them. Because of their great cost, the committee suggested that treatment for patients with ESRD should be covered by Medicare. A limited number of copies of the Gottschalk Report were made publicly available to the research community in November 1967 by the National Institute of Arthritis and Metabolism. And then nothing happened. Although the report galvanized the nephrology community, it was not widely disseminated, and the public was largely unaware of its recommendations and their implications. The Gottschalk Committee was not a public body but rather functioned in an advisory capacity to the Bureau of the Budget. The work of the committee was not publicly acknowledged by Mr. Schultze. Key congressional staffers and congressmen were not aware of the report, and they were preoccupied by other issues raised by the beginnings of the Medicare and Medicaid programs.

Realizing the Goals of the Gottschalk Report

Between the release of the Gottschalk Report and the congressional hearings that resulted in the establishment of the ESRD program, large dialysis programs developed at the University of Washington, regionally in Boston, at the Downstate Medical Center in Brooklyn, and at Georgetown University Hospital. Kidney transplant programs grew at Harvard, at the University of California, San Francisco, and at the University of Minnesota.

George Schreiner (1923–2012) was a larger-than-life figure, who became the leading U.S. practitioner of dialysis, from his position at Georgetown University, close to the power brokers of Washington, D.C.[12] Schreiner had treated patients with acute renal failure in the Korean War, and had worked as a fellow at NYU and Bellevue Hospital, where he studied with Homer Smith. Schreiner made Georgetown University a center for the study and treatment of patients with uremia. He served as the president of both the National Kidney Foundation and the newly formed American Society of Nephrology. Schreiner was a founder, in 1954, of the American Society for Artificial Internal Organs, the sponsor of the meeting where Scribner presented his patient, Clyde Shields, as evidence of the success of his dialysis treatment program. Schreiner, after serving as president of the NKF, became the chairman of its legislative committee. He hired Charles Plante, a neighbor, who had more than a decade of experience working on Capitol Hill, as the Washington representative of the NKF in 1969. Together they developed a plan to influence legislation, including requests for increased support for NIH funding of kidney disease research and establishing a Kidney Institute within NIH, as well as obtaining public funding for an ESRD treatment program.

Legislation had been proposed to support ESRD care in every Congress since 1965.[13] The legislation was supported by the two powerful Democratic senators from Washington State, Warren Magnuson and Henry (Scoop) Jackson. Magnuson had served in the Senate since 1944 and had been a strong proponent of the foundation, funding, and growth of the NIH and cancer care, as well as a supporter of the military and civil rights. Magnuson served on the Senate Commerce Committee, and in his final term, on the Senate Appropriations Committee. He is remembered in part by the naming of the NIH Clinical Center in his honor. Scoop Jackson became a senator in 1953 after serving for more than a decade in the House of Representatives. He supported the military, civil rights, health care, and environmental programs. Jackson vigorously opposed communism and the Soviet Union, focusing on the issue of lack of human rights in totalitarian states. A childhood friend of Jackson's became a patient of Belding Scribner's and began dialysis for ESRD in 1967. John Tower, Republican senator from Texas, joined them in support of funding for treatment of patients with kidney disease.

The Committee on Ways and Means of the House of Representatives was the locus of the taxation power of Congress as well as the committee with the ultimate purview over paying for health care, including through the established Social Security, and the newer Medicare and Medicaid programs. Legislation involving payments for health care must originate in Ways and Means before approval by the full House, after which it moves to the Senate for further consideration. The chairman of Ways and Means, the Democrat Wilbur Mills of Arkansas, had been in Congress since 1939, and had headed the committee since 1958. Mills had been crucial to the enactment of the legislation that created Medicare. Over yearly cycles, Ways and Means considered legislation related to taxation, Social Security, Medicare, and international trade and held lengthy public hearings on each matter. The committee at the time was open to hearing the testimony of individual citizens and advocacy groups on pertinent issues related to legislation under consideration.

How the ESRD Sausage Was Made

Congress was cognizant of the fact that legislation expanding coverage for health care had been blocked when the House and Senate had been unable to achieve compromise in 1970. Dr. John Merrill of Harvard and Dr. John Najarian from the Gottschalk Committee, then at the University of Minnesota, testified on June 2, 1970, at a meeting of the Subcommittee on Public Health and Welfare of the Committee on Interstate and Foreign Commerce of the House of Representatives.[14] The contents of the Gottschalk Report had been briefly introduced by Edward G. Biester Jr., congressman from Pennsylvania.

Merrill reminded the committee of his claim to have performed the first treatment in the U.S. of a patient with renal failure using an artificial kidney in 1948. He described the current course of a patient's illness and treatment of patients with kidney failure in Massachusetts. The patient was treated with maintenance dialysis while waiting for a kidney transplant, a procedure that involved an uncoordinated patchwork of state, municipal, and local agencies. Merrill opined that if a coordinated care system supported financially by the federal government existed, "the rewards, both economic and medical, to the community, I think, obviously will be enormous."

Najarian told the committee that 8 million people in the U.S. had kidney disease and that approximately 50,000 died each year from the illness. He said "about 70 percent of these young people are under the age of 35." Najarian reviewed that the Gottschalk Committee had "determined that approximately 7,000 to 10,000 of these patients could be successfully treated each year with either dialysis or transplantation." Najarian noted that originally only patients between fifteen and forty-five years of age without another illness besides kidney disease were considered for treatment but that currently patients as old as sixty-five had received transplants. He explained that current medical and technical advances had extended the age criteria, and now patients with diabetes, an important cause of kidney failure, could benefit from therapy. Najarian concluded:

> This means Mr Chairman, that 20 to 25,000 patients are dying needlessly in the United States, simply because we cannot implement the

program set out in the Gottschalk report. . . . To my knowledge, this unconscionable situation has never presented itself to medicine before, when a treatment modality has been available and not been given to the people because of lack of funds to implement the programs envisioned.

Schreiner followed Najarian, introducing himself as the president of the NKF. After complaining about "'doctor beating' [being] the second most popular sport" in the press, he noted that the first patient treated with dialysis in Seattle, Clyde Shields, was still alive ten years later, at the time of the hearing. He made a blunt and impassioned plea for the establishment of a U.S. program to treat patients with kidney failure:

I don't think you will find a group of doctors, such as the nephrologists, who feel so frustrated that there is not in this Nation a planned, systematic approach to the health field. Sweden has a national program, and Norway and Britain, for treatment of kidney disease. And the United States, which has been a leader in every other field of medicine and led in the research in this field, does not have at this moment anything like a systematic, planned approach to kidney disease. . . . Another 10 years will see the anniversary of a half million Americans who have died unnecessarily. . . . What is needed is a primary system, an organization that will sort of father this along, and, secondly, facilities and training money. . . . We don't have a big foundation to help. But, such as it is, we are committing all of our financial and human resources to this. We really need help. And as far as I am concerned, the place to get it is from you gentlemen, and we appreciate your interest.

Schreiner and the others addressed questions about the costs of an ESRD program, estimating that it could be accomplished at about $15 million a year and that costs were decreasing over time. The group suggested that the mortality associated with treatment was about 15% the first year, and 10% each year thereafter. They noted that transplantation and home dialysis would result in decreased costs. They estimated 40% of patients placed on dialysis would be alive after five years. When asked about physician costs, they opined that their services were often free of charge, but that insurance reimbursed a professional fee of $150 per dialysis session. The physicians felt that manpower would not be an issue as the field expanded. They were thanked by the committee for their testimony, and the legislative efforts, for the time being, went nowhere.

President Richard Nixon had proposed health initiatives in a message to Congress in February 1971, perhaps to garner support for his reelection. Thereafter, the Ways and Means Committee of the House of Representatives passed HR1 in 1971 and then held hearings on national health insurance in October and November. The Senate was not interested in establishing broad and comprehensive health insurance but did support insurance for catastrophic health costs and the expansion of existing Medicare and Medicaid efforts. HR1 was concerned with Social Security, Medicare, and welfare reforms, particularly with the expansion of Medicare benefits for the disabled. The Senate reviewed HR1 in July and August 1971.

On November 4, 1971, the Ways and Means Committee held hearings, as part of its work on national health insurance, on end-stage renal disease, including testimony from members of the National Association of Patients on Hemodialysis (NAPH). Shep Glazer, a dialysis patient from New York and the vice president of NAPH, William Litchfield, a dialysis patient from Houston, Texas, and June Crowley and Abraham Holtz, dialysis patients from New York, participated. Peter Lundin, a medical student in California who was also a dialysis patient and a member of NAPH, who later became a nephrologist at Downstate Medical Center of the State University of New York in Brooklyn, also testified.

The day before the hearing, at a press conference under the auspices of NAPH in New York, Glazer declared his intention to be dialyzed in the presence of committee members. According to Rettig, John M. Martin, chief counsel to the Ways and Means Committee, in consultation with William Fullerton, a committee staff member for health, facilitated the event.[15] The NKF opposed this approach, and Glazer had been discouraged from taking this tack by Schreiner. However, Glazer called Schreiner the evening before the hearing and asked if a dialysis machine could be provided for his treatment at that time. Schreiner, in his capacity as an NKF member, was unwilling to attend but sent

a machine and a Georgetown nephrology fellow, Dr. James Carey, to the Long-
forth House Office Building to supervise Glazer's treatment. As in any treatment during which complications might occur, Carey was instructed that if
difficulties supervened, he was to stop the dialysis by clamping the blood tubing connecting the patient to the dialyzer in order to cut off blood flow to the
machine. And the instruction proved necessary. During the procedure, Glazer
developed an abnormal heart rhythm, and the treatment was discontinued
shortly after it was started.

Glazer testified:

> I am 43 years old, married for 20 years, with two children, ages 14 and
> 10. I was a salesman until a couple of months ago until it became neces-
> sary for me to supplement my income to pay for the dialysis supplies. I
> tried to sell a non-competitive line, was found out, and was fired. Gen-
> tlemen, what should I do? End it all and die? Sell my house for which I
> worked so hard, and go on welfare? Should I go into the hospital under
> my hospitalization policy, then I cannot work? Please tell me. If your
> kidneys failed tomorrow, wouldn't you want the opportunity to live?
> Wouldn't you want to see your children grow up?[16]

A week later, Schreiner and Dr. William Flanigan of the University of
Arkansas testified before the committee in favor of the legislation on behalf of
the NKF.

Mills supported a bill to amend the Social Security Act (rather than
Medicare or Medicaid) in December 1971 to "assure that any individual who
suffers from chronic renal disease will have available to him [sic] the necessary life-saving care and treatment for such disease and will not be denied
such treatment because of his [sic] inability to pay for it," perhaps in part to
bolster his presidential ambitions.[17]

In January and February 1972, the Senate Finance Committee held hearings on HR1, and discussions continued until the fall. No ESRD provision had
been added to either the House or Senate language. Plante and Schreiner consulted Senator Russell B. Long, a Democrat from Louisiana and chairman of
the Finance Committee, Senator Herman Talmadge, a Democrat from Georgia

and member of the Subcommittee on Health, and Senator Vance Hartke, a Democrat from Indiana. Dr. E. Lovell (Stretch) Becker, president of the NKF, met with Long in February 1972. On February 22, Hartke, with Alan Cranston, Democratic senator from California, introduced S. 3210 "to . . . provide the establishment and operation of community programs for patients with kidney disease . . . and to provide financial assistance to individuals suffering from chronic kidney disease who are unable to pay the costs of necessary treatment" to amend the Public Health Service Act.[18] During the summer of 1972, the Republican platform endorsed a plank covering renal disease treatment, possibly at the request of Mamie Eisenhower, a member of the NKF board.

On September 26, 1972, the Senate Finance Committee produced an almost 1,300-page bill agreeing with proposals to extend Medicare coverage to people with disabilities. At the end of the report, a section titled "Additional Views of Senator Vance Hartke" added, "We have the opportunity now to begin a national program of kidney disease treatment assistance administered through the Social Security Administration, and I propose that we take that opportunity so that more lives are not lost needlessly."[19] On Saturday, September 30, 1972, fifty-two senators voted in favor of Hartke's amendment, while Wallace Bennett, a Republican from Utah, James Buckley, a Republican from New York, and Sam Ervin, a Democrat from North Carolina, opposed it. Forty-five senators were absent. In Rettig's report of an Institute of Medicine committee that considered the entitlement amendments (titled *Origins of the Medicare Kidney Disease Entitlement: The Social Security Amendments of 1972*), the consensus was that the previous agreement on coverage of disability allowed the provision for treatment of uremia to go forward.

A House-Senate conference committee in mid-October subsequently agreed to the Senate amendment, adding Section 2991 pertaining to kidney disease to the Social Security Amendments of 1972. The language allowing disability coverage and the treatment of kidney disease had been crafted by committee staffers. The legislation was signed by President Nixon on October 30, 1972, just before his reelection to office. The new law authorized Medicare to cover ESRD treatment for patients under sixty-five years of age.

Because of the short time frame between the introduction of Hartke's amendment and the passage of the House-Senate conference committee legislation, cost estimates were based in large part on data provided by the NKF, and government analyses were hurried. Compromises were rapidly reached regarding waiting periods, which were supposed to decrease program costs.

The Gottschalk Report estimated about 1,000 people were treated with dialysis at the time of its delivery in 1967. The United States Renal Data System has records on 1,752 people who started dialysis before Medicare coverage began, but these counts are necessarily incomplete, since the findings depend on claims and payments made. The first patients covered by the legislation began treatment on July 1, 1973. Rettig has estimated that by 1972, 10,000 people in the U.S. needed dialysis or kidney transplantation for ESRD. The physicians who testified for the Ways and Means Committee quoted $15 million a year as the costs for the dialysis program, while they acknowledged professional fees of $150 per treatment had been paid by insurance, or total costs of $22,500 a year for patients dialyzed three times a week. Hartke envisioned costs of $75 million initially and $250 million after four years for an ESRD program. These estimates assumed a high proportion of the patients would receive kidney transplants and that transplantation would be successful over the long-term. Hartke forecast that many of the patients would be able to return to work.

To obtain coverage for dialysis treatment for ESRD, a physician would have to certify the patient did not have sufficient kidney function to sustain life and that there was no prospect of recovery of kidney function. It was implicit that the patient was healthy enough to sustain the rigors of a treatment during which a portion of his or her blood was outside the body. The initial experience from Seattle and elsewhere suggested that the program would be small and that most of the patients would have kidney disease but not heart disease or diabetes. Most of the patients would be under sixty-five years of age. How many of the patients would be men was never explicitly stated, but the language used suggested that this would be a therapy for traditional breadwinners. Use of home dialysis would markedly reduce costs as patients would provide the rent, labor, and supervision of the procedure. Transplantation, much cheaper than dialysis in the long run, would grow as an alternative modality, and therefore, costs would decrease for the program over the years.

What Happened after the Law Was Passed?

The enactment by Congress, in the Social Security Amendments of 1972 (P.L. 92–603) of Section 299I, and the implications of the law following Nixon's signature, ushered in a new era. The birth of the ESRD program occurred at the same time as the birth of the subspecialty of nephrology. The ESRD program was characterized by the treatment of a large number of patients who otherwise would die, the development of a government bureaucracy involved in the care of the patients and the payment of nephrologists, and the explosive growth of nephrology as a field. The first board examination in nephrology, recognizing it as a subspecialty, took place in 1972. The founding of the ESRD program placed nephrologists into two camps—the dialyzers and the physiologists—who sustained an uneasy coexistence through the 1970s and 1980s. Each side felt it exclusively wore the mantle of the profession.

There are, at last count, more than 800,000 ESRD patients, according to the 2022 United States Renal Data System Annual Data Report. Presently, substantially more than 80% of ESRD patients start therapy with hemodialysis. More than 100,000 people in the U.S. become new ESRD patients each year. Less than one-third are treated with kidney transplantation, and less than 10% have dialysis at home. Currently, almost 39% have diabetes, and more than half the patients starting ESRD therapy are over sixty-five. Total costs for the ESRD program are more than $50 billion a year.[20] How we got to this point and what the prospects for the future are, are considered in a later chapter. Whether the growth of the ESRD program fulfilled the promises made to patients in a hearing room of the House of Representatives is examined from the perspective that half a century of implementation can provide.

Belding Scribner served as the president of the American Society of Nephrology from 1978 to 1979. Belding Scribner and Willem Kolff were honored with the Albert Lasker Award in 2002 for making dialysis a feasible therapy for patients with acute renal failure and end-stage renal disease. The Nobel Laureate Dr. Joseph Goldstein quoted Isak Dinesen's observation about the role of humans as artful machines for the conversion of the red wine of Shiraz into urine, and invoked Claude Bernard and Homer Smith before noting the achievements of Kolff and Scribner, culminating in contributions that "revolutionized the treatment of kidney disease, saving and prolonging the useful lives of millions of people. . . . What is the artificial kidney but an ingenious machine of Kolffian cellophane and Scribnerian Teflon for turning, with infinite artfulness, death into life?"[21]

Scribner, therefore, was not only the inventor of the device that allowed chronic dialysis to come into being but also an advocate for the development of the national ESRD program and a pioneer in bioethics, allowing members of the community to work with physicians to make decisions about allocating scarce resources to save the lives of desperately ill patients. For these achievements, Scribner is memorialized by an award given annually in his name since 1995 by the American Society of Nephrology that honors "one or more individuals who have made outstanding contributions that have a direct impact on the care of patients with renal disorders or have substantially changed the clinical practice of nephrology."

Belding Scribner died in 2003, shortly after receiving the Albert Lasker Award. According to his obituary in the *New York Times*, written by the eminent physician-journalist Dr. Lawrence K. Altman, Scribner's body was found floating near his houseboat. Scribner had had osteoporosis and heart disease and used two canes to walk. A spokesperson for the University of Washington said, "The presumption is that for some reason he lost his balance and drowned." The *Times* hailed Scribner as a "medical pioneer" in the fields of dialysis care and bioethics.

A study several years ago suggested a split in the age of nephrologists at about the age of forty-five.[22] Those starting training in nephrology today, born at the end of the 20th century, do not know of Belding Scribner, Willem Kolff, John Merrill, or George Schreiner. The more than three-quarters of a million people in the U.S. currently sustained by the ESRD program, as well as their compatriots worldwide, and many of the patients who started therapy after July 1, 1973, do not know now, or did not then know, their names either. But they owed the quantity and quality of their lives after starting therapy with dialysis to these people.

5

---- ✦ ----

KIDNEY TRANSPLANT DONORS, RECIPIENTS, AND NOBEL PRIZE LAUREATES

The story of kidney transplantation can be told by considering the histories of patients transplanted during different medical eras as the field developed. The illnesses and treatments of Ruth Tucker, Richard Herrick, Brian Kampschroer, Sally Satel, and countless others illustrate the marked advances in the therapy of uremia over the period of a lifetime. Their medical histories, discussed in this and later chapters, inform early and contemporary practices in kidney transplantation. Progress was marked by setbacks and seemingly insurmountable barriers as well as dramatic breakthroughs. In many instances, the heroism and sacrifice of individual patients—who may have faced death while confronting new challenges individually with their physicians or through participation in clinical trials—were fundamental to ultimate success. Physician-scientists battled failure, skepticism, and incredulity, sometimes at the cost of their personal and professional reputations. Kidney transplantation over the past more than seventy years has been a triumph of medical science, resulting in the provision of health, longevity, and well-being to hundreds of thousands of people across the world, acknowledged by the award of several Nobel Prizes. The implementation of these advances, nationally and globally, has also been characterized by bias and inequities in access to a life-extending treatment and shortages of the resources needed to provide optimum therapy.

Early Kidney Transplantation Efforts

Transplantation of a healthy organ into the body of a patient with a dire disease had been a long-term goal of medicine, since at least the start of the 20th century.

Early attempts at transplantation included surgical approaches to replacements of skin, corneas, and thyroid glands. In the late 19th and early 20th centuries, a widespread interest developed in gonadal transplants to provide recipients with vim, vigor, and eternal youth. Generalized clinical success in humans with such treatment was not achieved. Blood transfusion, however, represented an early accomplishment in transplantation. Red blood cells, white blood cells, and plasma could be transferred to a person in need, such as someone who sustained critical blood loss. Researchers realized early on that the body's reactions to tissues transplanted from another human might engender a cascade of responses that could both reject the organ as well as result in harm to the recipient's other organs, possibly even culminating in the death of the patient. The mediators of the response were unclear, but investigations centered on the clotting and immune systems. In the case of blood transfusions, harmful reactions could be avoided if blood typing, a classification system identifying compatible red blood cells, was used. Compatible blood could be used for transfusions without causing a catastrophic immune response, resulting in injury to the recipient. Dr. Karl Landsteiner won the Nobel Prize in Physiology or Medicine in 1930 after developing the blood typing system that led to safe transfusions, in reality the transplantation of cells with fluids.

Transplanting kidneys, not to mention livers, lungs, or pancreases and other solid organs, proved to be a much more difficult task. Rejection of foreign tissue introduced into the body of a host was a major barrier to the success of transplantation, especially at a time when the understanding of the immune system and its protean responses was largely incomplete. At the end of the 19th century, inadequate surgical technique also represented a challenge to the restoration of organ function by replacement of a body part by transplantation.

At the beginning of the 20th century, Dr. Emmerich Ullmann (1861–1937), a Viennese surgeon, successfully transplanted kidneys between dogs and from a dog to a goat using prosthetic tubes to make connections between the blood vessels.[1] Ullman placed the transplanted kidneys in the neck of the recipient animals. One animal was reported to survive for five days after transplantation. That same year, 1902, Dr. Alexis Carrel (1873–1944), at the time a French surgeon, developed a new technique for connecting blood vessels, which he termed anastomosis. Carrel was able to perform surgery on animals, as Ullman had. Carrel pioneered surgery using an intra-abdominal approach to kidney transplantation. After removing a dog's kidneys, Carrel was able to transplant a kidney into a new host. The animal lived for ten days. In kidney transplants between dogs and cats, Carrel noted immune cell infiltration into the transplanted kidneys in microscopic examinations. Carrel's studies earned him the Nobel Prize in Physiology or Medicine in 1912, "in recognition of his work on vascular suture and the transplantation of blood vessels and organs." Carrel continued experimentation with inserting organs by performing anastomoses of their blood vessels with those of the recipient. From the failures of those transplants, Carrel identified rejection as a response to the procedure, noting the invasion of transplanted tissues by white cells as well as delineating the role of thrombosis, as described in his Nobel Prize acceptance lecture. Carrel spent the bulk of his later career at New York's Rockefeller Institute.

Research reported in the French literature in 1906 by Dr. Mathieu Jaboulay (1860–1913) and colleagues from Lyon and in German by Dr. Ernst Unger (1875–1938) and colleagues in 1910 described various attempts at kidney transplantation from both animals to humans and humans to humans with lack of success. The transplanted kidneys did not function and the human recipients did not survive. Dr. Yuri Voronoy (1895–1961), a Ukrainian surgeon, transplanted a kidney from a deceased sixty-year-old man into a young woman with kidney failure from mercury poisoning in 1933, using the blood vessels in her right groin. The donor and the recipient did not have matching blood types. Unfortunately, the operation was unsuccessful, and the recipient died two days later. Voronoy continued his research, but the reports of his failed efforts in the non-English literature nevertheless stimulated further work in kidney transplantation after World War II had ended.

Dr. Gordon Murray (1894–1976), a surgeon at Toronto General Hospital and the University of Toronto, addressed the multiple problems of surgical approaches and immunological responses in transplantation models in both humans and animals over an extended period of time beginning in the 1940s. After graduation from the University of Toronto in 1921 and undertaking various postgraduate training positions, including stints in London, England, and New York, Murray joined the faculty at the University of Toronto and was appointed a staff member of Toronto General Hospital in the late 1920s. As a young faculty member, Murray became interested in a range of pioneering surgical approaches and techniques in several fields, including corrective esophageal, orthopedic, and rectal procedures. He reported the results of his early attempts at kidney transplantation in animals in 1940.[2] Transplantation in his hands was partially a model to study the clotting system.

Gordon Murray's early attempts and success with heparin as an anticoagulant, however, inspired him to conceive of an "artificial kidney." As described by Dr. Vivian C. McAlister in 2005,[3] Murray's design somewhat resembled the dialysis apparatus Dr. Willem Kolff had developed for clinical use in the Netherlands during World War II. Starting in 1945, and continuing over the next year, Murray and his colleagues Dr. Edmund Delorme and Newell Thomas worked on models of dialysis machines. In addition, they performed many experiments on animals, developing models of uremia and measuring the amount of chemicals removed from the blood by dialytic techniques. Murray ultimately performed dialysis in December 1946 in a twenty-six-year-old woman who developed acute renal failure after an attempted abortion. As in many clinical situations, it is unclear from the report the extent to which dialysis treatments, compared to the patient's spontaneous recovery of kidney function, contributed to the beneficial ultimate outcome. Nevertheless, this work constituted an important clinical advance. Murray and colleagues published their findings, including the clinical case report, in 1947 in a paper titled "Development of an Artificial Kidney."[4] They quoted Kolff's work, outlined in a book by him and Van Noordwijk, *The Artificial Kidney*, published in the Netherlands in 1946. Murray, however, maintained that they had only heard of Kolff's results recently and that the Toronto group's advances had been made "simultaneously and independently."

In addition, Murray made early efforts in the field of kidney transplantation, in animal models, using dogs as recipients. Murray and colleagues started a series of kidney transplants from deceased donors to humans in 1951, using surgical approaches remarkably similar to those employed today. Their results were published in 1954.[5] Kidney transplants were performed by Murray and colleagues in at least four patients, but three of the patients described died in less than two weeks. The fourth patient, who had Bright's disease, had surgery on May 2, 1952, and survived for at least fifteen months. It was unclear, however, whether the transplant was critical to that outcome, since important details regarding kidney functional tests had not been provided in the paper.

Although Murray envisioned many of the issues confronted by modern transplant physicians and scientists, he was unable to bring these efforts to fruition. Institutional politics, personality clashes, and funding dilemmas ultimately impeded Murray's progress in achieving his long-term goals in kidney disease research. Murray turned to other, perhaps more fruitful, fields of investigation for the rest of his career. McAlister praised Murray as a visionary and "Canada's greatest surgical pioneer, to whom history has been most unkind"[6] in a review of Shelley McKellar's biography of the surgeon, *Surgical Limits: The Life of Gordon Murray*.

The Peter Bent Brigham Hospital: Next Steps and New Competition in Kidney Transplantation

Similar scientific and medical efforts were beginning simultaneously in Boston. The Peter Bent Brigham Hospital was founded in 1913 to lead research efforts in clinical medical care. The first two physicians in chief at the Brigham, Dr. Henry Christian (1876–1951) and Dr. Soma Weiss (1898–1942), had abiding interests in kidney disease. Dr. George Thorn (1906–2004) had done extensive research in diseases of the adrenal gland and in therapy of patients with adrenal hormones. He was recruited as physician in chief at the Peter Bent Brigham Hospital in 1942 after the untimely death of Dr. Weiss and served in this capacity until 1972. Thorn expanded his purview from endocrine and metabolic derangements to include studies of kidney disease after reports of kidney failure due to crush injuries emerged in publications from England during and after World War II. The institution established a major focus on kidney disease, transforming the expertise and perspective of both its Departments of Medicine and Surgery. In the 1940s, two surgeons at the Brigham, Drs. Charles Hufnagel (1916–1989) and David Hume (1917–1973), had been studying transplantation in dogs. At Thorn's urging, in the late 1940s Hufnagel and Hume surgically attached the kidney of a deceased patient to a vein and artery in the arm of a young woman with acute renal failure following an infection. The patient's illness, although not associated with trauma, reminded the physicians of the occasional recoveries in cases of renal failure that had recently been reported in Britain. The Brigham physicians hoped that if the patient could be tided over during a period when the kidneys "shut down," perhaps her kidneys would recover as the infection was being treated. The Brigham patient survived, but the case was not reported in the medical literature at the time. The clinical details of the patient's course still remain murky—including the precise date of the surgery. It is not certain whether the patient's own kidneys recovered or the transplant truly provided critical kidney function in the absence of native kidney function. Nevertheless, the patient survived.

In 1947 Dr. Willem Kolff of the Netherlands visited Boston, at the invitation of Dr. Thorn, to discuss the dialysis technique he had invented for the treatment of acute renal failure. Thorn asked a young physician at the Brigham, Dr. John P. Merrill, who was hoping to start a career in academic medicine, to undertake research in kidney disease—with emphasis on acute renal failure, transplantation, and dialysis. Brigham investigators were able to reconstruct Kolff's apparatus from blueprints. The design of the Kolff-Brigham artificial kidney subsequently was widely shared among hospitals in the United States.

In 1950, in the *Annals of the Royal College of Surgeons*, Dr. William J. Dempster of the Department of Surgery of the Postgraduate Medical School in London reported on an animal model of renal transplantation.[7] Dempster reviewed the history of kidney transplantation in animals and described his own experiments. He had removed kidneys from the abdomen and transplanted them into the necks of dogs. In careful studies, Dempster reported various aspects of the physiology of the autotransplanted kidneys. He concluded that although the transplanted kidneys showed evidence of damage to the distal tubules, removal of kidneys and their replacement in the same animal in a different vascular bed could sustain life over the short term. He experimented with radiation and the administration of cortisone to modify the response to organ transplantation. Dempster and colleagues went on to publish many papers on transplantation in animal models and humans over the next three decades.

On June 17, 1950, Dr. Richard H. Lawler and colleagues of Little Company of Mary Hospital in Chicago transplanted a kidney into a forty-four-year-old woman, Ruth Tucker, who had polycystic kidney disease. Her blood type was AB, Rh negative. Her serum creatinine concentration (S[Cr]) at an unspecified time before the operation was 1.8 mg/dL, suggesting mild to moderate impairment of renal function. The donor was a forty-nine-year-old woman with Tucker's identical blood type who had cirrhosis of the liver and had died of gastrointestinal bleeding. The surgical team members had experimented with kidney transplants in animal models, but they were evidently unaware of the work that had taken place in humans in Toronto, at the Brigham, or in France. Lawler and colleagues were aware of advances in red blood cell typing and of the need for tissue compatibility to prevent immune cells infiltrating the transplanted kidney, resulting in subsequent loss of function, as well as the importance of speed in performing the surgery. The surgeons used an intra-abdominal approach to organ placement, anastomosing the transplanted kidney to Tucker's left renal vein and artery, after removing the large native polycystic kidney. The ureter of the donor kidney was anastomosed to the patient's ureter. Tucker was able to eat on the fifth postoperative day. She was able to leave her bed twenty days after the operation. Tucker was discharged twenty-nine days after the surgery. In August, her S[Cr] was 1.2 mg/dL, suggesting an overall improvement in kidney function. The data do not rule out the possibility of an intercurrent episode of acute renal failure following the surgery affecting her own or the transplanted kidney or both. After hospital discharge, Tucker was able to resume full activities, including, the team noted, taking automobile trips, going to meetings and banquets, and dancing.[8]

In *JAMA*, in September 1951, the team supplied further information about the patient's subsequent course.[9] Tucker had a second operation performed on April 1, 1951. At that time, the transplanted kidney was smaller, about four by three by two centimeters, but blood supply was still present. The authors described the transplanted kidney as "still definitely alive, but apparently not producing urine." The team had become aware of the work of Servelle and colleagues from Paris, France, reported in *JAMA* in May 1951 and of Dr. Rene Küss and colleagues in Paris.[10]

Ruth Tucker died of heart disease and pneumonia almost five years after the operation. Lawler taught at Cook County Hospital, the Cook County School of Medicine, and the Stritch School of Medicine of Loyola University in Chicago. He died in July 1982 at the age of eighty-six without performing any other kidney transplants.

In a letter to *JAMA*, published on May 26, 1951, a correspondent reported on the efforts of Servelle, Soulié, Rougelle, and colleagues in kidney transplantation from Paris, France. The results had been presented at the meeting of the Medical Society of Paris Hospitals on January 26, 1951. Their animal studies seemed to have had limited success. They then reported the case of a twenty-two-year-old woman with severe kidney disease ("hypertensive azotemic nephritis" with five grams of urinary albumin excretion a day) who was transplanted with the kidney of a convicted criminal who had just been executed by guillotine. The letter documented the event in full:

> The donor's kidney was taken within minutes after the execution, immediately perfused with Ringer's solution and kept at constant temperature till arrival at the hospital, where a second surgical team had prepared the patient. . . . The renal vein was anastomosed end to end; then the renal artery was anastomosed terminolaterally on the external iliac artery. After removal of arterial clamps, the artery pulsates and dilates; thus blood circulation is resumed through the kidney. The urethra is connected with the skin (a urethral catheter in its interior); urine then flows drop by drop. The postoperative condition was normal for 48 hours: there was 20 cc. of urine on the first day and 30 cc. on the second. On the third day, acute pulmonary edema appeared, which subsided under the influence of bloodletting and cardiotonics associated with oxygen. . . . On the 19th day, the urinary secretion of the grafted kidney reached 600 cc. per day. . . . A very slow subcutaneous injection of isotonic sodium chloride solution was given; the first 150 cc. was well tolerated, but, by the end of the administration of the 250 cc, shock

with pallor, fall of blood pressure, and other deleterious changes occurred, improved on administration of citrated blood but reappeared later and provoked death. At autopsy it was observed that the grafted kidney was normal both in volume and in appearance; the other kidney had the volume of a tangerine. Notwithstanding the fatality (for which the injections of the saline solution were partly responsible) the authors believe that such transplantation may be helpful.

The letter goes on to note that at the same meeting, Drs. Charles Dubost (1914–1991), Jean Hamburger (1909–1992), and colleagues reported two other cases of kidney transplantations. One patient was a forty-four-year-old woman with previous renal tuberculosis, who had high blood pressure, edema, and high circulating levels of urea. On January 12, she had a kidney transplanted, attached to her body using the iliac artery and vein in her groin. Urine drained through an ostomy (a conduit with an exit hole) made through her skin. A second patient, a twenty-year-old woman with chronic glomerulonephritis and failing kidney function, had a kidney transplanted using similar surgical techniques. The correspondents noted that "It is still too early to foretell the future in these two cases; the authors will report results later."

Rene Küss (1913–2006), the son of a surgeon, graduated from the University of Paris School of Medicine, served in the French navy, and assisted General Patton's troops during World War II. Küss was decorated by the French government for his military service. As a urologist, Küss served at the Cochin Hospital. He published papers on hematuria, or blood in the urine, associated with tuberculosis infection in the late 1940s. Küss, with colleagues, contributed a paper titled "Some Attempts at Kidney Transplantation in Man" in 1951, in a French surgical journal. Dr. Nicholas Tilney notes in *Transplant: From Myth to Reality* that Küss commented that the work of Lawler and colleagues

had an extraordinary impact on those of us in France who were doing experimental transplantation. He gave us the reason to believe that transplant surgery was possible in human beings. . . . We were so anxious to apply the experience we gathered working on dogs to human beings that we used Lawler's success as an excuse to begin kidney transplants in man.[11]

Dubost, in collaboration with Dr. Jean Hamburger and other colleagues, reported on the function of kidney grafts in man in 1951 in a paper published in Paris. Hamburger went on to report various attempts at kidney transplantation in humans, with Dr. Gabriel Richet and others, in the French literature from 1953 onward. Hamburger maintained a strong interest in irradiation as the modality of immunosuppression. So in the early days of kidney transplantation, European-American cross-talk facilitated a synergistic interest in moving forward with experimental kidney transplants in humans.

The Brigham Moves Forward—or Does It?

In 1955, the Brigham team presented their progress in human kidney transplantation over the previous several years to the world. In a long paper published in the highly regarded *JCI* by the team of Hume, Merrill, Miller, and Thorn entitled "Experiences with Renal Homotransplantation in the Human: Report of Nine Cases," members of the Departments of Surgery and Medicine collaborated to review their work, primarily in patients who received kidney transplants between 1951 and 1953.[12] Some of the cases had already partially been reported in abstract form. Looking over the paper—with its succinct description of cases, its photographic figures illustrating the kidneys, and the table of patient characteristics and outcomes, one is reminded of Richard Bright's "Medical Cases" and "Tabular View" in *Guys Hospital Reports*.

The authors first noted:

All of the recipients were patients in the terminal stages of severe, advanced renal failure. The risks were fully discussed with the patients and their families, and the uncertain outcome made clear. In several instances the function of the transplant was maintained for a surprisingly long period of time. All of the patients ultimately succumbed to their disease ...

. . . It was felt observations of the biologic response to kidney homo-transplantation in man might yield information that could not be obtained by animal experimentation alone. Data might be acquired which would suggest new lines of approach to the homotransplant problem and these could then be evaluated at the level of the laboratory animal.

Our results appear to indicate 1) that the disease of the patient can, under some circumstances, influence the course of the transplant, 2) that it is possible to perform renal homotransplants in the human that survive and function for far longer periods of time than those recorded for any experimental animal, and 3) that the rejection of the human homotransplant is not always comparable to that seen in the dog.

The Brigham investigative surgical team chose to implant the transplanted kidney into the thigh of the recipient because such an operation was deemed to be less traumatic and extensive, although it presented several challenges to the surgical team as well as to the patient, including the possibility of bleeding into the leg. The operative approach usually necessitated the construction of a uret-erostomy, by which the ureter drained out of a stab wound made in the leg into an external collection device. The authors acknowledged that their work and the surgical approach had been influenced by the French transplant teams. John Merrill had observed their work firsthand during travels to Paris.

Their conclusions were grim and sobering, and gave pause to physicians and innovators as well as patients with severe kidney disease. Kidney trans-plantation had been performed in nine patients. Five of the patients had no measurable kidney function after the procedure. Four of the patients experi-enced resumption of kidney function, with urine output from 37 to about 180 days after surgery. All the patients died, although one patient—Gregorio Woloshin, a physician who had undergone a slightly different surgical proce-dure in which the transplant kidney had been wrapped in plastic—survived about six months after the operation. Their conception of a "surprisingly long period of time" strikes us as almost insulting today. The authors wrote:

Renal homotransplantation has no place in the therapy of human patients at this time. Our own further studies in this field await the outcome of problems now under investigation in the experimental animal. We feel that it will prove valuable, as new data is accumulated in the laboratory, however, to continue to investigate the problem of human renal homotransplantation in light of these advances. Biological rejection in the human does not seem to be as violent, at least as regards renal transplantation, as that found in the experimental animal.

The research efforts of the Brigham team had been supported by grants from the Bristol-Myers Pharmaceutical Company, Eli Lilly and Company, the Lasdon Foundation, and the NIH. In a note at the end of the paper, the authors acknowledged the work of Gordon Murray and his team in Toronto, published previously in 1954 in the *American Journal of Surgery*.

In 1953, David Hume left the Brigham and began military service during the Korean War. Dr. Joseph E. Murray (1919–2012), a surgeon who had performed skin grafts in burned patients during his military service, joined the Brigham team in 1951. Murray attended the College of the Holy Cross, where he studied philosophy and English. He graduated with a degree in the humanities in 1940 and then matriculated at and graduated from Harvard Medical School. Murray served as an intern at the Brigham, and worked in the plastic surgery unit of Valley Forge General Hospital, which involved skin grafting, while serving in the army during World War II. After the war, Murray finished his surgical residency at the Brigham and pursued further training in New York, until returning to Boston. Murray continued the laboratory experiments started by Hufnagel and Hume with kidney transplantation in dogs at the Brigham, using an abdominal approach to surgery. The new team's efforts in human kidney transplantation were not marked by success.

Murray's work with his colleagues in animal models was published in *Plastic and Reconstructive Surgery* in 1953, in the *Proceedings of the Society for Experimental Biology and Medicine* in 1953, and in *Surgical Forum* in 1955.[13] Kidneys had been transplanted into the abdomen of dogs, the renal vessels had been anastomosed to an artery and a vein in the recipients' pelvises, and the ureters had been attached to the bladders. Several of the animals survived for relatively long periods of time—days and weeks.

It appeared that by early 1955, kidney transplantation in humans had reached a dead end, in places as disparate as Toronto and Paris, as well as Boston. The problem of curbing the effects of the immune system with clinically useful forms of immunosuppressants was overwhelming, and posed an apparently insuperable barrier to progress in the field. Everything changed, however, by the next year.

Twins at the Brigham

In late 1954, twenty-three-year-old Richard Herrick developed symptoms of uremia. Herrick had scarlet fever at the age of five but evidently recovered without incident. He had served in the Coast Guard, but about fourteen months before his first admission to the Peter Bent Brigham Hospital, he developed "puffiness about the eyes . . . and some elevation of blood pressure was noted." Herrick had protein and blood in his urine, and its ability to become concentrated was impaired. His blood urea nitrogen (BUN) level varied between 70 and 100 mg/dL, suggesting a relatively severe decrease in kidney function. Herrick was treated with blood transfusions for anemia and improved somewhat. Five months after a prolonged stay at the Public Health Hospital, Herrick was readmitted for three days, appearing chronically ill, with high blood pressure and evidence of injury to the small blood vessels of the eyes, and perhaps elsewhere, presumably because of hypertension. Six weeks later, Herrick was again admitted to the hospital with nausea, vomiting, headache, and muscle aches. The patient had high blood pressure and severe anemia. His BUN was now extraordinarily elevated at 185 mg/dL. His nausea and vomiting persisted, and he had a generalized convulsion. Herrick became drowsy and disoriented and continued to have seizures. These symptoms and laboratory evaluations were all consistent with a diagnosis of advanced chronic kidney disease and severe uremia, at that time an uncurable and untreatable medical illness.

In recollections long after the operation, Ronald Herrick, Richard's brother, said he had told Richard's doctor, after hearing the grim prognosis, "Doctor, I'd give him one of my own kidneys, if it would help." As Murray recalled the story in an issue of *Harvard Medicine*,[14] Herrick's physician at the Public Health

Hospital, Dr. David C. Miller, reportedly told Ronald that transplantation would be impossible because of rejection but suddenly realized he was talking to his patient's identical twin. Miller later discussed the possibility of kidney transplantation with Dr. Merrill at the Brigham. Herrick was transferred to the Brigham on October 26, 1954, to consider the possibility of kidney transplantation. On admission, Richard was described as being "extremely disoriented." Herrick received a dialysis treatment, using the Kolff Brigham apparatus, and improved. He became more lucid and was able to tolerate feedings. Ronald agreed to provide a kidney to Richard with the knowledge that he would have to undergo an arduous operation in order to recover the living organ in a usable state. Skin grafting was performed between the twins to determine if rejection might occur. Building on Murray's previous experience with skin grafts, the Brigham physicians hypothesized that if the brothers were genetically identical, their identical immune systems might not be a barrier to the survival of a grafted kidney. They confirmed that Richard was an identical twin, because he had shared a placenta with and was able to accept a skin graft from his brother, and they had the same blood type, eye color, and fingerprints. Ronald had undergone examinations to show that he was free of disease, that his kidneys were normal, and that he had no evidence of infection.

Richard Herrick was discharged from the Brigham in the middle of November, but he was readmitted December 12, 1954, because of experiencing symptoms of congestive heart failure. Herrick's blood pressure was extremely elevated at 220/146 mm Hg, he had severe swelling reaching to his knees, and examination of his chest revealed fluid in the lungs. Richard was literally dying of kidney disease. Murray described that extensive consultation and discussions with the patient, his brother, and clergymen of various denominations occurred regarding the newly raised ethical quandaries entailed in subjecting a family member to the rigors of an extensive operation that, while aiding his brother, would not provide any benefit to Ronald. When Ronald asked if he would be provided with medical care by the hospital over the course of his life after the donation, his surgeon, Dr. J. Hartwell Harrison, responded, according to Murray, "Of course not." Harrison then assured the donor that all the physicians involved in the procedure would always be there to take care of him as well as his brother. The matter was settled informally, as a matter of trust, but not legally. Such issues for living donors still have not been adequately resolved at the present time.

In a primitive form of informed consent documentation, and in an expression of fraternal devotion, Murray recalled that notes had been passed between the twins in their hospital beds. The evening before the operation, Richard wrote to Ronald: "Get out of here and go home." Ronald, the donor, reportedly replied in a note, "I am here, and I am going to stay."

The recovery of a healthy left kidney from a living donor, and the implantation of that kidney into a uremic recipient occurred during simultaneous operations in two adjacent operating rooms at the Peter Bent Brigham Hospital on December 23, 1954. Murray led Richard's surgical team. He used the technical approaches he and colleagues had developed in animal studies over the previous years. Murray decided to implant Ronald's kidney into Richard's pelvis, behind the covering of the peritoneum, anastomosing the transplanted kidney's vessels to the hypogastric artery and the iliac vein, allowing the ureter to be implanted into Richard's bladder, ensuring normal urination. This approach contrasted with previous kidney transplant procedures at the Brigham, in which the ureter emerged directly from the skin, draining into a catheter.

Dr. Harrison led Ronald's surgical team. The operation to remove Ronald's normal kidney started at 8:15 a.m. At 9:53, Ronald's kidney was brought into Murray's operating room, where Richard was sedated and receiving spinal anesthesia. The implanted kidney was attached to its arterial supply in Richard's body at 10:40 a.m., and the veins were connected at 11:15. Richard's new kidney immediately assumed a normal, pink appearance, and Richard began to have a normal flow of urine. The operation took three and a half hours.

The postoperative course of the donor was described as "uneventful," and Ronald was discharged two weeks after the surgery. Richard continued to produce urine after the surgery. He gained eleven pounds, but he had no edema or swelling. His blood pressure, BUN, lungs, and heart were normal. Richard Herrick was discharged on the thirty-seventh postoperative day. Richard and Ronald Herrick, Drs. Murray and Merrill, and their team had made medical history.

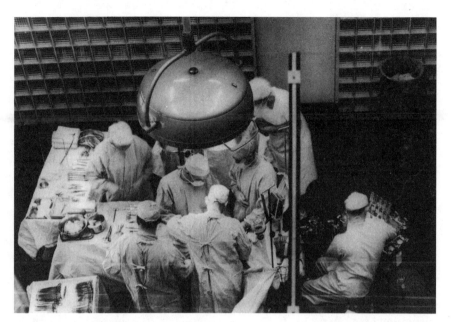

Figure 4. The world's first successful kidney transplant, on December 23, 1954, at the Peter Bent Brigham Hospital, Boston, Massachusetts. From left to right: Dr. Daniel E. Pugh, Dr. Joseph E. Murray, Dr. John L. Rowbotham (1st assistant), Dr. Edward B. Gray, Jr. (2nd assistant), Elizabeth A. Comiskey (circulating nurse), Dr. Leroy Vandam (anesthesiologist). The patient is Richard Herrick, receiving a kidney from his twin brother, Ronald. Source: Brigham and Women's Hospital Archives, with permission.

A year after the successful procedures, Drs. Merrill, Murray, Harrison, and Guild wrote about the survival of the donor and recipient twins in a landmark case report published in volume 160 of *JAMA*.[15] The article was illustrated by a figure showing the position of Ronald's implanted kidney in relation to its new blood supply and drainage into Richard's bladder. Renal function was similar in Richard and Ronald and was near normal levels in both of the twins. The authors considered why one identical twin would have glomerulonephritis, while the other did not, and whether the transplanted kidney would maintain its level of function and be free of infection over many years. The authors concluded, however, that kidney transplantation between identical twins was technically and immunologically feasible and that long-term outcomes, after a year, were excellent for both donor and recipient.

Richard met his wife-to-be, a nurse supervisor, in the recovery room, after his successful transplantation. They subsequently married and had two children. Unfortunately, Richard's glomerulonephritis recurred in the kidney transplanted from his brother, and he died of kidney disease and heart failure eight years after the transplantation at the age of thirty-one in March 1963. Ronald married Cynthia Barnes in 1959 and taught mathematics for thirty-seven years. He also managed farms in New England. In 2011, Joseph Murray, at the age of ninety-one, wrote in the *American Journal of Transplantation* (*AJT*) of his appreciation of the sacrifice made by Ronald Herrick, who had just died, in giving up a kidney for his brother, Richard, fifty-six years before.[16]

What about Patients Who Didn't Have a Twin?

This medical achievement—the successful transplantation of a kidney from a healthy identical twin to his brother who was dying of uremia—was astounding in many ways. It was critical, however, that it not be a one-off. Kidney transplantation between twins could not be a solution for the thousands or perhaps millions of people dying from uremia across the globe. Murray went on to perform transplantation between twins, but also considered the thornier problem of kidney transplantation between unrelated humans.

Proper modes of immunosuppression between patients with different genetic makeups and tissue antigen characteristics would be necessary to allow transplants to remain functioning in the bodies of recipients without rejection. Immunosuppression would have to maintain a fine balance—between dampening the host response and disabling the immune system to such a great extent that common or uncommon viral, fungal, or bacterial infections would pose untreatable, lethal complications. Murray's team knew that irradiation of animals could modify the immune attack function of animals, allowing them to accept skin grafts and the transfer of cells from various donors. Merrill had military experience as a flight surgeon in the 509th Bomb group, which carried out the atomic bombing of Hiroshima and Nagasaki in 1945. Merrill understood the potential lethal effects of irradiation as well as its therapeutic potential to dampen patients' immune responses. The downside of radiation was that the treatment could destroy rapidly generating cells, such as the white blood cells, the body's first responders that were key to the immune response as well as the appropriate short-term reaction to infections.

Therefore, radiation could be a clinical tool or the cause of a lethal outcome. The team decided to use radiation as the approach to immunosuppression in humans who desperately needed kidney transplants.

The results of their studies at the Brigham were reported in four papers published between 1960 and 1963, in the *Annals of the New York Academy of Science*, *Surgery*, the *Annals of Surgery*, and the *NEJM*.[17] The outcomes in humans were generally disastrous. By 1962, twelve patients at the Brigham, all terminally ill with almost complete lack of kidney function, had been given total body irradiation of different magnitudes. Eleven of the twelve patients had died. Two of the patients died from the effects of high doses of radiation before having a chance to receive a transplant. In most patients, the transplant did not last more than two weeks. Some of the patients never regained kidney function. The anatomical and histologic analyses the team presented began to define the characteristics of rejection of kidneys in humans. If the radiation was too intense, the patient died of its complications. If it was too meager, radiation did not provide protection from rejection of the transplanted kidney. In stark technical medical terms, it was damned if you did and damned if you didn't. In the only optimistic note, one patient was alive and well three and a half years after irradiation and transplant. What had made the difference was not well understood, but in that one case, the donor and the recipient were nonidentical (technically known as dizygotic and popularly as fraternal) twins, and the recipient had been treated long-term with cortisone, a steroid medication. The investigators determined that this set of twins did not completely share the genes that made transplantation between identical human twins possible, although the genetics of transplantation had not been well elucidated at that time. It was only manifestly evident that the odds were against patient survival with radiation. Radiation was not a viable clinical therapeutic tool in humans. Patients with kidney failure who needed transplants required better, safer, and more effective immunosuppressive treatments.

Over the next several years, the Brigham team reported progress with kidney transplants between identical twins. They also wrote a hopeful article on their successful efforts with kidney transplantation between nonidentical twins (published in 1960 in the *NEJM*),[18] but more generalizable approaches were needed if kidney transplantation was ever going to become a practical alternative long-term treatment for patients with advanced kidney disease. It was assumed that some kind of genetic interrelationships—perhaps a set of histocompatibility genes shared between the nonidentical twins, leading to better acceptance of donor tissue—was responsible for the sanguine outcomes.

In the *Encyclopaedia Britannica*, in 1961, the article on transplantation by the distinguished surgeon Sir Michael Francis Addison Woodruff (1911–2001) of the University of Edinburgh, who had written a paper on successful kidney transplantation between identical twins in the *Lancet* in 1961,[19] summed up the current state-of-the-art: "Homotransplantation of a whole kidney is unjustified unless an identical twin is available as a donor, because the transplant is unlikely to function for more than a few weeks and a patient can be maintained on an artificial kidney for this period. Several instances of successful transplantation of a kidney from an identical twin, however, have been reported."

Immunosuppression Using Pills

Gertrude Elion was born in New York City in 1918. Her parents were Jewish immigrants from Europe. She excelled as a student, finishing high school at the age of fifteen. Elion graduated summa cum laude with a degree in chemistry from Hunter College in 1937. She received an M.Sc. degree at New York University in 1941. Although academically qualified, as a woman, she was unable to obtain further training to attain a Ph.D., as was common in those times. Elion worked in various research and commercial enterprises before joining a laboratory at the pharmaceutical company Burroughs Wellcome, in Tuckahoe, New York, under the supervision of Dr. George H. Hitchings (1905–1998). Hitchings was interested in developing molecules that had specific targets in cellular pathways that could achieve precise pharmacologic as well as therapeutic goals. Elion and Hitchings focused on drugs that could disrupt pathways involved in DNA synthesis, causing a decrease in the ability of the body to generate rapidly reproducing cells, such as the various types of white blood cells. The drugs 6-mercaptopurine (6-MCP) and azathioprine, developed in their laboratory at Burroughs Wellcome, interfered with the synthesis of purines, molecules necessary for the formation of DNA and RNA from nucleotide building blocks. As expected, the drugs impaired the body's ability to synthesize the white blood cells that mediated the human immune repose. Gertrude Elion received the Nobel Prize in Physiology or Medicine in 1988, along with Hitchings and James Black. The Nobel Committee cited the three for the

> development of new drugs which have become essential in the treatment of a number of different disorders. . . . The research work carried out by Black, Elion and Hitchings has had a more fundamental significance. While drug development had earlier mainly been built on chemical modification of natural products they introduced a more rational approach based on the understanding of basic biochemical and physiological processes.

Roy Calne was born in 1930 in London, England, and graduated from Guy's Hospital Medical School. Calne published a paper in the *Lancet* in February 1960 on immunosuppression of kidney transplantation in dogs using 6-mercaptopurine.[20] In October 1960, Calne wrote a response to a letter received by the *Lancet* commenting on his paper, posted from the U.S. By that time, Calne and his family had sailed to America on the *Queen Elizabeth* so he could start work with Murray at the Brigham as a Harkness Fellow at Harvard. Calne had obtained the position with Murray with the help of the distinguished British immunologist, Dr. Peter Medawar, who won the Nobel Prize in Physiology or Medicine in 1960. Calne joined Murray in his research efforts between 1960 and 1961, bringing a new perspective on tackling the immune system to the team's studies. They published two papers on medical immunosuppression in animal models of kidney transplantation.[21]

In the *NEJM* in 1963, Murray, Merrill, and colleagues reported their experience using only drugs to suppress the immune system of kidney transplant recipients.[22] The investigators had been informed by the work of Calne and colleagues as well as studies by Zukowski, Lee, and Hume, who had demonstrated the beneficial effects of immunosuppression in dogs receiving kidney transplants, using 6-mercaptopurine, in several contemporary papers.[23]

The operations they described had been performed between 1961 and 1963. Thirteen cases were presented. Two women and eleven men received kidney transplants. The Brigham team used 6-mercaptopurine in the two earliest patients in their series and later prescribed azathioprine, or Imuran, as the immunosuppressant. There were five cadaveric donors. Three of the recipients of these kidneys had no renal function. One patient had a kidney that survived 26 days, but in the other recipient, the graft lasted for more than a year, as of the time of publication. Five patients received kidneys from infants who had hydrocephalus, where a kidney was removed to allow the formation of a shunt that would drain fluid from the brain into the child's bladder. One of these kidneys failed to function. Other recipients of the infants' kidneys had function from 3 to 160 days. In the last cases in the series, the team transplanted kidneys from a mother, a brother, and an unrelated adult living donor into patients with kidney failure. At the time of publication, these kidneys had functioned from 40 to 110 days in patients treated with Imuran.

A twenty-three-year-old student from Tulare, California, had been treated with repeated doses of amphotericin B for pulmonary coccidiomycosis, a fungal disease, and later for meningitis caused by the persistent fungal pathogen. Kidney injury was a dreaded side effect of therapy with the only effective, clinically available antifungal agent, amphotericin B. By the time of transplantation, the student had almost no kidney function and a very elevated BUN. He had a dramatic decrease of BUN after receiving a functioning allograft from his mother. The patient was treated with Imuran and azaserine (an alkylating agent that inhibits purine and DNA synthesis at a site distinct from azathioprine) and later with actinomycin C. The particular drug combination had been suggested by the results of Murray's previous experiments in dogs. After a rocky postoperative course, the patient's BUN decreased to normal.

A thirty-five-year-old printer had had gout and hypertension for at least eight years. In December 1962, he had a BUN of 148 mg/dL and a very elevated blood pressure of 180/90 mm Hg. He was treated with intermittent peritoneal dialysis. The patient's relatives were evaluated for histocompatibility, but none was a perfect match, using contemporary testing methods. Ultimately he received a kidney from his brother. The transplanted kidney functioned immediately, and the patient produced nine liters of urine over the first eighteen hours after the procedure. The patient was treated with Imuran and azaserine and later with actinomycin C. His BUN returned to normal within three days.

Another patient, a thirty-nine-year-old father of nine children, had polycystic kidney disease, which had reached the stage of uremia. An unrelated woman who had many compatible blood types with the patient volunteered to donate one of her kidneys to him. After the operation, the patient produced 30 liters of urine in three days, and his BUN declined from 245 to 15 mg/dL over forty-eight hours. The patient was treated with Imuran and azaserine, and later with actinomycin C.

In contrast to the 1962 paper in the *Annals of Surgery*, Murray and Merrill's 1963 *NEJM* paper told a different tale. The authors felt that immunosuppressive drugs could be used safely in humans undergoing kidney transplantation. Drugs provided a potential advantage over radiation since the doses could be decreased or the drug could be discontinued if complications such as depression of the white blood count or infections supervened. The team treated rejections variably with different combinations of steroids and actinomycin C. They noted that selection of kidney donors, including living altruistic volunteers, would pose logistic and ethical issues, as the use of immunosuppressant drugs disseminated. They wrote that "so-called 'tissue typing' or the selection of closely compatible donors is not too highly developed. . . . It does not seem advisable to advocate indiscriminate transplantation utilizing kidneys from adult, living volunteers at this time. However, when careful supporting laboratory work is available, a cautious approach in the use of a living volunteer for a carefully selected recipient may be justified."

In the first truly hopeful note the investigators had conveyed since 1955, the members of the Brigham kidney transplantation team concluded:

> Although at present there is good evidence that chemical suppressive agents may be temporarily effective many questions remain unsolved. The eventual status of these homografted kidneys, the length of time for which the drug must be continued, whether or not the possibility for rejection diminishes with the passage of time and whether the original kidney disease will develop in the homograft are all unsolved problems. The total immunological potential of the host is not known when one is considering the course of his future lifetime. However, this report permits a note of cautious optimism in a problem that ten years ago was considered almost insoluble.

The authors had outlined a course of research that could last for decades. They expressed their appreciation to Dr. George Hitchings, who had provided them with advice regarding the use of the immunosuppressant drugs in their patients, at the opening of new possibilities for people with kidney failure undergoing transplantation. Gertrude Elion was not mentioned.

Shortly thereafter, in September 1963 in the *Lancet*, Woodruff and colleagues published their series of kidney transplants performed using Imuran as the immunosuppressant drug.[24] Clinical investigation of kidney transplantation in humans using immunosuppressive drugs in various doses and combinations, under different protocols, began to spread to other U.S. transplant centers, including the Medical College of Virginia in Richmond under Dr. Hume, who had left Harvard, the University of Colorado, led by Dr. Thomas E. Starzl, and the University of California, San Francisco, newly established by Dr. John S. Najarian in 1963. A new era in transplantation had begun.

Starzl (1926–2017) (who was to become an international leader in organ transplantation over the next several decades) and colleagues reported on their experience with kidney transplantation in October 1963 in *Surgery Gynecology and Obstetrics*.[25] They used azathioprine as maintenance immunosuppression and treated rejection with high dose steroids acutely, with excellent results in ten patients. This regimen, with certain additions (such as the inclusion of steroids and other treatments in the initial and maintenance phases), became the basis of therapy for patients receiving kidney transplants for almost the next twenty years, with exceptions in certain medical centers.

The National Research Council (NRC) convened a meeting to review the current status and the future of kidney transplantation, held in Washington, D.C., on September 26 and 27, 1963, before Starzl's paper was published. Clyde F. Barker and James F. Markmann reported on the NRC meeting in 2013 in *Cold Spring Harbor Perspectives in Medicine*:

> About 25 individuals including most of the world's active transplant clinicians and scientists assembled in Washington to review the status of human kidney transplantation. The results presented by these acknowledged experts were extremely discouraging. Less than 10% of their several hundred allograft recipients had survived as long

as 3 months.... Of patients treated with total body irradiation, only 6 had approached or achieved 1 year survival.... Hope was expressed that immunosuppressive drugs might be more effective. Murray reported his first 10 patients treated with 6-MP and azathioprine instead of irradiation.... One had survived for a year, although at the time of the conference it was failing. The others died within 6 months. Thus, at this point, drugs seemed no more effective than radiation. The mood at the conference was so gloomy that some participants questioned whether continued activity in human transplantation could be justified....

The gloom was dispelled by only one presentation given by Tom Starzl, a virtually unknown newcomer to the field, who was invited to the conference as an afterthought. He described a new immunosuppressive protocol that had allowed 70% 1-year renal graft survival. He had more surviving patients than the rest of the world's better-known participants combined. At first, his audience was incredulous ... but eventually Starzl's unprecedented results had to be believed because he had brought with him charts detailing the daily progress of each patient—including laboratory tests, urine output, and immunosuppressive drug doses.... Starzl's innovation based on his consistent success in reversing homograft rejection in dogs was to add prednisone to azathioprine.... This presentation caused a sensation.... In fact, the impact on those present was extraordinary. They would have been still more impressed if they could have known that half a century later, some of the patients Starzl described would be off immunosuppression with the same functioning allografts.... The outlook for renal transplantation was completely changed by Starzl's report.... Many of the conference attendees promptly visited Starzl in Denver to learn how to adopt his immunosuppressive protocol.... The news of the breakthrough spread quickly by its publication 5 weeks later.... Before the NRC conference, there had been only three active renal transplant centers in North America (Boston, Denver, and Richmond). As the effectiveness of Starzl's innovative immunosuppression became known, within a year 50 new transplant programs began in the United States.[26]

How Do We Get the Kidneys We Need For Our Patients?

Francis D. (Franny) Moore (1913–2001) grew up in Illinois and Wyoming and graduated from Harvard College with an A.B. in 1935. While in college Moore was the president of both the *Harvard Lampoon* and the Hasty Pudding Club. He received his M.D. from Harvard Medical School in 1939. Moore did his surgical residency at the Massachusetts General Hospital. Moore soon became the surgeon in chief at the Peter Bent Brigham Hospital, at the age of thirty-five, in 1948, a post he held until 1976. He was the Mosely Professor of Surgery at Harvard Medical School. Moore was interested in metabolic and nutritional aspects of surgery and postoperative care. Like a nephrologist, he was focused on the chemical composition of the body's fluid compartments. Moore used radioactive tracers to determine in which compartments water and electrolytes were sequestered and followed changes in their distribution during the course of surgery and recovery and during episodes of medical stress. Moore published a multi-part series entitled "Common Patterns of Water and Electrolyte Change in Injury, Surgery and Disease" in the *NEJM* in 1958.[27] He also considered the common problems related to the surgical treatment of duodenal ulcers and breast cancer. Moore's book *The Metabolic Care of the Surgical Patient* was published in 1959 and guided the training of surgical residents for decades.

Moore's greatest contribution was arguably the nurturing of the surgical transplantation team at his hospital, in collaboration with members of the Department of Medicine, primarily the internist Dr. George Thorn, his protégé John Merrill, and their associates. Moore became a celebrity as transplantation became more clinically applicable. He was pictured on the cover of *Time*, on May 2, 1963, in surgical scrubs and cap, with his mask hanging below his chin. The article celebrated the advances made in surgery over the previous three decades, including reliance on multidisciplinary science and cooperation with other physician specialists, culminating in an era where "surgeons now make a routine performance of lifesaving procedures so radical that they were almost unimaginable a few years ago." The new science of transplantation was given pride of place in the piece, and Murray's successful twin transplant procedure was revisited, with Hume put into the limelight. (Curiously, Starzl was not cited at all in the story.) Although the article mentioned famed surgeons of the past, and contemporary leaders in the field, it focused on and lionized Moore.

> The grey-gowned figure in charge looks like a visitor from another planet. Between skull cap and mask, his head sprouts a startling pair of binocular spectacles. His hands move with confident precision and his even voice snaps with authority, but his very words seem part of an alien language—a communication designed solely for his colleagues.... Because of his own contributions to surgery's body of basic knowledge, his phenomenal ability to recall the right things at the right time and to make the right decision in the operating room or at the patient's bedside, Francis Moore ranks as one of the half dozen greatest surgeons.

Moore published the first edition of his book *Give and Take*, a review that described his personal view of transplantation, in 1964. Later, in 1995, he published a memoir, *A Miracle and a Privilege*. At the end of his career, Moore considered health policy issues in many papers published in high-impact journals. In his obituary in the *New York Times*, former president of Harvard Derek Bok said, "He stands out in my mind as one of the three or four people who were most likely to articulate what the medical school stood for and what doctors ought to be.... It was people like that who really helped define standards of conduct for doctors."

Moore and colleagues wrote about the state of the art of cadaveric kidney transplantation in the *NEJM* in 1964.[28] In those early days of transplantation, the paper dealt with decisions regarding which decedents were suitable as organ donors. The crude nature of these first medical evaluations is brought out by considerations of patients who had had "serum hepatitis" (now characterized by viral subtypes identified on molecular bases), emphasizing the rudimentary level of diagnosing the presence of viral infections and determining suitability of these dying or dead patients for providing organs for patients in need. In the bulk of the paper, medicolegal issues were at the forefront. Knowing the time limits diminished blood supply and retrieval of organs imposed on outcomes, the authors noted, on pathophysiologic grounds, patients "who are dead on arrival, or within a few minutes afterward, cannot be used for their critical tissues, because the transplantation team will have insufficient time to arrange the transplant." The transplant physicians had already learned that patients dying of central nervous system disease were prime candidates for cadaver donor status. The authors acknowledged that patients dying from cardiovascular causes "are usually hypothermic, but the conditions of death, with repeated resuscitative attempts and prolonged shock, may restrict their usefulness to the donation of non-critical tissues." The authors recommended the infusion of chilled solutions into kidneys that had been procured for transplantation. They stated interhospital systems for "tissue salvage, preservation, transportation and transplantation" were necessary and would need to be developed. The authors emphasized that potential cadaveric donors should be cared for by a completely different team from those taking care of the presumed recipient. They noted that in Massachusetts, the next-of-kin held the ultimate authority regarding the use of organs from a deceased donor but reported that laws pertaining to the donation of organs varied across the states. Clearly the law, as well as ethical principles, had to catch up with new medical realities. The authors envisioned a card carried by people during their lifetimes that would authorize donation of organs at their deaths.

Henry Beecher and Brain Death

It would take the work of another Harvard physician, from a different discipline and Harvard hospital, to make donations of kidneys from patients who had suffered neurologic catastrophes available to those suffering from kidney failure. Henry K. Beecher (1904–1976) started life with the surname Unangst but changed it in the 1920s. By 1927, Beecher had received his undergraduate education and a master's degree in physical chemistry from the University of Kansas. Although Beecher had planned to go to Europe to pursue graduate studies in chemistry, he matriculated at Harvard Medical School in 1928 and graduated in 1932, cum laude. Beecher pursued postgraduate work in anesthesiology, returning to practice at the Massachusetts General Hospital. Beecher was appointed the Henry Isaiah Dorr Professor of Anesthesia Research at Harvard in 1941.

Beecher became a preeminent American expert on the subject of pain. On Christmas Eve in 1955, he published a review article in *JAMA* titled "The Powerful Placebo."[29] The paper had implications for the science of the placebo, noting that a substantial subset of patients had clinically meaningful responses to an inert substance. The article also had importance in bolstering clinical trials science, affirming that to show the effect of a drug in a patient population, randomized and preferably placebo-controlled trials were necessary. In 1957, Beecher published an article, "The Measurement of Pain: Prototype for the Quantitative Study of Subjective Responses," summarizing eleven principles for the study of pain and its treatment by analgesic medications. Although the responses to pain were necessarily subjective, Beecher recognized that quantitative measures could be employed in research on pain, emphasizing the use of pharmacologic and psychologic tools in its evaluation.

In 1959, Beecher published a report to the Council on Drugs of the American Medical Association, entitled "Experimentation in Man" in *JAMA*.[30] The paper attempted to provide some "rules" to guide clinical research after the horrors of medical experimentation during World War II by Nazi scientists had been revealed. Beecher outlined a medico-legal and ethical framework for the conduct of research by physicians, emphasizing the critical importance of truly informed consent and the use of an appropriate control group. He highlighted that research was distinct from treatment. Beecher argued that medical research in humans be viewed as a societal benefit. Beecher quoted Pope Pius XII on ethical medical research principles. The paper delineated vulnerable groups whose members should not be coerced into research, for example, prisoners and children. In 1961, Beecher published a review article in *JAMA*, "Surgery as Placebo: A Quantitative Study of Bias."[31] The paper called for carefully controlled, double-blind experiments to evaluate the results of novel surgical approaches to treat disease, especially when subjective responses were outcomes. Beecher concluded the article by considering ethical issues engendered by surgical treatments. The academic anesthesiologist had become an expert in the evaluation and quantification of pain, on the extent that placebos influenced therapeutic responses and in clinical trial design, as well as a pioneer of medical ethics.

Dr. Guy Alexandre, from Belgium, a research fellow in surgery at Harvard Medical School, supported by the Belgian-American Educational Foundation

Inc., had trained with Joseph Murray at the Brigham, succeeding Roy Calne, also serving as an assistant in surgery at the Peter Bent Brigham Hospital. Alexandre participated as a coauthor on several of Murray's early clinical and research studies, including the dismal paper in the *Annals of Surgery* in 1962 on "modified recipients" who received radiation to downregulate the immune response, as well as their seminal paper on immunosuppression with drugs, published in *Transplantation* in 1963. Alexandre returned to Europe and continued work in kidney transplantation, contributing to the literature until 2004. As Dr. Joshua Mezrich points out in *How Death Becomes Life: Notes of a Transplant Surgeon*,[32] Alexandre described a patient who had sustained head injury and was in a comatose state, in June 1963. The patient was "areactive" and was diagnosed with "coma depassé." Alexandre recounted that the chair of surgery proceeded to remove a kidney from the patient while the heart was still beating. The kidney was subsequently used for transplantation. Mezrich further recounts a conference held in London in 1966, called by Woodruff and attended by Murray, Calne, and Starzl, which considered ways to increase the kidney donor pool. Alexandre reported in "nine cases we have used patients with head injuries, whose heart had not stopped, to do kidney transplantations." Attendees were surprised by this controversial approach and did not endorse the practice. Murray returned to the Brigham.

Beecher continued his work in ethics and published a landmark report in the *NEJM* in 1966, "Ethics in Clinical Research."[33] The article was intrinsically controversial, presenting case studies recounting breaches of ethics in research studies that had been published in prominent medical journals. Beecher described these papers as presenting "troubling practices ... from leading medical schools, university hospitals, private hospitals, governmental military departments ... governmental institutes (the National Institutes of Health), Veterans Administration hospitals and industry." The paper had originally been rejected by *JAMA*, but Beecher submitted it afterward to the *NEJM*, where it was extensively criticized, revised, and rewritten before publication. It was published as a "Special Article," accompanied by a short unsigned editorial emphasizing that research ends did not trump the means of human clinical research, and that informed consent and the evaluation of the potential benefit of the research were paramount criteria for ethical studies. Beecher's paper emphasized that obtaining true informed consent from patients was critical. Beecher observed that "thoughtlessness and carelessness, not a willful disregard of the patient's rights, account for most of the cases encountered. Nevertheless, it is evident in many of the examples presented, the investigators have risked the health, or the life of their subjects."

In 1967 and 1968, the confluence of ethical imperatives, the growing need for donated organs for patients with kidney and heart disease, and the call for a more specific, clinically useful definition of death as technologies to support life in critically ill patients developed came to a head. In a remarkable piece of historical investigation, Dr. Eelco F. M. Wijdicks published, in *Neurology* in 2003, source material related to the establishment of clinical criteria related to a new concept, "brain death."[34] Wijdicks, a neurologist at the Mayo Clinic in Rochester, Minnesota, obtained access to and reviewed Beecher's papers from Harvard, in the Countway Library of Medicine, with the concurrence of the dean of Harvard Medical School, and interviewed Drs. Joseph Murray, Raymond Adams, and Ralph Potter, of the Harvard faculty, about discussions that had taken place more than twenty-five years earlier. The process of policymaking can be said to have started in September 1967 with a letter Beecher wrote to Robert H. Ebert, M.D., the dean of Harvard Medical School. Beecher asked Ebert to call a meeting of the Standing Committee on Human Studies to consider a paper he was writing titled "Ethical Problems Created by the Hopelessly Unconscious Patient." The subject was an increasing problem in the newly formed intensive care units that had many critical implications for patients and their families as well as physicians and hospital administrators. Beecher wrote,

As I am sure you are aware, the developments in resuscitative and supportive therapy have led to many desperate attempts to save the dying patient. Sometimes all that is rescued is a decerebrated individual. These individuals are increasing in numbers over the land and there are a number of problems which should be faced up to.

The meeting at Harvard was called to order on October 19, 1967. Correspondence ensued thereafter between Murray and Beecher. Beecher thanked

Murray for his contribution to the meeting and for his support. Murray, in his reply to Beecher, emphasized two key concerns stemming from the discussions: considerations regarding "the dying patient" and, as a "second and distinct" issue, the need for organs for transplantation. Shortly thereafter, Beecher wrote another letter to Ebert, using Murray's arguments, suggesting the dean form a subcommittee to act on the issues, followed by another letter to the dean in which he suggested committee members. On January 4, 1968, Ebert sent letters to selected faculty members, convening an "ad-hoc committee." The first meeting of what Beecher called the "Ad-Hoc Committee to Examine the Definition of Brain Death" was scheduled for March 14, 1968. The committee worked on several drafts of a report between April and June 1968 and sent their final report to Dean Ebert on June 25, 1968. Wijdicks described in detail the intellectual, scientific, clinical, legal, and practical elements of horse trading that determined the final language and structure of the report and suggested the committee worked hard to dissociate issues related to transplantation from the definition of brain death. Not surprisingly, given his field of expertise, Wijdicks outlined the key roles the neurologists played in the final wording of the document.

In June 1968, Beecher, as sole author, published, as a "Special Report" in the *NEJM*, a paper entitled "Ethical Problems Created by the Hopelessly Unconscious Patient."[35] The article addressed many of the historical, clinical, theoretical, theological, and policy issues critical for the work of the committee Dean Ebert had constituted. Beecher considered seriously issues (as well as definitions) of life and death in the paper that might be the basis for clinical as well as ethical discussions and reviewed differences of opinions and controversies in the field. Beecher recounted the criteria Alexandre had used in Belgium to move forward with retrieval of the organs of "unconscious patients with head injuries, whose hearts had not stopped" but who were considered dead by the clinicians. Beecher reported on the objections that Calne and Starzl had made at the conference regarding the approach to organ procurement in Belgium, since its proceedings had been published. Beecher also considered "The Prolongation of Life," a statement on medical care of the desperately ill by Pope Pius XII. His paper came to two conclusions. First, "a time comes when it is no longer appropriate to continue extraordinary means of support for the hopelessly unconscious patient." Second, "a strong case can be made that society can ill afford to discard the tissues and organs of hopelessly unconscious patients so greatly needed for study and experimental trial to help those who can be salvaged."

The report of the Ad Hoc Committee of the Harvard Medical School to Examine the Definition of Brain Death was published shortly thereafter as a special communication in *JAMA* in 1968, entitled "A Definition of Irreversible Coma."[36] The committee was a blue-ribbon panel composed of eminent clinicians and scholars, all Harvard faculty, and chaired by Henry K. Beecher. Members of the committee included neurologists, a physiologist, an expert in health-care law and ethics, a psychiatrist, a "neurochemist," a neurosurgeon, a sociologist, and a theologian. John Merrill and Joseph Murray served on the committee as well. Reflecting the times, the committee was constituted without any women.

The report began with an explanation of its charge.

Our primary purpose is to define irreversible coma as a new criterion for death. There are two reasons why there is a need for a definition: (1) Improvements in resuscitative and supportive measures have led to increased efforts to save those who are desperately injured. Sometimes these efforts have only partial success so that the result is an individual whose heart continues to beat but whose brain is irreversibly damaged. The burden is great on patients who suffer permanent loss of intellect, on their families, on the hospitals, and on those in need of hospital beds already occupied by these comatose patients. (2) Obsolete criteria for the definition of death can lead to controversy in obtaining organs for transplantation.

The two aims of the report mirrored the conclusions of Beecher's *NEJM* paper on the "Hopelessly Unconscious Patient." The report outlined the clinical characteristics needed to make a diagnosis of irreversible coma and reviewed legal aspects of the declaration of death. Toward the end of the paper, the authors stated:

In this report . . . we suggest that responsible medical opinion is ready to adopt new criteria for pronouncing death . . . in an individual sustaining irreversible coma as a result of permanent brain damage. If this position is adopted by the medical community, it can form the basis for change in the current legal concept of death. No statutory change in the law should be necessary since the law treats this question essentially as one . . . to be determined by physicians. The only circumstance in which it would be necessary that legislation be offered in the various states to define "death" by law would be in the event that great controversy were engendered surrounding the subject and physicians were unable to agree on the new medical criteria.

It is recommended as a part of these procedures that judgment of the existence of these criteria is solely a medical issue. It is suggested that the physician in charge of the patient consult with one or more other physicians directly involved in the case before the patient is declared dead on the basis of these criteria. In this way, the responsibility is shared over a wider range of medical opinion, thus providing an important degree of protection against later questions which might be raised. . . . It is further suggested that the decision to declare the person dead, and then to turn off the respirator, be made by physicians not involved in any later effort to transplant organs or tissue from the deceased individual. This is advisable . . . to avoid any appearance of self-interest by the physicians involved.

The report is a combination of review article and a compendium of diagnostic criteria as well as a call for policy and legal change rather than for a research initiative. In some ways, it can be read as more concerned with protecting doctors than patients. The proposed changes in policy the report suggested are justified by claims about burdens on patients, families, and hospitals, including the use of precious beds by the comatose. To some extent, the ends are outlined in the beginning of the paper, highlighting the need for better criteria to allow the more efficient procurement of organs for transplantation to relieve patients' suffering rather than considering ethical principles. The ends would justify the new means of electroencephalographic criteria of death. The authors did not assert or prove that brain death was synonymous with classic determinants of death such as the absence of a heartbeat over a substantial amount of time. To be meaningful, and to change clinical practice, the report needed the entire medical and patient communities to endorse its conclusions. And the committee pleaded with the medical community to accept its views and eschew "controversy."[37]

Although brain death became a widely agreed-on criterion for death, which allowed physicians to withdraw the means of life support and transplant teams to procure organs from patients with beating hearts, acceptance was not uniform across time or communities. In 1970, Moore, in a *NEJM* editorial entitled "Changing Minds about Brains," commented on a piece published previously in the *Journal* by neurosurgeon John Shillito.[38] Moore suggested some key revisions to the neurologic criteria outlined in the report on brain death published in *JAMA*. In addition, Moore reconsidered his report in *Give and Take* of the dim view of retrieval of organs from neurologically impaired patients with beating hearts that participants had expressed in the Ciba Symposium in 1965. Endorsing the new concept of brain death, he noted, "How rapidly thinking has changed!" Moore brought up the issue of clinicians fundamentally changing the culture of practice. "'What do we do when they change their minds?' At least we can be thankful that they do—and are willing to admit it."

Robert D. Truog, Thaddeus Mason Pope, and David S. Jones considered the legacy of the Report in *JAMA* in 2018.[39] They noted that several medical organizations, such as the English and Scottish Health Ministries, the World Health Organization, and the World Medical Organization, acknowledged the concept of brain death contemporaneously. Kansas adopted the Harvard criteria in 1970. Other states followed, adopting specific criteria for determining death. The President's Commission for the Study of Ethical Problems in Medicine and Biomedical and Behavioral Research proposed a definition of death in 1981. The Uniform Determination of Death Act, from 1981, provided a model, standard criterion for use across the U.S., stating, "An individual who has sustained either (1) irreversible cessation of circulatory or respiratory functions, or (2) irreversible cessation of all functions of the entire brain, including the brainstem, is dead." The concept of brain death allowed the procurement of organs that might have improved in quality compared to those obtained during previous decades. Truog and colleagues noted, "The procurement and allocation of organs have had widespread public admiration and support, with few cases of controversy or dissent." Although issues regarding death in some rare cases may still be unresolved or disputed,[40] Beecher would have been pleased. A 2021 article in the *NEJM* by Dr. David Greer, though outlining advanced techniques of diagnosis and verification, basically reaffirmed the principles regarding brain death that had first been promulgated so many years before.

The Genetics of Transplantation and Matching by Tissue Types

Dr. Benjamin Barnes, a surgeon at the Massachusetts General Hospital in Boston, published a paper on the overall survival of patients with kidney transplants in the *NEJM* in 1965,[41] summarizing the experience of these early days, primarily before drugs were used to suppress the immune systems of recipients. Barnes analyzed almost 495 cases of patients with kidney failure who had been transplanted, evaluating long-term outcomes according to the source of the donated kidney. Barnes classified kidney donations from (1) an identical (monozygotic) twin, (2) a mother or father, (3) a sister or brother, including a dizygotic (or fraternal) twin, or other relative, (4) a spouse or living unrelated donor, or (5) what was then termed a cadaver donor. There were only thirty-three recipients of kidneys from identical twins. Not surprisingly, the survival of these kidneys donated by identical twins was excellent, for that time, estimated at 60% through eight years of follow-up. Barnes showed that survival of kidneys transplanted from siblings was almost as good as that from identical twins over a follow-up period of up to six years (about 58%), and that these kidneys fared better statistically than those exchanged between a parent and a child, as well as the kidneys provided by cadaver or unrelated donors.

Barnes could not identify the cause of the difference in survival between the groups but speculated that the interaction between the genetic relatedness of donors and recipients and the need for greater immunosuppression in donor-recipient pairs that were less closely genetically related might have played roles in determining outcomes. Selection of donors applied by the medical and surgical staff might also have affected the findings. Barnes noted improvements over the previous decade in organ preservation and surgical techniques as well as in immunosuppressive therapies and the treatment of organ rejection and infections in transplant recipients. He mentioned that kidney transplantation outcomes might be determined by genetic factors, such as seen in the H2 compatibility system present in mice. Barnes implied that better knowledge regarding the immunogenetics underlying transplant biology was truly necessary.

All these early studies suffered from being sets of case series rather than randomized controlled trials (RCTs). For example, how could investigators know azathioprine was truly superior to 6-MCP as a drug in the absence of the head-to-head comparisons mandated by randomization? Randomized trials, if well-powered (meaning that they have enough participants) can provide patients and physicians with clear answers to important clinical questions about the advantages and disadvantages of specific medical interventions. The lack of controlled comparison data was a problem in evaluating new therapies in the early era of kidney transplantation that impeded the unbiased scientific assessment of the outcomes of the procedure, especially compared to other ESRD treatment modalities, such as dialysis. The effects of many of the factors involved in transplantation (such as organ transportation time and preservation medium and aspects of patients' medical backgrounds) remained unclear. Lack of definitive answers to important clinical questions, garnered from well-designed randomized controlled trials, continues to hamper the provision of optimal patient care to transplant recipients.

The first successful kidney transplant had involved the ne plus ultra of transplantation, a living related donor—and an identical twin at that! Early experiences in France and at the Brigham involved experimental transplantation between relatives with different degrees of kinship. But "closeness" between relatives could not yet be defined immunologically. Several of the early Brigham procedures had involved kidneys obtained from altruistic living unrelated donors. Better immunosuppressive techniques and better immunologic matching held the promise of making transplantation a more reasonable as well as attractive alternative to dialysis for ESRD patients.

Understanding the genetics of the immune system that posed such a barrier to transplantation between any two people who were not identical twins developed slowly, initially between 1958 and 1970, but to a certain extent, the increase in knowledge continues through today. In 1958, Dr. Jean Dausset

(1916–2009), of Paris, France, a physician specializing in hematology who was interested in the biology of antibodies, identified an antigen in the blood he called MAC, which interacted with antibodies in various human serum samples he tested.[42] Subsequently, MAC was determined to be the first discovered antigen of the Human Leukocyte Antigen (HLA) classes discovered. These antigens were the protein flags on the transplant kidney that signaled the degree of similarity or difference between the donor of the transplant kidney and the recipient detected by the immune system of the host. Concordances and differences between the manufacture of these antigens by donors and recipients might predict whether the recipient would mount an immunologic response to reject the transplanted organ or allow the transplant to successfully function in the body. Over time, standardized antibodies were developed and shared between "tissue typing" laboratories connected with transplantation centers to identify antigens of the HLA A, HLA B, and HLA DR groups. If the donor and recipient shared the two HLA A antigens, the two HLA B antigens, and the two HLA DR antigens, that indicated a six-antigen, or "perfect," match. Perfect matches are extremely rare between members of the general population because there are so many HLA antigens corresponding to so many different versions of the genes. But in a very large population, such as in the U.S., identifying a perfect match between a patient on the waitlist and an unrelated deceased donor happens occasionally enough to be noticed. Dausset received the Nobel Prize in Physiology or Medicine with Drs. Baruj Benecerraf and George Davis Snell in 1980 for "discoveries concerning genetically determined structures on the cell surface that regulate immunological interactions."

The proteins (or antigens) of the HLA system are coded by genes located on chromosome 6. These genes are usually inherited together on the chromosome—one set from the father and one from the mother. This finding may have explained, in part, the early survival curves generated by Barnes. A child is a half immunogenetic match of a parent, and the chance of the survival of the graft is based on that similarity. Sisters and brothers of a patient waiting for a transplant may inherit the same immunogenetic makeup and be immunologically identical one quarter of the time, be half matches (receiving one set of genes from the mother and a different set of genes from the father—or vice versa) half of the time, or be completely immunologically different (receiving the set of genes from the mother and the father that the patient did not get) a quarter of the time. The early results of improved survival of sibling transplants compared to parent or child donations may have been the result of screening efforts with skin grafts—so siblings would only be half matches or perfect matches. (Siblings with no matches would be eliminated from consideration.)

In 1966, Paul I. Terasaki, Ph.D. (1929–2016), of the University of California, Los Angeles (UCLA), and colleagues, in a small study of cadaveric kidney transplant recipients, showed HLA matching was associated with better clinical outcomes.[43] Terasaki, born in the U.S.A., had as a high school student been interned, with his family, for three years at the Gila River Relocation Center in Arizona during World War II. He completed his undergraduate and master's studies and was awarded a Ph.D. at UCLA in 1956. He then did postgraduate work in the immunology of transplantation in London with Professor Peter Medawar. After returning to UCLA, in 1964, Terasaki and colleagues developed a method for identifying tissue types, by mixing donor lymphocytes and recipients' sera in a uniform fashion that soon became the nationwide standard. Terasaki and Dr. Ramon Patel followed up with a clinically important study, using sera and data from donors and patients from many of the nations' transplant centers, published in 1969 in the *NEJM*,[44] on the poor outcomes of kidneys transplanted when the recipient had preformed cytotoxic antibodies reacting against the donor's cells. Terasaki's laboratory was involved in the development of the Collins solution that allowed better preservation of kidneys for transplantation for long-distance shipping. Terasaki started a national transplantation registry in 1970. Terasaki initiated collaborative research with many transplant clinicians but most preeminently with Dr. Starzl. Terasaki and Starzl began to study the long-term implications of tissue typing in Starzl's transplant recipient patient population.

As interest in transplantation grew, technologies and practices disseminated, and outcomes of kidney transplantation improved, it was realized that sharing information about deceased donors' histocompatibility status across multiple sites might result in better allocation of kidneys, a scarce resource. Terasaki started an organ sharing program in 1967 in Los Angeles. This was followed by the establishment of the Boston Interhospital Organ Bank in 1968.

In 1969 the Southeastern Organ Procurement Foundation (SEOPF) was founded in Richmond, Virginia, by Dr. David Hume while he was on the faculty of the Medical College of Virginia and Dr. Bernard Amos, a physician and immunogeneticist at Duke University who had served on the Gottschalk Committee. SEOPF brought together transplant physicians, surgeons, nurses, and immunologists, as well as administrators and donor organizations, in one group. The foundation aimed to "enhance access to transplantation, improve quality and outcomes, and increase organ donation by facilitating collaboration between transplant centers and professionals by providing education, training and sharing of best practices." SEOPF, which received funding from the U.S. Public Health Service, coordinated organ sharing between medical centers in the southeastern United States, including Washington, D.C., using methods enhanced by computer programming. The computerized system had been called the United Network for Organ Sharing since 1977. Eventually the system expanded to involve transplant centers throughout the entire U.S., as a new organization, devoted to the matching and sharing of organs for transplantation across the nation. Taking the same name, the United Network for Organ Sharing (UNOS) came into being in the early 1980s. UNOS was awarded the U.S. government contract from the Department of Health and Human Services to serve as the National Organ Procurement and Transplant Network (OPTN) in 1986, under the auspices of the National Organ Transplant Act (NOTA) of 1984. NOTA called for the establishment of a national network to supervise organ allocation between medical facilities and to collect information about organ donors and transplant candidates and recipients. In addition, UNOS received authorization to establish the Scientific Registry of Transplant Recipients (SRTR), a data analytic and dissemination group. UNOS matching systems, reflecting different points assigned to such factors as waiting times and HLA compatibilities, determined the priority of individual patients to receive kidneys. Today, UNOS coordinates the sharing of thousands of organs between 251 transplant centers across the U.S. SEOPF has become the American Foundation for Donation and Transplantation.

In 1970, Terasaki's career changed when he attended The Hague International Transplant meeting in the Netherlands. He presented data there showing that, in larger populations, the results of HLA matching between donor and recipient did not correlate with the outcomes of kidney transplantation and that "mismatched transplants could function well." Terasaki's presentation created a furor, as it went against the conventional wisdom that had grown up, largely based on his own research: that HLA matching mattered. Terasaki's paper was the only one not published in the proceedings of the conference. The NIH investigated his laboratory. Only subsequently, over time, was it appreciated that his findings had been correct. Today, Terasaki is posthumously celebrated as one of the founding fathers of kidney transplantation.

Matching systems became the standard of care for both allocating precious kidneys from deceased donors to patients on the waitlist and determining which family members were eligible to give a kidney to a sick relative, in the hope of improving the outcomes of kidney transplantation, by diminishing the chance and severity of rejection. But the role of HLA matching, in a new era of better immunosuppression, organ preservation and sharing, would have to be rigorously confirmed in the context of large samples of patients from different backgrounds, with a range of clinical characteristics that could also determine outcomes.

By the mid-1970s, kidney transplantation had hit its stride. Most medical centers associated with medical schools had started kidney transplant services. Immunosuppression generally consisted of azathioprine and maintenance oral steroids, which were tapered over time as possible. Some centers pioneered and used protocols adding antilymphocyte therapies. Episodes of acute rejection were treated with high doses of steroids, administered for relatively short periods. Organ sharing across the country was facilitated by UNOS and its computer infrastructures, air transport systems, technical advances in cooling methods for kidneys destined for transplantation, and the development of solutions for infusion into those kidneys, which enhanced their viability over longer periods of time.

Kidney Transplantation Epidemiology

Dr. Henry Krakauer (1939–2006), a physician working at the NIAID, at NIH, was interested in the development of new technologies and the allocation of scarce resources, as well as the cost-effectiveness of novel therapies. Krakauer was born in Poland shortly before the German invasion at the start of World War II. He arrived in the U.S. in 1951, and became a naturalized citizen in 1958. He entered the NYU School of Medicine in 1960 and graduated in 1964. Rather than pursuing a clinical internship, Krakauer used a U.S. Public Health Service scholarship to obtain a Ph.D. in Physical Chemistry at Yale. He was studying the energy relationships in building blocks of DNA and RNA. Thereafter, he joined the faculty of Washington State University, where he pursued studies in the biochemistry of transplant immunological molecules. Krakauer entered public service in the Genetics and Transplant Biology Branch of the NIAID in 1980. In 1981, he participated in the Program in Health Policy, Planning, and Regulation of the Executive Programs in Health Policy and Management at Harvard. Krakauer brought this unique background, in the absence of special training in internal medicine, nephrology, or epidemiology, to the question of treatment of ESRD patients, a large entitlement program financed primarily by the U.S. government.

In 1980, Krakauer began to write about issues related to kidney transplantation, in his role as a government official. He and colleagues published a landmark paper in the *NEJM* in 1983,[45] delineating for clinicians how the ESRD program, financed by the government, worked to change the lives of people with advanced kidney disease after its ten years of existence.

For people in the U.S. who started therapy for ESRD in 1977, the chance of one-year survival for those who received a kidney from an unrelated donor was 87%. Their three-year survival rate was 79%. The comparable values for those who received a kidney from a related donor were 94% and 89%. The kidney graft survived 52% of the time at one year and 40% of the time at three years in the group who received a kidney from an unrelated donor. The values for those transplanted with a kidney from a related donor were higher, 70% and 61%, respectively. In contrast, one- and three-year survival in patients treated with dialysis for ESRD was 82% and 57%, respectively. Of the 16,501 ESRD patients in the cohort, almost 89% were treated with hemodialysis and only a few more than 10% received transplants. Approximately 60% of the transplanted ESRD patients received a cadaveric kidney.

Krakauer and colleagues suggested that transplant patients had better survival than dialysis patients but acknowledged that the design of their study, using retrospective, administrative data, could not definitively answer the question of whether transplantation or dialysis conveyed enhanced survival in a set of patients matched at the outset for key clinical characteristics. The groups of patients treated with different modalities of therapy were dramatically different in terms of age and race, among other clinical and sociodemographic characteristics.

Key questions regarding these findings were posed by Dr. Robert G. (Robin) Luke, a graduate of the medical school at the University of Glasgow in Scotland and a distinguished nephrologist, then at the University of Alabama, who provided an editorial review on the Krakauer paper and an accompanying paper on the long-term outcomes of ESRD patients treated by the Seattle group in the same issue of the *Journal*.[46] Luke contributed a brief but masterful overview of the different therapeutic options currently available for ESRD patients. He pointed out that transplantation seemed to be the most desirable treatment modality, but noted the results were not optimal, and that the availability of kidneys for the many patients who desired renal transplantation was limited. Luke acknowledged that many patients had contraindications to receiving a kidney transplant and that infection was always a potential problem in immunosuppressed hosts. He carefully outlined the short- and long-term complications of kidney transplantation. Luke also turned his attention to issues related to survival. Only a prospective, randomized controlled trial could answer the question of whether dialysis or transplantation provided greater length (and quality) of life. Given the constraints of the treatment and limited access to transplantation, and the fact that patients might be quite unwilling to base their treatment decisions on the toss of a coin, such a perfect randomized trial was unimaginable. Administrative data comparing the outcomes of similar patients would have to suffice for the time being. Luke concluded by relating that improved access to care, better patient/physician communication, and clear informed consent procedures before deciding on a course of therapy were essential to progress in ESRD care and outcomes.

Putting People First!

As success in kidney transplantation improved, the attention of physicians, patients, and families turned to the experience of patients. One could focus on quality as well as quantity of life. Dr. Roberta G. Simmons (1937–1993) studied the psychologic reactions to kidney transplantation in donors and recipients. Simmons did her undergraduate work at Wellesley and received a Ph.D. in sociology from Columbia University in New York. Simmons was a professor of sociology and psychiatry at the University of Minnesota. The wife of a transplant surgeon at the University of Minnesota, Richard L. Simmons, M.D., she had access to living related donors, starting during the early days of transplantation. Simmons died at the age of fifty-five after battling breast cancer for fifteen years. Her work, published between 1971 and 1990, pioneered early interest in the psychosocial adaptation of kidney donors and the recipients of renal transplants.

Dr. Renée C. Fox (1928–2020) set out to understand the cultural, sociologic and psychologic landscape of transplantation during its early developmental stages from a varied number of perspectives. Fox, born in New York City, graduated summa cum laude from Smith College in 1949. Her undergraduate work was interrupted by a bout of polio. Fox went on to receive a Ph.D. in sociology from Radcliffe College of Harvard University, working in the Department of Social Relations. Her thesis examined interrelationships between patients with tuberculosis and the physicians who cared for them while performing research. Her book, describing the intertwined medical and social culture of the physicians and their patients, *Experiment Perilous*, was published in 1959. Fox taught at Barnard College and Harvard before joining the faculty of the University of Pennsylvania in 1969. During her time at Harvard, from 1951 to 1954, Fox was an observer on the metabolic research ward at the Peter Bent Brigham Hospital while dialysis was being developed and during the early experimental days of human kidney transplantation.

The Courage to Fail: A Social View of Organ Transplants and Dialysis, published in 1974, was researched and written by Fox in conjunction with Dr. Judith P. Swazey, born in 1939, a historian of science, then of the Socio-Medical Sciences Department at Boston University Medical School. Swazey graduated from Wellesley College and received her Ph.D. from Harvard. Fox and Swazey had participated in the Harvard University program on technology and society in 1968. They decided to study "organ transplantation and chronic hemodialysis," representing medical fields in the midst of therapeutic innovations that were at the beginning of mature phases of technological development. They planned to study the medical researchers, in tandem with their patients, to understand better "the social and cultural dynamics of medical research with human subjects."

Their book provided perspectives of patients and family members, as well as transplant physicians and staff, from which the authors sought to illuminate the human side and social consequences of these medical procedures. The study was portrayed as an anthropologic expedition. Difficult problems related to ethics, including limited access to scarce resources, the interfamily dynamics associated with kidney transplantation and donation, as well as the refusals of potential donors to provide a kidney to family members in need, were explored. The authors concentrated on the anthropological concept of "gift exchanges" and the challenges of living with uncertainty, viewed from both professional and patient viewpoints. Fox and Swazey reviewed the early as well as contemporary history of kidney transplantation at the Brigham and elsewhere. Their judgments were well-documented and nuanced. Fox and Swazey cited the work of Merrill, Murray, and Moore frequently throughout the text. They quoted, usually approvingly, from *Give and Take*. The authors cited a portion of the text of Moore's update of *Give and Take, Transplant: The Give and Take of Tissue Transplantation*, published in 1972, on early controversies in heart transplantation, commenting that it was one of "the few censorious statements by a research physician" on the topic.

The Courage to Fail incited controversy in multidisciplinary circles. Dr. Francis Moore of Harvard Medical School, with two colleagues, Drs. Mitchell Goldman and Christopher Gates, reviewed *The Courage to Fail* in the *NEJM* in 1975.[47] Although *The Courage to Fail* had received some appreciative reviews, Moore, a patriarch of transplantation, damned it with faint praise. The reviewers suggested the authors of *The Courage to Fail* had insufficient appreciation of the similarities between typical medical care and therapeutic innovations, and provided an unrealistic portrait of the transplant surgeon as "something of a superman pioneering the therapeutic unknown." Fox and Swazey were criticized for failing to understand the lapses of the American early surgical innovators in heart transplantation. The review suggested that sociologists should take an "internship" rather than set themselves up as disinterested, scientific observers of medical practice. The reviewers compared the book's intellectual structure unfavorably with Paul Tillich's *The Courage to Be*. While not a complete dismissal, one could view the review as a shot over the bow in an interdisciplinary territorial war between social and medical scientists or perhaps a sour reaction to academics who had been invited to join a medical team and formed, as well as published, unwanted perspectives. From a contemporary viewpoint, one wonders if the male surgeons took umbrage at being assessed by women. Perhaps the authors of the review felt Fox and Swazey didn't sufficiently appreciate Moore's *Transplant: The Give and Take of Tissue Transplantation*. (Neither Fox nor Swazey was mentioned in the index of that book.) Dr. Robert McCabe of Columbia University provided a more measured review of *The Courage to Fail* in *JAMA* in November 1974.[48] However, he noted the authors had "unconvincingly drawn a sociologic portrait of the transplant surgeon, a type of research physician. They were unrealistically captivated by the excitement of heart transplantation, the boldest therapy ever undertaken by the medical profession." Erdman Palmore, Ph.D., of Duke University, in a review in the *AIM* in December 1974, found the book lacking in scientific rigor.[49]

An unsigned review in *Medical History* in 1976 was much more laudatory. Drs. Richard and Roberta Simmons reviewed the book in the *Journal of the History of Medicine* in July 1975 and provided a more generous viewpoint:

> For a reader interested in the contemporary history of medicine, we can recommend no book more highly than *The Courage to Fail* by Renée Fox and Judith Swazey. It is beautifully and clearly written; it is fascinating in its treatment of the history of one of the most publicized of the new medical technologies—organ transplantation and renal dialysis. Because of the great human interest with which many of the issues are presented and the large ethical problems raised, the book should appeal to a wide audience, both lay and professional.[50]

It would seem that the reaction to this book, which straddled academic and scientific disciplines, was predicated on the field of the reviewer. Interestingly, the generally more positive sociologist reviewers pointed out that Fox and Swazey had adopted the physician perspective rather than interviewing patients in depth.

A Patient from the 1980s

In 1983, Brian Kampschroer needed a kidney. He had had a long history of kidney disease, starting during his childhood. At the age of two, Kampschroer was diagnosed with an unknown disease. His bone structure was abnormal, and he had had several bouts of pneumonia before he was nine years old. He was treated with steroids from age seven. Around the age of twelve, he was told he had kidney disease due to abnormalities of the ureters draining his kidneys as a result of retroperitoneal fibrosis, a process of abnormal tissue growth. Brian's kidney function continued to slowly deteriorate over the next ten years. He eventually had surgery to divert and drain the outflow of the ureters. The operation forestalled the progression of kidney failure somewhat, but in his early thirties, Brian had to start treatment with hemodialysis when his kidney function deteriorated to the point it could no longer support his life. An arteriovenous fistula was placed in his left arm, and he began dialysis three times a week in September 1983. Describing the course of the days for a typical hemodialysis patient, Brian remembers,

> My life revolved around dialysis. The morning of dialysis I usually felt pretty bad, and the afternoon afterwards I still felt quite tired. The next morning I usually felt quite good, but by mid-afternoon I began feeling tired again. So, in the course of a week I felt fairly good for three of the seven mornings; the rest of the time I felt lousy, with no energy and no appetite. After several months, my nephrologists began talking with me about the possibility of a kidney transplant. . . .
>
> Having been involved with hospitals and medical procedures all my life, I was adamantly opposed to having any family member go through surgery for my benefit. I did say I would consider a cadaver transplant since it seemed my case was not urgent and I could wait for a kidney to be available. My family, all of them, began working on me to accept a kidney from one of them. My sister, both my brothers and my

parents all said they would happily give me a kidney. This was not a surprise since we had always been very close. I would also happily have given them whatever they needed as well. I just really did not want any of them to have to undergo the ordeals and risks of fairly painful surgery. During this time I researched kidney transplants and learned of the scarcity of organs and how lucky some patients were to have compatible family donors. With this information churning in my brain, with dialysis slowly wearing me down, and my family putting tremendous pressure on me to at least agree to have them tested, I finally conceded. In good conscience I could not take a scarce organ from another needy patient when I had an alternative.

My older brother, Kevin, who lives within two and a half hours of me, and my sister . . . both got tested. They were both perfect matches, and therein was another quandary. Both insisted each was best suited to donate. Now I had to choose. I had to choose a sibling as a donor when I really did not want either one of them to have such an ordeal. Agony. A telephone call from my mother's sister solved the dilemma. She devised a numbers game of chance over the phone where she chose a number from one to ten, as did Kevin and my sister. The one who came closest to my aunt's number would be the winner (or in my mind, the loser). Kevin chose the closest number. My sister rolled her eyes, certain the contest was rigged. Thus, I evaded what was probably the most fateful decision of my life.

During the months prior to the transplant, transplant coordinators, the unsung heroes of the whole transplant process, explained all the risks, the procedures, the life-changes and especially the medicines involved. It came as a surprise to me that one of the primary reasons for rejection of transplanted organs was the failure of patients to take their drugs as often as directed and in the manner directed. While I knew in my case that would not be an issue, because I had been taking daily, twice daily, thrice daily medications, even as needed pain medications, on my own responsibility since I was seven years old, and knew that at least one of the medications, prednisone, was keeping me alive, the coordinators were not convinced. . . .

. . . From my standpoint, the kidney transplant, squeezed into my lower right abdomen, was the easiest operation I had ever had, and I had had many. I was up and walking around within an hour of awakening. I visited Kevin and my worries and concerns were borne out. He was in great pain and quite swollen. Nevertheless, he grinned and made light of his torment. Between groans. He did recover well, however, as did I. It was a strange sensation to urinate again after four months of abstinence.

The anti-rejection drugs prescribed were Imuran and prednisone. I was already taking prednisone, so the dose was initially raised to 40 mg. The policy then was to keep a transplant patient isolated for a week or two. While I was isolated my prednisone was gradually decreased to 20 mg a day. Six months later it was 10 mg and two years after that 5 mg. My Imuran started at 200 mg and over the course of a year was reduced to 150 mg. It is now 125 mg a day. As new anti-rejection drugs proved themselves, my transplant surgeons and nephrologists tried them with me. After perhaps six months on cyclosporin, we decided there was really no reason to change from Imuran, which had been spectacularly successful for me. After all, at the time of my transplant the expected life of a transplanted living donor kidney was just five years, and we were past that deadline.

Kevin's kidney, now mine, is bigger than either one of my original kidneys. For many years after my transplant my creatinine and BUN were lower than it had ever been measured. My creatinine was usually between 0.8 and 0.9. After 37 years my creatinine is now usually between 1.2 and 1.3. From May 1st, 1984, until now, I have experienced not one episode of rejection.

Brian Kampschroer's story exemplifies the state of the art in kidney transplantation during the early 1980s, before the introduction of different, more potent, and safer types of immunosuppressive drugs were available to physicians and patients. It illustrates the changes in the experience of living donors over time. Brian Kampschroer's case shows the dramatic interaction of family dynamics when a family member is desperately ill, and everyone's altruism is tested. Ethical considerations and interpersonal history are thrust to the forefront of family relationships and medical outcomes during chronic illness and the search for a viable kidney, as Fox and Swazey and Simmons had described. Happily, Brian's story culminated in a superb outcome, for the donor as well as the recipient, over almost four decades. Finally, it is a saga of chronic, unrelenting, severe pediatric illness and individual fortitude in the face of medical adversity, during which new therapies allowed patients who would have previously died to live long, fulfilled lives. The story illustrates the generally long extension of life for younger kidney transplant recipients and for those who receive a perfectly matched kidney from a willing living family member under controlled medical conditions.

6

———— ✤ ————

HEMODIALYSIS MATURES

It's All About the Money

Was Dialysis Worth the Money?

Legislation enabling the establishment of the ESRD program was passed by Congress and signed into law in 1972 by President Richard M. Nixon, and dialysis patients in the U.S. began to be treated for uremia in July 1973 under its auspices. In 1972, it was estimated that about 10,000 people in the U.S. would need ESRD therapy. The patients envisioned to be part of the program were expected to have disease limited to their kidneys, such as glomerulonephritis or polycystic kidney disease. Patients with diabetes mellitus or heart failure were considered too sick for this kind of heroic treatment. In addition, elderly people would not be able to tolerate the stresses of hemodialysis. Doctors would never refer such frail patients for dialysis. Dialysis would rehabilitate people with uremia so that they could return to meaningful employment. The system might even pay for itself if patients were treated with home dialysis therapies, had kidney transplants, and were able to return to gainful employment. In 2020, the ESRD program covered more than 800,000 people at a cost of over $50 billion to the Medicare system, covering about 7% of total Medicare expenditures, for approximately 1.25% of the beneficiaries.

Controversy has raged over the system, starting after its first decade of existence. Was the relatively short survival time of patients provided by dialysis worth the societal costs? Was it in fact short survival, or in reality was it the extension of life for desperately ill patients for a meaningful period? Was the entitlement a good idea, or should entry into the ESRD program have been rationed and restricted only to certain patient subgroups? Did this lifesaving service grow too fast and accommodate the wrong kind of patient, covering people who were never meant to be treated? Were patients who received ESRD benefits too old and too sick and therefore people who would survive for only a short time? Should patients whose kidney function had declined to perilously low levels rather have conservative care and be made comfortable as uremia gently took their lives away? Or was dialysis indeed a wonderful, life-extending technology that consumed a lower and lower percentage of the Medicare budget over its half-century existence, as corporate dialysis providers became more efficient and nephrologists developed better therapeutic approaches? Was it worth letting an eighty-four-year-old grandmother live an extra year to put her holdings into order, achieve final goals, and say goodbye to her family?

The medical, ethical, and rationing arguments had always been both about patient choices as well as the money expended on the program. What remains unclear on the macroeconomic level, rather than from the perspective of individual patient care, is whether the negative considerations were stoked by the entry of Black patients and poor people into the program and the cost associated with their treatment.

In April 1973, the *NEJM* published "Survival of Patients Undergoing Chronic Hemodialysis and Transplantation," by Drs. Edmund G. Lowrie and colleagues, including Constantine L. Hampers and John P. Merrill, all of the Departments of Medicine and Surgery at the Peter Bent Brigham Hospital in Boston, Massachusetts.[1] The paper reviewed the outcomes of ESRD patients who had been given kidney transplants from living or cadaver donors, with those who had been treated with home hemodialysis in Brigham programs from 1964 until 1972. The results of three years' treatment of center hemodialysis patients from the Brigham program were also evaluated. There was no difference in survival between the 172 transplant patients who had received a kidney from a living donor and the 125 patients who had been treated with home hemodialysis before the legislation that enacted the ESRD program was signed into law. The authors acknowledged that the small size of the study limited its power to detect survival differences. Patients who had received a kidney from a cadaver donor did more poorly. Hemodialysis patients, with an average age of 44.3 years, were older than the transplant patients. The majority of patients had glomerulonephritis. Center hemodialysis patients had one- and two-year survivals of 92.9% and 86.1%, respectively. Three-year patient survival on hemodialysis was much lower, at 59.6%, probably due to selection bias, because of the many healthier patients in the program who had received kidney transplants in their first year or two of ESRD. The paper considered hemodialysis and transplantation outcomes before the legislation that enacted the ESRD program was signed into law, as well as transplantation results from the beginning of the era of immunosuppression with azathioprine, and as such is a landmark. Everything was to change after HR1. Several of the authors established or later worked for a company that would revolutionize dialysis care in the U.S. Funding sources for and conflicts of interest of the authors were not cited in the paper.

NMC and the Growth of Dialysis as a Business

In June 1978, Daniel S. Greenberg, in the Washington Report section of the *NEJM*, described changes in the ESRD program since its birth in 1973.[2] The proportion of people dialyzed at home in the ESRD program had decreased over time from about 40% to fewer than 10%. The costs of the program and the number of patients the ESRD program served had increased far beyond original estimates. The consensus was that the changes had occurred because financial disincentives to the less expensive home treatments had unwittingly been built into the original legislation. In 1977, legislation was considered in the House of Representatives aiming to direct half of dialysis patients to home therapies. As the bill advanced through Congress, the home dialysis goals were continually whittled away. Greenberg implicated the dialysis corporation, National Medical Care (NMC), in a lobbying effort to reduce regulatory requirements to enforce home dialysis goals.

The *Washington Post*'s Lawrence Meyer reported, in July 1977, that the initial debate on the new ESRD program legislation had started in the House of Representatives. The cost of the ESRD program was by that time estimated at a half billion dollars a year. Testimony suggested that there were between 30,000 and 34,000 patients undergoing dialysis at that time in the U.S. ESRD program. Dr. Eugene Schupak's testimony before Representative Dan Rostenkowski's Ways and Means Committee was described.

> One of the most outspoken opponents of the bill during the hearings was Dr. Eugene Schupak, president of National Medicare Care, Inc., a firm that operated 68 centers in 19 states and Puerto Rico and did $128 million worth of business in 1976, treating and selling medical supplies for dialysis patients.
>
> "The notion" Schupak said, "that since Congress is paying the bill, it can mandate the particular form of therapy to be rendered, if carried to its logical conclusion, would permit Congress to dictate or prescribe therapy for all diseases and medical disabilities, and, for all practical purposes, enable Congress to practice medicine."

Dr. Belding Scribner, the director of the not-for-profit Northwest Kidney Center, in Seattle, Washington, who testified to Congress before Schupak spoke, emphasized that conflicts of interest for physicians existed in referring patients to treatment facilities through which they could reap profits. Scribner stated:

> What started in 1960 as a noble experiment gradually has degenerated into a highly controversial billion-dollar program riddled with cost over-runs and enormous profiteering.... In addition, the present regulations have encouraged the rapid expansion of a very profitable business, selling in-center dialysis to the Government.... If you are successful in this attempt, you will benefit many dialysis patients who would be much better served by home than by in-center dialysis; you will save the taxpayer hundreds of millions of dollars each year; and you will set an important national example of effective cost control, without compromising quality in a federally funded health care program.

Congress intended to provide incentives to reduce costs and substantially favor home dialysis (rather than the relatively more expensive hospital-based or satellite center facilities) and kidney transplantation. Lobbying efforts by National Medical Care were implicated by *NEJM* correspondent John Iglehart in the failure of Congress to finalize legislation to achieve these goals. Richard Rettig was quoted in 1982 in the *NEJM* by Iglehart as characterizing the battle regarding the financing of the ESRD system between Seattle and Boston as "rivalry, if not enmity."[3] By the end of 1980, there were 63,214 ESRD patients. The number had increased two-and-a-half-fold since 1974. Expenditures in 1980 for ESRD patients were $1.4 billion, a figure that had risen fivefold between 1974 and 1980. Iglehart quoted from a Senate Financing Committee source that outlined goals for amendments by the Carter administration that would

provide incentives for the use of lower cost, medically appropriate self-dialysis, particularly home dialysis, as an alternate to high-cost institutional dialysis; eliminate program disincentives to the use of transplantation; provide for the implementation of incentive reimbursement methods to assure more cost-effective delivery of services to patients dialyzing in institutions and at home; develop a long-range objective, on the basis of the continuing review and judgment of professional peer review organizations, with respect to the most effective use of resources for treating renal disease; and studies for alternative ways to improve the program and for regular reporting to Congress on the renal disease program.

At that time, with few exceptions, hospital payments from the ESRD Medicare program were $159 per dialysis treatment, and independent facilities received $138 a treatment. The Carter administration favored a single rate system, which would perhaps achieve the goals outlined by the Senate Finance Committee. During congressional budgeting at the beginning of the Reagan administration, however, the legislature rejected this approach in favor of a dual-rate system approach. After NMC sent letters to hospitals, proposing to take over their dialysis patients if reimbursement rates were diminished by Congress (one of which was published in Iglehart's article), Senate Finance

Committee staffers feared that home dialysis would be greatly disadvantaged by a single-payer system. Iglehart reported that "the letter raised the question whether an aggressive company was striving to enlarge its segment of the market at the expense of home dialysis and at a reimbursement rate that might enable it to turn an excessive profit." Committee staff feared this kind of takeover of dialysis patients from academic units by NMC might limit use of the less expensive home dialysis. The government proposed new rates of $133 for hospital-based dialysis treatments and $128 for treatments taking place in independent dialysis facilities. Iglehart reported that NMC vigorously opposed the proposed two-tier government payment system. Dr. Constantine L. Hampers of NMC sent a six page letter to Secretary Richard S. Schweiker of the Department of Health and Human Services, rebutting the financial and care assumptions made by the department. Portions of the letter were quoted in the article.

Arnold S. Relman, M.D. (1923–2014), left his position as chairman of the Department of Medicine at the Hospital of the University of Pennsylvania in 1977 to assume the post of editor in chief of the *NEJM* and to join the faculty of Harvard Medical School. Relman received his M.D. from the Columbia University College of Physicians and Surgeons in 1946 at age twenty-two. After internship and residency at Yale, he joined the faculty at Boston University School of Medicine. In 1968, he joined the University of Pennsylvania School of Medicine.

Relman was interested in the relationship of kidney function to body fluid chemistry and acid-base balance before there was a real field of nephrology. He had published papers on these subjects since 1949. Relman was the editor of the prestigious *JCI* from 1962 to 1967. As president of the American Society for Clinical Investigation, he published a paper on "Academic Medicine and the Public" in 1969 in the *JCI*.[4] Relman lauded the role of federal funding, through NIH grants, which had resulted in advances in clinical medicine over the past two decades. He decried the recent decrease in funding because of the Vietnam War and called for greater federal support of medical educational activities. Relman warned that public expenditures entailed public scrutiny, and that urban medical schools and hospitals would have to assume greater responsibilities for indigent patient care. Relman argued that medical schools indeed did have social responsibilities. Medical research was a public function, funded with taxpayers' dollars, that had societal consequences. He opined medical schools and their hospitals needed to address flaws in the health-care system. Relman encouraged the members of academic medicine to embrace public policy issues.

Although his previous work had focused on kidney function in health and disease, by the 1980s, Relman had become a different kind of physician, with publication of papers on public health in addition to those in the basic scientific literature. Important articles on social aspects of medicine appeared under his byline in periodicals aimed at very different audiences, such as the *New York Review of Books*, the *Atlantic Monthly*, and the *New Republic*. As a prerogative of his editorial position, Relman published a Special Article in the *NEJM* in 1980 titled "The Medical Industrial Complex."[5] The title referred to President Dwight D. Eisenhower's valedictory warning to the U.S. populace in 1961 about the "military-industrial complex." Relman argued that business interests had become predominant in American medicine, involving commercial hospital chains, laboratory and diagnostic facilities, nursing homes, and home care services as well as dialysis treatment organizations. Relman felt doctors should not have financial conflicts of interest regarding the care of their patients and that salaried positions for American physicians would help to ameliorate their duties by focusing practitioners on patients rather than profits. He deplored the increasing role of financial over fiduciary considerations in medical care. Relman mentioned a single dialysis company by name in the paper:

> But one corporation, National Medical Care, soon became preeminent in the field. This company was founded by nephrologists and employs many local nephrologists as physicians and medical directors in its numerous centers around the country. It currently has sales of over $200 million annually and performs about 17 per cent of the long-term dialysis treatments in the country. It has recently expanded into the sale of dialysis equipment and supplies and the provision of psychiatric hospital care, and centers for obesity treatment, but its main business is still to provide dialysis for patients with end-stage renal disease in

out-of-hospital facilities that it builds and operates. According to data obtained from the Health Care Financing Administration, nearly 40 per cent of the hemodialysis in this country is now provided by profit-making units.

Earlier in the year, the journalist Gina Kolata had profiled NMC in two articles in *Science*,[6] marveling that the company had enough clout to hire Ronald Reagan's campaign manager as its lobbyist. At that time, Kolata estimated there were 48,000 U.S. dialysis patients. She described the procedures and economics of home dialysis and outlined its champions and detractors. Kolata quoted prominent nephrologists regarding the changes in the ESRD program that had taken place since 1973. ESRD patients were progressively getting older and sicker and could no longer be "rehabilitated." Kolata suggested depression was an important problem for patients enrolled in the contemporary dialysis population. Kolata explored the origins of NMC from the Department of Medicine at the Peter Bent Brigham Hospital. She attributed, quoting Dr. Constantine Hampers, part of the ascendance of NMC to its partnerships with academic nephrologists and their institutions across the country. Kolata reported that the government was again seeking to decrease reimbursements for dialysis and agreed with experts that such maneuvers would favor efficient business enterprises like NMC. Kolata noted in April that Dr. Edward Hager, chairman of the executive committee of NMC, was running for senator from New Hampshire. Hager lost the primary election (to Warren Rudman, who won the seat in November).

In 1981, Drs. Ed Lowrie and Gus Hampers, of National Medical Care, rebutted Bud Relman's editorial on the medical-industrial complex in the *NEJM* and made a full-throated case for vindicating capitalism in the care of patients with kidney disease, in their own Special Article in the *Journal*.[7] They wrote:

> The ESRD program has been highly successful in many ways, and there is a strong case to be made for the role of the profit incentive and the private marketplace—not only in the ESRD program but in the delivery of health care generally....

When the financial constraints of treatment were removed for patients, as Congress intended, the population undergoing dialysis changed from an educated, young, white and male one to a population that better approximates a cross section of American citizens. The number of patients increased and so did the program's costs.

Lowrie and Hampers wrapped NMC in an early antiracist banner. They noted that the Medicare payment system had imposed a limit of $138 on the cost of individual outpatient dialysis treatments and that the yearly cost of treatment of individual dialysis patients, given cost of living increases, had fallen over the initial years since the start of the ESRD program. Quoting data from the Health Care Financing Administration (HCFA), in early 1980, Lowrie and Hampers reported there were 44,591 ESRD patients, with an average age of 53.5 ± 16.0 (mean plus or minus the standard deviation of the mean) years. Those on dialysis had been treated for an average of 3.3 ± 2.2 years. Women made up 44.9% of the population. Black patients comprised 28.9% of patients, while White patients constituted 68.1% of the program. (The remaining 3.0% of patients were coded as "other.") The most common illness leading to ESRD was glomerulonephritis, with 27.3% of the population, followed by hypertensive kidney disease (19.6%), diabetes mellitus (10.7%), polycystic kidney disease (9.1%), and interstitial nephritis (9.0%), making up a subtotal of 75.7% of patients. (The case mix is dramatically different today.) At that time, about three-quarters of freestanding dialysis units were operating for profit. The authors quoted sources suggesting the treatment of patients in for-profit and not-for-profit units was similar. In complex arguments, they asserted physicians were economic actors and that ignoring that fact was "silly" or "foolish." Lowrie and Hampers opined that placing physicians on salary to reduce incentives to order higher-profit tests and procedures would limit productivity and reduce work efficiency. They attributed the successful cost containment in the ESRD program to be based, in large part, on physician profit sharing. Little did they (or Relman) realize that in the future, the majority of American physicians would be salaried employees, rather than private entrepreneurs, and that the ownership of dialysis units would pass from physicians to large corporations run by businessmen.

In the late 1970s, congressional staffers during the Carter administration had originally proposed a single pay rate for outpatient facilities and the more expensive and costly hospital facilities. As National Medical Care, responding to the possible effects of decreasing reimbursements for hospital-based units, proposed to provide management services for the hospital facilities, in effect buying previously independent academic dialysis units, congressional staffers and government bureaucrats became alarmed and realized a one-price-for-all scheme might disincentivize home dialysis therapies. NMC, in letters to the Secretary of the Department of Health and Human Services in 1981 (quoted by Iglehart), suggested that if fees were set too low, the company might have to close a substantial number of unprofitable units, potentially leaving patients adrift. While HCFA and the Department of Health and Human Services were considering new fee structures, a public relations war broke out between executives of NMC and Baxter Travenol regarding the care of dialysis patients if government funding proved inadequate to support NMC business interests. The CEO of Baxter Travenol, Vernon R. Loucks, generously agreed to take all the patients NMC would give up, neatly hoisting them by their own petard. Congress, however, ultimately enacted a dual-payment system. NMC lost its case for a single-payment system but succeeded in avoiding federal quotas for ESRD patients assigned to home dialysis.

The Beginning of NMC

National Medical Care (NMC) was founded in 1968, encouraged by Dr. John Merrill, in part to provide ongoing dialysis support for ESRD patients referred to the Peter Bent Brigham Hospital and awaiting kidney transplantation. Edward B. Hager, M.D., a St. Louis native (1931–2021), graduated from the Washington University School of Medicine and started his internship at the Brigham in 1955 and afterward left to meet his military service obligation in the army. He returned to the Brigham in 1960 to work as a renal fellow under Dr. Merrill. Hager covered dialysis services at the hospital, initially using Kolff's techniques, laboriously wrapping cellophane around the machine's drum holding the dialysis fluid. However, Hager was interested in technical innovations in dialytic care. He was successful in obtaining grant funding and gaining independent hospital privileges as a nephrologist, establishing himself on his own as a clinician. Hager wrote about peritoneal dialysis and complications of uremia and did bench research in kidney transplantation.

Eugene Schupak (1931–2008), from Brooklyn, New York, did his undergraduate work at Seton Hall University, in New Jersey, and graduated with an M.D. degree from the University of Chicago. Thereafter, Schupak did residency work at Cook County Hospital in Chicago. Schupak did postgraduate work in nephrology at the Cleveland Clinic with Dr. Willem Kolff in 1961, and then under John Merrill at the Brigham from 1962 until 1964. Schupak was sent by Merrill to Seattle to learn techniques of chronic, maintenance dialysis from Dr. Belding Scribner. He used the knowledge he gained in Seattle to set up a chronic dialysis program at the Brigham, and was also instrumental in starting the home dialysis program for Brigham ESRD patients in 1964. Schupak wrote about chronic and home hemodialysis and did clinical research on anemia in ESRD patients, primarily with Merrill. Schupak left the Brigham to join the faculty at the Downstate Medical Center in Brooklyn in 1964 but suggested his protégé, Dr. Gus Hampers, join the Brigham for training in kidney disease.

Constantine L. Hampers (1932–2021), a nephrologist, physician at the Brigham and a faculty member at Harvard Medical School was a cofounder, with Dr. Edward Hager, of National Medical Care. Hampers received his M.D. degree from the University of Pittsburgh in 1958, and did postgraduate training at Cook County Hospital and the Philadelphia General Hospital. He served in the U.S. Navy as well. Shortly after his graduation, and during his military service, Hampers had taken care of his father, who had become ill with acute kidney failure in Pittsburgh and was treated three times with acute hemodialysis. His father survived the acute illness. Hampers met Schupak at Cook County Hospital in 1961. Hampers started his Renal Fellowship at the Brigham in 1964, under the tutelage of Dr. John Merrill. Dr. Schupak had mentored Hampers in the operation of the Kolff-Brigham dialysis apparatus in 1963, before leaving the Brigham for Brooklyn. During his fellowship, Hampers met Hager, performed several bench research projects in kidney transplantation, and wrote papers with him. Hampers soon became the director of the Artificial Kidney Services at the Brigham. From the beginning of his career through 1968, Hampers published twenty-five papers on various aspects of kidney disease.

Hampers published extensively with Merrill, Hager, and Schupack. The first edition of the textbook *Long-Term Hemodialysis: The Management of the Patient with Chronic Renal Failure*, by Hampers and Schupak, was published in 1967. The second edition of *Long-Term Hemodialysis*, published in 1973, added Brigham nephrologists Drs. Edmund G. Lowrie and J. Michael Lazarus as coeditors.

Addressing the problem of limited space for chronic hemodialysis at the Brigham's chronic facility, Hager and Hampers negotiated with a businessman, Sam Saitz, to set up dialysis stations in an extended care facility in the Boston area in 1966, calling it the Kidney Center. They settled on a charge of $160 a treatment in what became an outpatient, or "satellite," dialysis facility associated with the Peter Bent Brigham Hospital. The venture was medically and financially successful. Thereafter, Hager and Hampers struck a deal with businessmen and lawyers to found National Medical Care to provide chronic outpatient dialysis to ESRD patients across the U.S. The company was incorporated on June 25, 1968, in the state of Massachusetts. With an initial investment of $1.5 million, the businessmen backing the enterprise received 51% of the stock, while Hager and Hampers shared 34%. Hager served as NMC's inaugural president and Hampers was the vice president of the company. A search for further funding diluted the ownership of the original physician stockholders but kept the fledgling company alive, enabling it to open ten dialysis centers across the country by 1971.

Meanwhile, Schupak, who had left Downstate and joined the staff at Mount Sinai Hospital in Manhattan, was attempting to set up a chronic, outpatient dialysis facility in New York City. Schupak had been successful obtaining federal grant funds from the U.S. Public Health Service to evaluate home dialysis services. He was not successful at engaging investors to finance an outpatient dialysis facility in New York City. At the same time, NMC was hoping to expand its operations across the country. Hager and Hampers contacted their old colleague Schupak, and the three worked out a deal whereby a new company, Bio-Medical Applications Inc. (BMA), was created to circumvent laws in New York State that limited corporate ownership of dialysis facilities. The Queens Artificial Kidney Center was established in 1970, and Schupak joined NMC as a major shareholder. Hampers became the executive vice president when Schupak assumed the vice presidency of NMC.

The model of the Queens Artificial Kidney Center was extended in Dallas, Texas, by Dr. Alan Hull, a nephrologist at the University of Texas Southwestern Medical Center, and Dr. Charles Swartz, a nephrologist at Hahnemann Hospital in Philadelphia, Pennsylvania. Both units became BMA operations. NMC attempted to recruit top-flight nephrology practitioners and allowed them to run their units with a minimum of interference. NMC or BMA units soon opened in Miami and Tampa, Florida, and in the Washington, D.C., suburbs.

A hagiographic picture of Hager, Schupack, and Hampers is painted by Tim McFeely, who served as corporate counsel of NMC from 1974 to 1989, in his 2001 book, *The Price of Access*.[8] McFeely consistently depreciated the work of Dr. John Merrill (who died in 1984) in comparison to the efforts of his former trainees, Hager, Schupak, and Hampers, who are portrayed most favorably. NMC grew into a large dialysis organization with units situated across the U.S. The initial commentary in the press, principally the *Boston Globe*, focused on the perhaps dubious ethics of for-profit medicine for ESRD patients. Supporters of NMC, including patients treated at its Boston center, made various responsive points in the press, including the notions that the company provided a unique service unavailable elsewhere that was saving patients' lives, that the quality of the care rendered in NMC units was unimpeachable, and that the business sector was a proper intermediary to provide efficient, affordable, and safe patient care. Arguments cited by McFeeley in support of the company in *The Price of Access* included that NMC reduced the strain on the limited moneys available from charitable and philanthropic sources and that the taxes on profits paid by the company redounded to the good of society. McFeeley portrayed the salutary role of NMC by comparisons to other familiar companies, such as Archer Daniels Midland, General Foods, Weyerhauser, or Levi-Strauss, which provided useful goods and services to the public and supported the economy.

The newspaper articles about NMC created a stir in Boston. As Dr. George Thorn retired from his post as physician in chief at the Brigham in 1972 and Dr. Eugene Braunwald, a distinguished cardiologist from the University of California, San Diego, succeeded Thorn as physician in chief and Hersey Professor of the Theory and Practice of Physic at Harvard Medical School, Hampers's yearly appointment to the medical staff was reconsidered. Ultimately, his appointments at the Brigham and at Harvard Medical School were not renewed.

In September 1975, the *New York Times* reported that NMC, under Dr. Eugene Schupak, then its president, proposed to take over dialysis services for a component of the New York City municipal hospital system. Schupak's legal counsel was Jack E. Bronston, who also at the time served as a New York State senator from Queens. (The *Times* pointed out that the federal dialysis budget for 1975 would be $300 million.) Schupak had previously been an associate professor of clinical medicine at the Mount Sinai School of Medicine and a nephrologist at the municipal New York Health and Hospitals Corporation Elmhurst Hospital in Queens and had set up a private dialysis unit in Long Island City. Hampers was now the chairman of the board of NMC. In 1980, Iglehart quoted NMC as being a $245.4 million business.

NMC under Pressure and the Growth of Other Dialysis Organizations

W. R. Grace purchased NMC in deals executed between 1984 and 1989, for a value estimated by the *Wall Street Journal* at approximately $360 million. Institute of Medicine (IOM) staff estimated, in *Kidney Failure and the Federal Government*,[9] that almost 20% of U.S. dialysis patients received care in one of the over 300 NMC units. Hampers was unsuccessful in an attempt to wrest control of NMC from Grace in a hostile takeover in 1995. The story, reported in the *New York Times*, described Hampers as a ruthless businessman. In 1996, Fresenius took over ownership of NMC from Grace and thwarted a takeover bid from Hampers, in a deal valued by the *Wall Street Journal* in Hagers's obituary at about $4 billion.

Fresenius got its start taking over a Frankfurt am Main pharmacy in the 18th century. In 1966, Fresenius established itself as a maker of dialysis machines and dialyzers. By 1979, Fresenius had produced a widely accepted dialysis machine, and in 1983, the company manufactured the newly popular polysulfone dialyzers, which were soon marketed worldwide. In 1996, Fresenius Medical Care was founded when it took over National Medical Care. By 1999, Fresenius had produced 100,000 dialysis machines. In 2003 Fresenius claimed to be the largest worldwide dialysis company, involved in the care of more than 119,000 patients and producing more than 50 million dialyzers a year. In 2019, Fresenius acquired NxStage Medical Inc., a pioneer in the manufacture of home dialysis machines, situating itself as a leader in home dialysis modalities.

Gambro was founded in 1964 in Lund, Sweden, by Holger Crafoord. Crafoord was a businessman who had met Professor Nils Alwall, a pioneer in dialysis techniques and dialyzer design, and decided a corporate investment in dialysis treatment was warranted. The new company specialized in manufacturing dialysis equipment, including dialyzers and dialysis machines. As Gambro grew and prospered, its products were sold in the United States. Gambro acquired providers of dialysis equipment, including Hospal in 1987 and COBE in 1990. Gambro expanded into managing dialysis facilities in the U.S., including buying dialysis units previously run on a nonprofit basis by medical centers. For example, George Washington University ended up selling its outpatient dialysis unit to Gambro in the 1990s. The benefits to the Division of Renal Diseases and Hypertension disappeared as the profits were largely appropriated by the Department of Medicine and the Medical School at George Washington University. Immediately thereafter, the ability of the members of the faculty of the Division of Renal Diseases and Hypertension to conduct research was limited. Baxter International completed its acquisition of Gambro in 2013.

DaVita Inc. came into being as the result of multiple corporate changes over time. Medical Ambulatory Care Inc., a subsidiary of National Medical Enterprises, was founded in 1979. (National Medical Enterprises is now the giant Tenet Healthcare.) In 1994, the majority of the company was taken over by DLJ Merchant Banking Partners. The company's name was changed to Total Renal Care Holdings Inc. After an initial public offering, the company went public in October 1995. In February 1998, the company acquired Renal Treatment Centers. In 1999, however, the company underwent turmoil, and its chief executive officer and chief financial officer resigned.

Shortly thereafter, Kent J. Thiry, who led the dialysis company Vivra, which had been purchased by Gambro, was named CEO. The company took the name DaVita Inc. in 2000. In 2005, DaVita acquired Gambro Healthcare, which had an extensive U.S. dialysis network. Thereafter, DaVita continued to grow and acquired dialysis facilities and health-care entities. However, multiple lawsuits were filed against the company, regarding billing irregularities and other issues, which were ultimately settled. In 2018, the company settled allegations that it violated the False Claims Act by improper billing of Medicare Advantage plans for $270 million. DaVita and Kent Thiry were indicted in 2021 on charges of labor market collusion. The indictment alleged that "DaVita and Thiry both participated in two separate conspiracies to suppress competition for the services of certain employees." Thiry faced up to $3 million in fines and up to ten years in prison. On April 15, 2022 a federal jury found DaVita and Thiry, its former CEO, not guilty of violating U.S. antitrust laws.

At this point, DaVita provides dialysis services for more than 200,000 U.S. patients at more than 2,800 outpatient dialysis units. DaVita also has an international presence, with more than 300 outpatient centers in 10 countries, serving more than 3,000 patients.

Sicker Patients and Shorter Treatment Times

In the decade following the initiation of the ESRD program, it had become apparent that older and sicker patients had been entering the dialysis program, despite the lack of reliable data from national registries. Individual dialysis unit medical directors noticed that the older patients with diabetes, with heart disease and peripheral vascular disease, who were now being treated could not tolerate longer periods "on the machine." The typical dialysis prescription was supposed to be four hours of center hemodialysis, three times a week, usually on a one-size-fits-all basis. On this regimen, the blood pressures of these frail patients dropped precipitously, and they became light-headed or woozy or lost consciousness completely, making the treatment perilous for the patient and a source of anxiety for physicians, nurses, and other staff members. Dr. Fred Shapiro, one of the pioneers of the concept of "satellite dialysis," or dialyzing patients in outpatient facilities not located within a medical center or hospital in 1968, was an author of a paper outlining the challenges involved in dialyzing the newer cohort of sicker patients in 1982.[10] These new patients had heart disease and abnormalities of the nervous system that prevented them from defending their falling blood pressures against the loss of fluid experienced during dialysis. Some of the treatment options included shortening dialysis treatments and scheduling more frequent short treatments, in addition to using drugs to raise blood pressures. Patients naturally liked the shorter treatments, as did dialysis administrators. For the latter, shorter treatments meant more patients could be treated, with equivalent bills submitted to Medicare, in a fixed number of dialysis stations over a given amount of time. But academic dialysis physicians worried that shorter treatments might compromise the short- and long-term health of ESRD patients, since removal of toxins in short procedures might be limited.

Beat von Albertini, M.D. (1944–2018), had been interested in improving the efficiency of dialysis treatments for many years. His goal was to provide the most dialysis for the patient in the shortest period of time. Educated in medicine in Europe, with a background in engineering, von Albertini pursued postgraduate renal fellowship training at Mount Sinai Hospital in New York City in the 1970s. In 1978, he was the senior author, with several distinguished Mount Sinai nephrology faculty members, of a paper entitled "High Flux Hemofiltration."[11] Von Albertini used two high-efficiency dialyzers in series to "turbocharge" the amount of toxins removed from each patient per unit time of treatment. Hemofiltration, or the related hemodiafiltration, techniques were common in Europe but almost nonexistent in the U.S.

Von Albertini, a young and vocal champion of patient care and dialysis techniques, ran into conflicts with the division chief at Mount Sinai, Dr. Marvin Levitt, an esteemed but old-school classical renal physiologist. Von Albertini left Mount Sinai to pursue research with a team of technically oriented physicians at the Wadsworth Veterans Administration Hospital in Los Angeles. Improving on the techniques of fast dialysis, they published two papers in 1984 in the *Transactions of the American Society for Artificial Internal Organs*.[12] Their thesis was that dialysis delivery comparable to that of four hours of conventional dialysis could be delivered by their methods in two hours. Whether such techniques were truly comparable to more conventional modes of therapy remained to be determined. Von Albertini moved to join Dr. Juan P. Bosch at the George Washington University School of Medicine in the late 1980s to pursue studies of "short dialysis."

In contrast to the first years after ESRD care became a Medicare-covered entitlement, intellectual leadership and patient care issues were increasingly being determined by the large dialysis organizations as they began and continued to purchase units associated with academic nephrology groups. Research administration groups within the dialysis organizations began to establish rules to approve and provide oversight for research projects proposed by nephrologists to limit the use of dialysis unit staff in research operations and to ensure that dialysis profits and operations were not compromised by research activities.

By 1981, physicians were concerned about the mortality statistics for patients treated with dialysis, and the medical implications of the shortened treatment times some patients received. It was not clear how to prescribe dialysis to maximize long-term outcomes for patients. Drs. Edmund Lowrie, of NMC, and Tom Parker, of the Dallas Kidney Disease Center, and colleagues addressed the issues of time and goals for laboratory tests for ESRD patients treated with hemodialysis in a randomized controlled trial of dialysis prescription, the National Cooperative Dialysis Study (NCDS), in the *NEJM* in 1981.[13] Participating centers enrolling patients into the study were drawn from leading dialysis programs. The authors noted that the "dose" of dialysis required by individual patients had not been scientifically determined and that patients of different weights with different clinical characteristics and presumably different metabolic requirements were often treated in the same fashion.

The NCDS evaluated two treatment times (about four and a half and three hours) and two (time-averaged) goals for blood urea nitrogen (BUN) concentrations (about 40 and 100 mg/dL). They used clever statistical techniques to result in four randomized groups representing the different treatment conditions. The different averaged BUN levels were achieved in the different groups of patients by using different dialyzers that cleared greater or lesser amounts of urea over a given time period. Patients with diabetes, severe heart disease, liver disease, lung disease, or systemic lupus erythematosus were excluded from participation in the study. The study was funded through a contract from the National Institute of Arthritis, Metabolism, and Digestive Diseases at NIH.

Not much was known about the effects of varying treatment time and BUN goals on hospitalizations and mortality when the study was designed. Therefore, the investigators had trouble planning the logistics of the study. Nevertheless, they ultimately achieved landmark research. The study team recruited only 151 patients in the four groups, which in retrospect was far too few participants to delineate meaningful differences in mortality over the observation period. The study was stopped by its safety committee when it was determined the high BUN group patients had the highest hospitalization rates.

The National Cooperative Dialysis Study had an important influence on clinical nephrology practice. Nephrologists were to keep the BUN of their patients at low levels. Since time appeared not to matter in this small randomized study, many practitioners balanced shorter treatment times with larger dialyzers to achieve BUN goals. BUN, however, is a complex parameter determined by many factors besides dialysis prescription, including diet, intercurrent illnesses, the use of certain medications, and the remaining kidney function of dialysis patients, for example. It was unclear if the BUN goal in the NCDS study was merely a surrogate for some other, unevaluated factor. The members of the NCDS team, in further studies, including a colleague of Dr. John Sargent's (an expert in the delivery and quantification of dialysis), Dr. Frank Gotch, proposed the use of Kt/V, a measure of the amount of urea removed by a particular dialyzer or during a specific treatment.[14] Payors and professional societies considered the use of Kt/V in determining payments and developing guidelines.

Were Inadequate Payments Driving Shorter Times, Less Treatment, and Worsening Survival?

In 1983, Dr. Henry Krakauer and colleagues published a definitive description of ESRD outcomes in the *NEJM*, using data from the Medicare system to assess practically the entire population of U.S. dialysis patients.[15] The survey consisted of patients who had started therapy under the auspices of the ESRD program from January 1, 1977, to December 31, 1980. The investigators compared patients treated with dialysis to those treated with transplantation. About 85.5% of the ESRD population were treated with dialysis. The number of new patients starting treatment for ESRD with dialysis (incidence) rose from 16,501 to 17,863 from 1977 to 1980, about an 8.5% increase. The authors showed that dialysis patients had poorer survival over time than kidney transplant patients. Mortality for dialysis patients was about 19% a year. Younger dialysis patients tended to live longer. One-year survival for the dialysis cohort, including patients who started treatment from January 1, 1977, to December 31, 1980, was 81% ± 0.2% (mean ± the standard deviation), while three-year survival was 56% ± 0.3%. Survival for dialysis patients did not improve between the cohorts that started in 1977 and 1980.

About 28.1% of the dialysis patients were Black. The investigators noted "the incidence of end-stage renal disease in blacks was out of proportion to their representation in the U.S. population by a factor of nearly three." (As we see in a later chapter, this disparity is still relatively unchanged.) Unlike Black patients with any other chronic illness, Black ESRD patients treated with dialysis, albeit probably younger, as a group had longer-lasting survival than those who were White. (This paradoxical finding is still largely unexplained.) Men and women treated with dialysis had comparable survival rates. The most common kidney diseases in the dialysis population were hypertensive kidney disease (about 10.8%) and glomerulonephritis (about 10%). Patients with diabetes at that time made up only about 9% of the ESRD dialysis program. Patients with polycystic kidney disease constituted about 3% of the population. The investigators pointed out that since this was an observational study, differences in outcomes between transplant and dialysis patients were subject to biases related to selection and treatment, as well as other factors, perhaps related to differences between the two populations at the outset, such as the ages of the groups considered. The authors noted that while age might account for differences in survival between dialysis and transplant patients, age did not fully account for the improved survival seen in Black compared to White dialysis patients.

The demonstrable lack of improved patient survival over the years distressed dialysis physicians. As acceptance policies broadened, and the population aged, many dialysis units shortened treatments to accommodate the unstable blood pressures of the new, sicker patients. In addition, the amount (or "dose") of dialysis to be administered to patients was unclear but was evidently related to the treatment time. The long-term consequences of these demographic and treatment changes highlighted clinical uncertainties and the lack of measures of quality for dialysis treatments became apparent. Clearly mortality was a solid, meaningful measure of quality of care, which could be evaluated across many dialysis centers. (But it was a measure that could not be acted on.) The Krakauer paper suggested the mortality of U.S. dialysis patients was not progressively improving. Some dialysis physicians claimed that the decrease of payments for dialysis treatments, enacted by the federal government in the later 1970s and the early 1980s, made giving optimal care too difficult and, as such, was putting patients at risk. Concerns were raised suggesting the number and type of staff (nurses compared to dialysis technicians), the number of dieticians and social workers available to each patient, and the presence of physicians during treatments were being limited by financial considerations (related to low government payments), resulting in worsening mortality statistics for dialysis patients. Dialysis physicians who claimed that decreases in reimbursements for treatments were putting patients at risk were treading on thin ice. Were those who complained more interested in profits than in patients and, therefore, skimping on patient care? Unspoken bitterness characterized some relationships between Medicare payer intermediaries, large dialysis organizations, and individual physicians.

Drs. Alan Hull and Thomas Parker, of Southwestern Medical Center and Dallas Nephrology Associates, convened the Morbidity, Mortality, and Prescription of Dialysis Symposium, held in a hotel in Las Colinas from September 15 to 17, 1989.[16] Parker and Hull, established dialysis clinicians, who had clear financial interests in dialysis operations, invited speakers from around the world who reported on individual survival statistics in their dialysis populations, the way the dialysis prescription was measured, and how dialysis was delivered. The Dallas nephrologists presented data demonstrating that the gross mortality of U.S. dialysis patients had increased, rather than decreased, during the previous decade. A key issue was whether the case mix—such as the proportion of elderly patients or those with diabetes mellitus, for instance— perhaps mandated by different and more contemporary national selection criteria, was a determining factor in the differences in mortality of dialysis patients seen between regions, dialysis organizations, or countries. Reports from the U.S., Australian, Japanese, French, Canadian, and German registries were considered. The conference determined the U.S. had the highest dialysis patient acceptance rate, and the highest mortality rate, of the different countries represented at the symposium. The conferees noted that practices in treating ESRD patients, including ages of patients accepted into programs and the proportions of patients transplanted, differed greatly between the countries represented. Higher rates of transplantation could remove "healthier" ESRD patients from the dialysis populations, leaving a sicker group remaining to receive dialysis. Criticisms from the conferees focused on lack of comparability of the data from different sources and lack of adjustment of mortality results for many characteristics of ESRD patients and care processes.

The conference was attended by a large number of academic dialysis nephrologists representing U.S. and foreign centers and registries as well as policymakers. (It was a very popular meeting. Juan Bosch and I attended from George Washington University.) It seemed to many attendees that the organizers were trying to make a perhaps not-so-subtle case that diminished reimbursements were, for a variety of reasons, resulting in poorer outcomes for American dialysis patients, especially compared to results from other countries. Perhaps lower reimbursements resulted in shorter treatments with diminished staffing and poor patient outcomes. Arguments were made that different dialytic techniques, such as hemodiafiltration, used in Europe, were associated with better dialysis patient outcomes. The heterogeneity in treatment practices made comparisons between patient populations, both within the U.S. and internationally, difficult. Many factors had to be considered in such analyses, including patient characteristics, treatment modalities, time devoted to treatment, the quality and extent of physician, nursing, technical, dietary, and social work staffing, as well as economic considerations related to reimbursement for physician care and dialysis unit management. These many factors could not be analyzed by the conference attendees. The proportion of patients in a population who were transplanted and criteria for and accessibility of transplantation were key in such analyses, and these patients could not just be "excluded" from evaluations. It was recognized that many of these factors were inextricably intertwined, rendering a search for "independent" parameters associated with outcomes problematic. How to measure the "dose" of dialysis was unclear, with proponents of Kt/V (a measurement of efficiency of removal of urea by dialysis) and "middle molecule clearance" (a measure of the removal of larger molecules that might be more related to uremic toxicity) at loggerheads.

Dr. Lowrie, of National Medical Care, emphasized morbidity and mortality related to poor nutrition and adequacy of dialysis, gleaned from the company's independent database, and suggested monitoring such intermediate measures might have an impact on outcomes. Dr. Paul Eggers of HCFA, which at the time administered the U.S. ESRD program, suggested that the current rates of morbidity and mortality in the U.S. were more related to changes in patient case mix over the previous decade and a half than to financial considerations. Eggers argued, in effect, that the dialysis population had become older and sicker over time, with more patients with diabetes being treated, as entry criteria had expanded to create a more accessible program. The organizers attempted to rebut that argument, noting that although the population of dialysis patients in most of the other countries had been increasing over the years, only in the U.S. had gross mortality increased as well. Accusations of self-interest followed many of the presentations. Dr. Richard Rettig of the IOM described a study in progress, including a blue-ribbon panel, that would deal with equity in the treatment of U.S. ESRD patients and evaluate the effects of changes in reimbursement rates on dialysis patient outcomes. Hull and Parker noted that data suggested dialysis times had been shortened in the U.S. in recent years, particularly compared to practices in other countries. These shortened times had been associated with, in some studies, greater patient mortality.

In addition, largely unmentioned, was the stark fact that the information on outcomes considered was the result of observational studies and comparisons of diverse observational studies covering different time periods. It was well known to clinical scientists that attributing causal relationships to findings could only be determined by randomized controlled studies. In the absence of randomized controlled data, causal inferences regarding treatment times, dose of dialysis, staffing levels, and extent of reimbursements could not be invoked. Therefore, sicker or more nonadherent patients might have had shorter treatment times, and their intrinsic characteristics, rather than treatment conditions, might have determined outcomes. In addition, the dose of dialysis prescribed might be much higher than the dose the patients received because of technical or other factors, including lack of patient adherence to the prescribed treatment time. The organizers called for improved quality assurance and quality control measures. Dr. Gotch cautioned that the prescription of dialysis solely based on BUN levels was fraught with controversy, since low

BUNs, as Dr. Lowrie had pointed out, might be a function of malnutrition rather than adequate dialysis.

When something goes wrong in American medicine, the IOM wants to know all about it and tell American political and scientific communities, as well as the general public, about the findings. In 1987, as part of the Omnibus Budget Reconciliation Act, Congress tasked the IOM to study and report on demographic and epidemiologic changes in the ESRD program, access to ESRD care, the quality of care provided by the program to patients, and the effects of reimbursement on quality of care. The IOM convened a panel of experts to assess these issues.

The chair of the Committee for the Study of the Medicare ESRD Program was Norman G. Levinsky, professor of medicine at Boston University. Levinsky was a renowned basic and clinical researcher in nephrology and was an expert in the field of acute renal failure in the presence of severe liver disease, the so-called hepatorenal syndrome. Other committee members included nephrologists (with pediatric, nutritional and dialysis organization provider expertise), nurses, an economist interested in policy and planning, and a social worker.[17]

The IOM study officer was Richard A. Rettig, Ph.D., who had been a student of administrative and regulatory aspects of ESRD as well as the outcomes of patients treated in the program. Rettig had been at the RAND Corporation from 1975 until 1981. He had produced a monumental report on the implementation of the ESRD program for HCFA in 1980. Rettig worked at the IOM from 1987 to 1995, directing various programs including the Council on Health Care Technology and studies of the ESRD program.

The committee conducted a series of public hearings, workshops, and focus groups related to its study tasks between 1989 and 1990 and incorporated the views of a wide range of stakeholders, including those of individual patients. The findings of the committee were released in 1991 in the book *Kidney Failure and the Federal Government*.[18]

The committee noted that reimbursement rates for dialysis services had not increased since 1973. In fact, federal reimbursement for dialysis services in absolute dollars had been lowered over the course of almost two decades and had been severely diminished, if adjusted for inflation, over time. The committee was concerned that reimbursement policy might have affected the quality of patient care as well as patients' outcomes, notably morbidity (hospitalizations, intercurrent complications, and well-being) and mortality. The committee acknowledged that there had been no research to date that had addressed these concerns definitively, and opined that such studies would necessarily be difficult to design and complete.

The committee recommended that Congress "extend the Medicare entitlement for ESRD treatment to all Americans, remove the three-year limit on Medicare eligibility of successful transplant recipients, and pay for immunosuppressive drugs for the period of a transplant patient's entitlement." In addition, the committee endorsed objectives for the ESRD program: "to guarantee access to treatment for all for whom it is medically appropriate; to provide care of high quality that achieves desirable health outcomes consistent with patient health status and current professional knowledge; to develop policies that steadily improve patient well-being and patient outcomes; and to manage the program prudently at the lowest cost compatible with adequate care." The committee acknowledged that these goals would require the outlay of additional federal funds. The committee further recommended the institution of a "quality assessment and assurance program" in addition to a "technical advisory committee." The committee recommended that reimbursement for dialysis services should be studied extensively and that in light of the lack of data, further decreases in reimbursement should not be considered.

NIDDK to the Rescue?

The Dallas Symposium and the IOM report focused policymakers and researchers on questions of whether federal reimbursement rates and care in a for-profit compared to a not-for-profit dialysis center were associated with patient morbidity and mortality. After the IOM report was released and discussed, the NIH convened a Consensus Conference to further address these issues, led by the NIDDK and the Office of Medical Applications of Research (OMAR) of the NIH. The planning committee for the Consensus Conference was led by NIDDK personnel.[19]

The academic members of the planning committee, a smaller group than the NIH participants, represented diverse constituencies, including nephrologists (such as Juan P. Bosch, M.D., of the George Washington University School of Medicine, C. Craig Tisher, M.D., of the University of Florida College of Medicine, and William Harmon, M.D., a pediatric nephrologist from Children's Hospital in Boston). The planning committee also included prominent voices from the world of for-profit treatment of ESRD patients.[20]

In a presentation at the Dallas Conference and in a subsequent paper published in 1990 in *AJKD*, Lowrie and Lew had established, from data derived from their large database on hemodialysis laboratory values and patient outcomes, that as in the general population, the level of serum albumin (a common protein found in the bloodstream in high concentrations) correlated with survival in dialysis patients.[21] It was not clear at the time, and indeed is still uncertain now, whether nutrition or inflammation is the more important determinant of this key laboratory measure in hemodialysis patients.

In September 1993, just before the NIH Consensus Conference met, the *NEJM* published an observational study of dialysis patients treated between October 1, 1990, and March 31, 1991.[22] The investigators came from the Brigham and Women's Hospital and National Medical Care Inc. (noted to be a subsidiary of W. R. Grace and Co. in the paper). The research was supported "in part" by a grant awarded to Dr. Owen by NIDDK. The study evaluated the simultaneous associations of serum albumin concentration and the urea reduction ratio (related to Kt/V, or "dose of dialysis") with survival in 13,473 hemodialysis patients. Life-Chem, a laboratory company associated with NMC, provided the laboratory values. Both a high urea reduction ratio (indicating a higher dose of dialysis) and higher hemodialysis patient serum albumin concentrations (thought to be related to nutritional status) were associated with improved patient survival. More than half the patients evaluated in the study had suboptimal urea reduction ratios and low serum albumin concentrations. Patients with diabetes, known for many years to have had higher mortality, tended to have low urea reduction ratios and low serum albumin concentrations. The authors noted the duration of dialysis was not associated with survival in this study. A key issue revolves around the use of the word *associated*. Since the study involved the collection of observational data rather than from conducting a randomized controlled trial, the authors could not prove that these factors caused changes in survival. It still could not be proved that the abnormal laboratory values "caused" the deaths. Critics noted that the sicker patients, including those with diabetes, might have had lower urea reduction ratios and serum albumin concentrations and the gross clinical situation of the patients may have determined the outcomes. Urea reduction and serum albumin concentrations were in fact "risk factors," whose effects had to be tested in clinical trials to prove causality. At the time, approximately 150,000 patients were treated with dialysis in the U.S. ESRD program. Nevertheless, the paper was on everyone's mind as the conference started.

The NIDDK, with OMAR, held an open, public conference from November 1 to 3, 1993, on the NIH campus to discuss the clinical consequences of the prescribed and delivered "dose" of dialysis, the time prescribed for dialysis, and the treatment of comorbidities such as hypertension, anemia, cardiovascular disease, and malnutrition in ESRD hemodialysis patients, in addition to considering the question of the quality of life of such patients.

The Consensus Development Panel at the meeting was chaired by Dr. Tisher. Other members of the committee were nephrologists, including one with pediatric expertise and one representing a dialysis organization, an expert in critical and nutritional care, a biostatistician, a nurse, and a patient representative selected by the National Kidney Foundation.

The NIH Consensus Conference Report was published in the prestigious *AIM* in 1994.[23] Among many recommendations, the panel noted "It is obvious that a randomized controlled study relating the dose of delivered dialysis to morbidity and mortality is of great importance." The panel also commented on the issues of reimbursement that had been brought up in the Dialysis Symposium and by the IOM report.

Current concerns about morbidity and mortality raise issues regarding the present uniform reimbursement system for dialysis, especially in the area of nutritional and psychosocial support systems. Linking direct reimbursement for such care to important outcomes such as serum albumin levels, mean blood pressure, and measurement of fractional urea clearance during dialysis should be explored.

The panel noted the newer, more expensive polysulfone membranes might be associated with better patient outcomes for several reasons. The panel summarized the state of the art and made several conclusions and recommendations, including suggesting earlier referrals of CKD patients to nephrologists before the need for ESRD care (in part to create vascular accesses and preclude emergency "catastrophic" initial treatments), enhancing patient quality of care by employing multidisciplinary care teams, evaluating the dose of dialysis provided in relationship to patient outcomes, and prescribing appropriate dialysis doses. They advocated addressing patients' cardiovascular risk factors, evidence of malnutrition, and delivering stipulated levels of Kt/V to patients until RCTs established best treatment parameters.

The panel had briefly touched on psychosocial issues related to adaptation to chronic treatment for ESRD patients. The panel had outlined an impressive, comprehensive, and lengthy list of studies that should be undertaken in the population of patients treated with dialysis and in those with chronic kidney disease. The implicit assumption was the panel called for more spending on dialysis research by federal agencies, not including the NIH, as well as favoring randomized controlled trials to answer some of the key questions raised by the conference attendees.

Often, a conference or workshop at NIH is a harbinger of a Request for Applications for research proposals. On December 17, 1993, the NIDDK published a call for applications in the NIH Guide, RFA DK 94–004, "Morbidity and Mortality in Hemodialysis Patients: Full-Scale Trial." The RFA acknowledged that a separate group of investigators had previously produced a protocol for the study. The study would be a

prospective, multicenter, randomized, two-by-two factorial clinical trial of increased delivered hemodialysis as measured by the formula KT/V ((K is the dialyzer urea clearance (ml/min), t is the treatment time (min), V is the body urea distribution volume (ml)) and high-flux dialysis. The objectives of the study are to reduce mortality and morbidity in hemodialysis patients. Mortality due to all causes is the primary outcome. Secondary outcomes include rate of non-access (vascular) related hospital admissions, cardiovascular events including myocardial infarction, acute angina, and congestive heart failure, occurrence of severe infections, and decline in serum albumin.

The study would be funded at $3.65 million a year for seven years. Awards would be made before September 30, 1994. It was anticipated that fifteen Clinical Centers would be funded to recruit nearly two thousand patients. John W. Kusek, Ph.D., would oversee the study for NIDDK.

Applications were submitted and reviewed. Ultimately, the Cleveland Clinic was chosen as the Data Coordinating Center. Fourteen clinical centers devoted to recruiting patients, delivering the treatments, and following the outcomes in patients received funding and completed the trial. Dr. Garabed Eknoyan of Baylor College of Medicine in Houston, Texas, was appointed the chair of the steering committee by the NIDDK. The NIDDK also appointed a group of distinguished researchers to the External Advisory Committee.[24] The study took approximately seven years to perform, and recruitment was a constant issue during the first five years of the trial. Patient enrollment started in March 1995 and finished in October 2000. Ultimately, 1,846 patients participated in the study. It was called the Hemodialysis Study, or, colloquially, the HEMO trial.

The NIDDK and the External Advisory Committee received the study results from the Data Coordinating Center in the fall of 2001 for a meeting on November 9. All the usual risk factors for hemodialysis patients were associated with participant mortality and survival in the trial, so the study looked valid. Astoundingly, against all expectations, neither the administration of a very high Kt/V nor the use of high flux dialysis membranes made a difference in the mortality of hemodialysis patients. The staff at the NIDDK were momentarily dejected. However, Dr. Josephine Briggs, director of DKUHD at NIDDK at the time, quickly realized that this "null" or "negative" result had important implications (as should any well-designed clinical trial addressing a salient medical question when the proper way to treat a patient was unknown). There was a silver lining to this cloud, although its messaging was critical. An optimistic reading of the data suggested the federal money was well spent and that the status quo was acceptable. Patients had not been harmed by contemporary dialysis practices. The way American nephrologists had been treating U.S.

hemodialysis patients was correct. Notwithstanding popular beliefs, originating in hype, medical and scientific marketing, and the puffery of individual clinicians and investigators based on observational data, neither higher doses of dialysis than usual or use of newfangled, expensive membranes affected important patient outcomes. Although there were some salutary effects of the interventions in two different subgroups of patients, the ultimate implication was that the organizers of the Dallas Symposium on Morbidity and Mortality had been wrong. Randomized controlled trials were absolutely necessary to establish clinical guidelines for important practices. Case mix probably accounted for the differences between results from the U.S. and other countries. The HEMO study turned out to be a definitive landmark trial. Dialysis reimbursements were not increased, and a randomized controlled trial of higher payments for better dialysis for patients was not contemplated. In fact, the NIDDK began to plan the next trial for hemodialysis patients almost immediately. Dr. Paul Eggers left HCFA in 2000 to join the NIDDK as an expert in the structure and epidemiology of the ESRD program. He later became the project scientist for the Frequent Hemodialysis Network

The paper describing the HEMO study appeared in the *NEJM* in 2002.[25] Many of the recommendations of the consensus panel still hold true today, and it still holds true that they may not be achieved for all patients.

7

---- ❖ ----

A TRIUMPH OF MOLECULAR BIOLOGY AND THE EXCESSES OF CORPORATE GREED

Amgen, one of the first biotech companies, launched the revolution in molecular treatment of patients with kidney disease and anemia by synthesizing erythropoietin, a hormone that had been, for almost one hundred years, biologists' holy grail. Erythropoietin, made by the kidneys, responded to anemia by increasing the synthesis of red blood cells by the body. The work of the company forever redirected patient care in a spectacular simultaneous feat of molecular biology and clinical medicine. The success of the biosynthesis of erythropoietin, however, let loose a corporate feeding frenzy resulting in a plethora of epo-like drugs with competing claims and varying prices as well as aggressive treatment recommendations that were not always in patients' best interests.

Blockbuster Medical News at an Italian Conference

Attendees at the fifth Capri Conference in September 1986 were startled by the presentation of an exciting, important, and totally unexpected scientific finding in a small but well-known medical meeting that had usually been characterized by bonhomie and good food along with the presentation of incremental research advances. The meeting was hosted by Professore Carmelo Giordano, a nephrologist interested in chronic renal disease who was renowned for the Giordano Giovanetti diet for people with advanced kidney failure.

This meeting took place almost fifteen years after the U.S. government committed to payment of dialysis costs for ESRD patients, regardless of age or need. Dialysis treatments and techniques had diffused around the high-income world, and patients with kidney disease no longer needed to starve themselves to ward off death. The conference took place in Naples at the Castel D'Ovo, overlooking the Bay, and on the legendary, flower-bedecked isle of Capri, where the venue was accessed by funicular. Attendees stayed at luxury hotels on the promenade in Naples, dined on linguini con vongole, and quaffed Lacryma Christi. One night, a piano was shipped from the island of Ischia to Capri so a musician could give a concert for the conference attendees and their spouses or friends at a buffet in the garden of an ancient villa. Dr. Thomas Starzl was one of the attendees. I, a nobody as a lowly assistant professor of medicine at George Washington University, attended the conference as well, to present a paper on zinc and vitamin D metabolism in an animal model of chronic kidney disease (now dubbed CKD).

Joe Eschbach presented work at the conference that would appear months later in the *NEJM*. Eschbach, in a short oral presentation using Kodachrome slides shown through a Carousel projector, told an amazing scientific and clinical story. He briefly mentioned that the hormone erythropoietin had been synthesized by a startup biotech company called, at the time, AMGen. (No one at the conference had ever heard anything about AMGen then.) A clinical trial involving fewer than thirty patients with kidney disease showed a dose-related increase in hematocrit (the proportion of red cells in the blood) in response to higher administered doses of the synthetic erythropoietin. ESRD dialysis patients did not need as frequent blood transfusions during the trial. Although there were some side effects, like increased blood pressure and, rarely, seizures, these were said to be mild and unusual. We all wondered when this therapy would be available. Eschbach said the sponsor was seeking FDA approval. Eschbach easily won Giordano's prize for the best abstract presented at the meeting. The more business savvy nephrologists made notes to look up this company when they got home (there was no internet) and buy stock in AMGen.

Joseph W. Eschbach, M.D., had worked in the field of erythropoietin for many years. He had been primarily interested in the anemia of ESRD patients. Eschbach was born in 1933 in Detroit, Michigan, and graduated from Otterbein College in Ohio in 1955 and Jefferson Medical College in Philadelphia in 1959. He completed residencies in Seattle and Detroit and then undertook training in Seattle at the University of Washington in nephrology. As a fellow working under Dr. Belding Scribner at UW, he was challenged to begin studying the treatment of anemia in dialysis patients. Eschbach joined the UW medical faculty in 1970 and in 1975 became a clinical professor of nephrology. He worked at the Northwest Kidney Centers in Seattle, the successor to Scribner's Seattle Artificial Kidney Center, eventually directing its home dialysis program. Eschbach was active on the faculty through 1994. During the 1970s, working with Dr. John Adamson, he studied the biology of anemia in a large animal model (sheep).[1]

John W. Adamson received his bachelor's degree from University of California, Berkeley, in 1958, and his M.D. from University of California, Los Angeles, in 1962. Thereafter, he finished internship and residency at the University of Washington and started fellowship training in hematology in 1964. He was interested in red blood cell biology, iron metabolism as it related to erythropoiesis, and erythropoietin itself. One of his early papers, from 1968, was "The Kidney and Erythropoiesis."[2] In addition to the well-known senior hematologist Clement Finch, another coauthor on the paper was Joseph Eschbach.

Clinical Correlates and Early Studies

Although dialysis had been readily available in the U.S. for more than a decade, the early experience in Scribner's group pointed out that many complications occurred in patients kept alive by dialysis. Shana Alexander's simple concept of the kidney as merely a filter was dead wrong. Many of these consequences of kidney failure were noted in Scribner's first and long-standing patient, Clyde Shields, as well as in most of the patients undergoing pioneering dialytic therapy in the 1960s and 1970s in Seattle. Patients often developed crippling bone disease, termed renal osteodystrophy. Patients also typically had severe anemia at the start of ESRD therapy, and if the disease was chronic and slowly progressive, anemia might have been a problem for many years. Eschbach, Adamson, and Scribner, as well as other colleagues, published their experience with anemia in ESRD patients in Seattle in the *NEJM* in 1967.[3]

Physicians had known for many years that kidney disease was associated with anemia. It was not uncommon (as doctors like to phrase it) to meet a new patient who had never been sick in her life but who presented with the very recent onset of severe fatigue and listlessness. No other history might be elicited. Physical examination could show pallor of the conjunctivae (the lining of the inside of the eyelids). There would be no evidence of an enlarged spleen. Rectal and vaginal examinations for signs of blood loss would be normal. The doctor might say, "I suspect anemia; I'm not sure about the underlying reason. We'll have to do some tests." Both the patient and the physician might be surprised at the extremely low hematocrit and hemoglobin concentration, prompting amazement that the patient could walk, work, or think. The physician would immediately think about a source of undiscovered bleeding (there would be none) or destruction of red blood cells, which might prompt an immediate request to view a blood slide. But there would be no evidence of red blood cell destruction (hemolysis) or a disease like leukemia or lymphoma. The physician might think that the bone marrow had stopped making red cells (erythrocytes). The doctor would be crafting mental plans for a referral to a hematologist for a bone marrow biopsy to make a definitive diagnosis. And then at the end of the lab report would be the clear but unsuspected answer. The serum creatinine concentration (S[Cr]) would be 9.0 mg/dL (normal is typically less than 1.3 mg/dL), suggesting a severe decrease in renal function, probably due to chronic kidney disease. The doctor would wonder if she had done or ordered a urinalysis. Of course she had. And of course, it was normal. Or pretty normal. (Whew!) The physician would think about scheduling an ultrasound to confirm whether the kidneys were shrunken, consistent with chronic kidney disease, or conversely that they might be enlarged and covered with cysts, signifying polycystic kidney disease. (Had she performed a really good abdominal examination? Might those kidneys have been palpable?) She would mentally cancel the referral to the hematologist and initiate consultation with a nephrologist. ("Let him do the ultrasound!") The doctor would start to formulate questions regarding possible causes of kidney disease not evaluated at the first visit, and prepare to quickly start a discussion of the unfortunate implications of the findings. But besides glibly attributing the anemia to kidney failure, why did this patient lack red blood cells? What were the real mechanisms underlying this complication of an entirely different organ system disease?

Physicians had long posited that the kidneys made a hormone that supported red blood cell development. Clinical evidence was abundant regarding the concurrence of anemia and renal failure. Scientific evidence came from experiments where rodents and other animals had had their kidneys damaged or surgically removed. A fall in the proportion of red blood cells in the blood, commonly termed hematocrit, would invariably follow. If plasma from animals that had been made anemic by means not involving the kidneys was transferred to anemic or normal animals, their red blood cell counts would rise. If the anemic donor animal had had its kidneys removed, the plasma transfer experiment would not work, and the recipient's hematocrit would not increase. The plasma from nephrectomized animals had lost the ability to increase the red blood cell (RBC) count. L. O. Jacobson, Eugene Goldwasser, W. Fried, and L. Plzak definitively showed the kidneys were the source of a substance that promoted RBC production in a short paper in *Nature* in 1957.[4]

For many years scientists had tried to isolate the substance controlling the production of RBCs. If one could figure out what the substance was, perhaps it could be given, as a drug or medicine, to patients with kidney disease to treat their anemia. The analogy to insulin for patients with diabetes comes to the forefront. At that time, however, technical ability did not match scientific desire. Researchers, however, could come up with a name for the suspected hormone. Dr. Paul Carnot, a French scientist (1869–1957), called it hemopoietin in 1906. In 1905, Carnot posited the existence of a circulating hormone that enhanced synthesis of erythrocytes. In experiments in rabbits that had been subjected to bloodletting, Carnot and C. Deflandre in 1906 implicated hemopoietin as a factor in the response.[5] By the late 1940s, the substance had been renamed, although not identified. In 1948, E. V. A. Bonsdorff and E. Jalavisto linked the RBC synthetic response to residence at high altitude and reviewed the literature on the phenomenon from 1882 until 1948.[6] They showed, like other investigators, that plasma from fifteen patients with "circulatory or respiratory insufficiency," injected into the abdomens of thirty-one normal rabbits, resulted in an increase in RBC count and reticulocyte count (a measure of newly released red blood cells) compared to the values in seven rabbits that had not had such injections. They cited erythropoietins as the name for such substances.

In 1985, Eschbach and Adamson published a review article in *Kidney International*, summarizing the state of the science until that time.[7] Much was known about a hormone that had been recently purified and genetically sequenced. Eschbach and Adamson shortened erythropoietin to "Ep" for the paper. They noted that erythropoietin deficiency correlated with the severity of anemia, and the diminution of kidney function. Eschbach and Adamson linked anemia in dialysis patients to early notions of disruption of the perception of quality of life, a construct that had recently been developed by social scientists. Erythropoietin activity was not restored by treatment with peritoneal or hemodialysis. They acknowledged other causes of anemia in ESRD patients, including renal bone disease, which limited bone marrow capacity (where red cells are made and mature), as well as iron deficiency and inability to use iron supplements. They decried the dismal state of treatment for the anemia of kidney disease: male reproductive hormones (androgens—primarily testosterone) and transfusions, which were associated with unacceptable side effects. They almost casually finished the article by noting that a new therapy might be at hand. Biotechnology companies had

> isolated the human structural gene for Ep. . . . The gene has been expressed, and biologically active material from recombinant sources should be available for testing in patients soon. This is a major advance for a number of reasons, but is of particular importance to patients with severe anemia and ESRD. Once animal and human trials for safety and efficacy satisfy the governmental regulatory agencies, recombinant Ep should be available for therapy trials.

They concluded their article with a prescient sentence about clinical trials of the hormone in uremic patients: "Only through careful physiologic studies will it be possible to determine the optimal red cell mass in such individuals." The article does not comment on possible conflict of interest with commercial entities.

The Next Step for EPO: A New Paradigm for Pharma

During the Civil War, a nascent American pharmaceutical industry supplied opioids developed in Germany to Civil War soldiers. In the 19th century, the general populace was exposed to cocaine and opioids, as patent medicines. These drugs provided lucrative markets for casually purchased products laced with chemicals that induced dependence in patients, a surefire formula for enhancing profits. Pfizer and Squibb in Brooklyn, the brothers Wyeth in Philadelphia, Parke and Davis, and Eli Lilly all started their firms, giants of industry, through the middle to the end of the 20th century, before 1900. The next great wave of pharmaceutical growth began with U.S. government support for the development of penicillin during World War II. In the 1950s, firms such as Merck, Pfizer, and Lederle gained corporate prominence when they brought antibiotics to market. Merck synthesized an adrenal hormone, cortisone, in the mid-1950s. The release of more potent corticosteroids soon followed, changing the therapy and course of autoimmune and rheumatologic diseases as well as that of patients with adrenal insufficiency, or Addison's disease.

The era of clinically useful antihypertensive medications emerged in the mid-20th century. The early antihypertensives were created from plant derivatives. More effective drugs were soon developed, based on sulfonamide antibiotics. An important therapeutic advance was the release of thiazide and loop diuretics in the late 1950s, allowing physicians to approach the problem of sodium overload as a factor underlying hypertension in most patients. In the 1960s and '70s, as neuroscience blossomed, drugs based on modulators of the nervous system were developed. These advances in antihypertensive therapeutics occurred in parallel with the development of psychotherapeutic drugs, including the major and minor tranquilizers, cancer chemotherapeutics, and drugs designed for patients with diabetes (sulfonylureas such as tolbutamide [Orinase] and chlorpropamide [Diabinese]), which increased the ability of the failing pancreases to release insulin.

Perhaps the most important developments in antihypertensive therapeutics after the 1960s were the angiotensin-converting enzyme (ACE) inhibitors. This class of drugs originated from studies of snake venom, which can be profoundly effective at lowering blood pressure, to the point that it can result in shock and death. Pharmacologists realized that the ACE was involved in this response, and drug development centered on the design of antagonists to this protein. Modifying this enzyme would change the balance of angiotensin II, a potent blood vessel tightener, or vasoconstrictor, one of the factors contributing to high blood pressure. The first drug of this class to reach patients was Captopril, marketed by Squibb in the 1980s. These advances were followed by the release of a variety of calcium channel blockers later in the 1980s and angiotensin II receptor blockers (ARBs) in the 1990s. The advent of well-tolerated, effective antihypertensive medications, as well as the release of a new class of effective antihypercholesterolemic drugs, the statins (starting in 1987 with lovastatin), triggered a wave of large cardiovascular trials, often supported by industry. The success of these trials resulted in the improvement of public health, validated by an increase in longevity in developed countries and a decrease in death rates from cardiovascular diseases as well as an increase in pharmaceutical industry profits. These drugs were extensively used in the care of patients with CKD. In addition, lovastatin and the ACE inhibitors and ARBs dramatically improved laboratory abnormalities and outcomes in patients with kidney disease.

H2 blockers, for the treatment of peptic ulcer disease, revolutionized care by focusing on receptor biology. These drugs all radically changed the therapeutic landscape and improved the clinical course and outcomes for patients with potentially fatal or untreatable diseases. The technology boom saw the development of clinically useful oral contraceptives as well. Yet all these drugs were created using traditional biochemical methods, by modifying plant molecules or preexisting drugs or compounds.

None of these drugs, however, was synthesized using the tools of molecular biology. Industry had previously looked for compounds with biologic activity that might be useful in treating human disease from a large group of potential organic candidates in soil. Scientists continued to make slight changes in the chemistry of drugs found in natural settings, which allowed the extension of patents and acquisition of exclusive and long-lasting marketing rights for pharmaceutical companies. Now industry was poised to consider the biology of receptor interactions with circulating biochemicals and use molecular techniques to synthesize hormones as "designer" drugs.

The next great chapter in pharmaceutical history began with the development of biotechnology firms. The start of the ESRD program took place almost at the same time as the birth of the molecular biologic pharmaceutical era. After the description of the helical nature of DNA in 1953 by James Watson and Francis Crick, standing on the shoulders of Rosalind Franklin and Maurice Wilkins and building on the work of an army of proto-molecular biologists of the 1930s and 1940s in the U.S. and Great Britain, industry was ready to move forward. Twenty-five years of incremental as well as transformative scientific work culminated in the ability of researchers to link the amino acid structure of proteins to the DNA nucleotides that served as their templates and to locate specific DNA, encoding unique proteins (or hormones) in "libraries," or collections of human DNA.

Scientists dreamed the synthesis of normal human hormones and enzymes that might become blockbuster drugs could be accomplished using the tools of molecular biology, rather than by cumbersome and time-consuming biochemical methods. The discovery of insulin by Frederick Banting and Charles Best in 1922, isolated from dogs' pancreases, led to its manufacture and distribution for the use of patients by Eli Lilly and Company and revolutionized the care for people with diabetes, dramatically improving outcomes, especially for younger patients whose bodies were unable to produce any insulin at all. The insulin was made from pigs and cattle, biologic primary sources. Animal pancreatic tissues were ground up, and the bioactive insulin was isolated and purified for patient use. Countless animals died to provide the insulin to treat patients with diabetes. In 1951, Frederick Sanger elucidated the fifty-one amino acid structure of insulin. Sanger, the only person to have won two Nobel Prizes in Chemistry, received the prize in 1958 for this achievement and in 1980 for work on DNA sequencing.

The biotechnology firm Cetus was founded in 1971, about a century after the leading pharmaceutical houses were established in the U.S., by Ronald E. Cape, Peter Farley, and Nobel laureate Donald A. Glaser. The company focused on recombinant DNA technologies, the development of monoclonal antibodies, diagnostic gene expression technique processes, and the polymerase chain reaction for use as a molecular tool. The company manufactured β-interferon, an immune molecule thought to have antiviral and anticancer properties that could be useful in clinical practice, and interleukin-2, another immunoreac-tant that supported the growth and function of T-lymphocytes.

Genentech was founded in 1976, by Robert Swanson, a financier, and Her-bert Boyer, a biochemist at University of California, San Francisco, and a leader in the new field of molecular recombinant biotechnology. Boyer had worked on a project to produce the hormone somatostatin in 1977. This was a molecular biologic feat, although somatostatin was a small peptide, composed in one form of only one chain of fourteen amino acids. Biogen was founded in 1978 by a group of eminent scientists in the field of molecular biology and focused on producing interferon.

Applied Molecular Genetics (also initially known as AMGen), which was to become Amgen in 1983, was established in 1980 by two venture capitalists, William K. Bowes (1926–2016) and Sam Wohlstadter. Dr. George Rathmann was recruited from Abbott to serve as the CEO. Rathmann hired Fu-Kuen Lin, Ph.D., to join the new company. Bowes served as the first treasurer and chairman.

The first drug developed using recombinant DNA technology was insulin. Rat insulin gene sequences had been identified by Ullrich and colleagues, reported in *Science* in 1977,[8] and by a competing group from the Joslin Research Laboratory and the Peter Bent Brigham Hospital in 1978 by Gilbert and col-leagues in the *Proceedings of the National Academy of Sciences.*[9] In 1978, human insulin was synthesized using recombinant DNA technology by David Goeddel and colleagues at Genentech.[10] The production of the two insulin amino acid chains was directed by synthetic, recombinant DNA, developed in the labora-tory, using the molecular machinery of *E. coli* bacteria as a factory for the man-ufacture of bioactive proteins. Genentech entered into a marketing agreement with Eli Lilly and Company to distribute the new/old drug/hormone Humulin. The recombinant insulin, Humulin, was approved by the FDA in 1982. Sales started in 1983.

After advances in harnessing molecular biology to produce insulin in bac-teria using molecular means, biotechnology firms looked for the discovery and manufacture of novel hormones.

To study a biologically active compound, researchers must isolate it and characterize its biological properties and chemical structure. This was done for insulin but proved elusive for erythropoietin. In the 1970s, scientists were still quantifying its levels by a technique called bioassay. A bioassay would measure a biologic response and back calculate the concentration of the substance, perhaps a hormone, that would induce the physiologic result. Standardization, laboratory practice differences, and batch-to-batch variations posed problems in quantification with these approaches.

For instance, to study erythropoietin (or EPO), an animal would be made anemic by interfering with a red blood cell forming pathway not involving the kidneys—using severe iron deficiency, for example. It was presumed that erythropoietin synthesis would be increased as a result of the physiologic derangement and that levels of EPO in the animals' bloodstreams would rise. The investigator could use plasma from the anemic animal and assess the response of erythrocyte progenitor cells in a Petri dish compared to plasma from a group of normal animals with normal circulating hemoglobin levels using a technique called a bioassay to estimate the amount of the erythropoietin in the plasma. The technique was roundabout, and somewhat imprecise, but useful for getting papers published. It was not clear how such information would help people with kidney diseases and anemia. They needed a hormone like insulin that would prevent them from having the symptoms that overworked their hearts into congestive failure and limited their quality of life. And that drug could not be associated with severe side effects.

Consequences of Treating Anemia in Patients with Kidney Disease before EPO

Patients with severe anemia have weakness, fatigue, and breathlessness, and because of these limitations, have poor quality of life. Some of these symptoms mimicked those of uremia, as well as clinical major depression. Dialysis patients often had to be treated with multiple blood transfusions, sometimes receiving two units of packed red blood cells a week during their treatments. A price had to be paid for this therapy of a symptom, not a cure. Blood transfusions can result in iron overload when the iron in the transfused RBCs cannot be used efficiently, as is the case in patients who lack the capacity to produce erythrocytes. Iron overload, or hemochromatosis, can occur as a result of a genetic disorder or can be a consequence of multiple blood transfusions. The iron from the erythrocytes in the transfused blood that cannot be used in the bone marrow to make RBCs then deposits in the heart, the liver, and the pancreas, resulting in the development of heart failure, cirrhosis, and diabetes. So long-term transfusions are not a good treatment option. A physician could tell a lot about the state of iron overload in a patient by checking the serum ferritin. High ferritin levels indicated iron overload. And the ferritins in dialysis patients treated with multiple transfusions were sky high.

Blood transfusions were also complicated by viral and other infections, since it was hard during the early days of dialysis to efficiently screen for hepatitis A and B viruses and other pathogens that might have contaminated blood products. Furthermore, an infection known as "non-A, non-B hepatitis" was not yet definitively linked to a unique virus, hepatitis C, until the late 1980s. In addition, there was concern that transfusions might sensitize patients to foreign proteins and therefore compromise any future kidney transplantation.

Besides providing dialysis patients with the building blocks of RBCs, such as folic acid, other vitamins, and iron, it was known that testosterone, because of its ability as an anabolic steroid to enhance protein synthesis, might be useful to improve the anemia caused by ESRD. (That's the same drug/hormone bodybuilders use, legally or illicitly, to bulk up their muscle mass.) By the 1960s, several investigators had shown that androgens had a place in the treatment of patients with various types of anemia. John R. Richardson and Morton B. Weinstein reported in 1970 that testosterone enanthate, given intramuscularly for up to forty-four weeks to fifteen ESRD dialysis patients, resulted in a clinically significant increase in hematocrit, red cell volume, and iron utilization.[11] Laboratory scientific studies showed testosterone analogs could cause an increase in red cell progenitors.

In 1973, an experiment where 150 mg of testosterone propionate was given to maintenance hemodialysis patients twice a week was reported by Walter Fried and colleagues.[12] Five patients who had no kidneys because they had been surgically removed (or had "undergone nephrectomies") and six patients with some renal tissue remaining participated. Packed red cell volume and plasma erythropoietin levels, ascertained by a bioassay, increased in those with kidneys, but there was no similar response in anephric patients. The authors concluded testosterone increased RBC production by increasing erythropoie-tin production by the kidneys. Adamson and Eschbach published their experi-ence with testosterone supplements to treat anemia in patients with kidney disease in 1973 as well.[13] Testosterone therapy took off nationwide. Male and female ESRD patients were given injections of a testosterone analog, nan-drolone decanoate (Deca-Durabolin), on an intermittent basis. It sometimes worked the way it was intended. Nevertheless, often a cost was exacted for a therapy that did not quite hit the mark. The side effects were often unendur-able, especially for women, who underwent unwanted masculinization, including acne and hair growth in unwanted places, such as their faces. Some men developed enlargement of breast tissue. Abnormalities in liver enzymes, clotting factors, and the development of sleep disorders were attributed to tes-tosterone therapy in ESRD dialysis patients. More recently, some studies have demonstrated mortality risk from testosterone administration in other popu-lations. The situation regarding anemia and its treatment in ESRD dialysis patients was simply untenable but could not be fully addressed by scientific or clinical methods during the first fifteen years of the ESRD program. Dialysis could keep people alive but could not allow them to feel well.

Identification and Synthesis of Erythropoietin

In 1977, Takaji Miyake, Charles K. Kung, and Eugene Goldwasser of the Univer-sity of Chicago reported that they had purified and characterized erythropoie-tin.[14] They used urine from patients with aplastic anemia, a group of dreaded, often incurable bone marrow diseases in which erythrocyte production is markedly diminished. In these diseases, circulating erythropoietin levels rise to very high values in order to stimulate consistently unresponsive bone mar-row to make erythrocytes. Urinary levels of erythropoietin had been shown, using bioassays, to rise as a concomitant of the increase in circulating levels in several animal models. The urine of these patients was thought by investiga-tors to be a source of highly concentrated human erythropoietin for their stud-ies. The researchers used contemporary state of the art biochemical techniques to purify the molecule, including ion exchange chromatography, gel filtration, and absorption chromatography.

In 1984, Sylvia Lee-Huang of New York University described the cloning of erythropoietin DNA.[15] Lee-Huang isolated RNA from human renal cell cancer tissue, in which the synthesis of erythropoietin was increased. She used antibodies directed against protein products, which she developed, to identify specific erythropoietin-encoding RNA. Lee-Huang used these specific RNAs to synthesize cDNA probes to identify the erythropoietin gene. The research was supported by NIH. The erythropoietin gene sequence was not published in this report.

In February 1985, in a letter to *Nature*, Kenneth Jacobs, Miyake, and colleagues reported the cloning of the human erythropoietin gene, using the structure that had been elucidated by their teammate Miyake and colleagues almost a decade before.[16] The erythropoietin, extracted from the urine of humans with aplastic anemia (where it was in plentiful supply), was used to generate small stretches of its presumed DNA (known as oligonucleotides). These sequences, the so-called targeted oligonucleotides (oligos), could be inferred from the amino acid sequence of a given protein. The test oligos were then used to identify the human erythropoietin gene in a collection of human genomic sequences (also known as a "library"). The recombinant cDNA that had been identified by the oligos was inserted into a transformed African green monkey kidney cell system, which synthesized erythropoietin. The synthetic, or recombinant, erythropoietin was confirmed by different methods to be virtually identical to the substance previously identified by Miyake and colleagues.

In essence, the investigators were able to use the erythropoietin gene they identified to manufacture erythropoietin in a cellular system without the use of an animal. The manufactured hormone was for all intents and purposes identical to the human substance. Allergic reactions occasionally occurred in patients treated with porcine or bovine insulin as a result of their immune reactions to these peptides, which differed slightly from the human molecule. Identity of the manufactured product with the human hormone would be important, as hormones obtained from animal organs might be relatively or completely inactive in humans, in addition to being capable of eliciting allergic reactions in susceptible patients. The paper illustrated the structure of the human erythropoietin gene. It was not lost on the research team that this

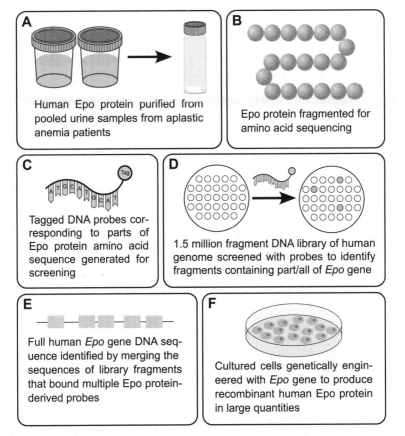

A Human Epo protein purified from pooled urine samples from aplastic anemia patients

B Epo protein fragmented for amino acid sequencing

C Tagged DNA probes corresponding to parts of Epo protein amino acid sequence generated for screening

D 1.5 million fragment DNA library of human genome screened with probes to identify fragments containing part/all of Epo gene

E Full human Epo gene DNA sequence identified by merging the sequences of library fragments that bound multiple Epo protein-derived probes

F Cultured cells genetically engineered with Epo gene to produce recombinant human Epo protein in large quantities

Figure 5. Cartoon depicting the process involved in identifying the erythropoietin gene and synthesizing human erythropoietin in an artificial cellular system. See text for details. Image courtesy of Erik Koritzinski.

process might be used to create a drug to treat patients with anemia if the disease process was based on lack of the hormone, such as was the case in patients with advanced kidney disease. (Interestingly, hormone replacement would not help patients with aplastic anemia. In that case, the bone marrow was resistant to the hormone, explaining the high circulating and urinary levels of erythropoietin.) The research was supported by a Japanese commercial entity, Chugai Pharmaceuticals. The Genetics Institute was later identified in a *NEJM* review article on erythropoietin as a biotechnology firm.

Just a few months later, in November 1985, Fu-Kuen Lin and colleagues, in the *Proceedings of the National Academy of Sciences*, also announced the cloning and expression of the human erythropoietin gene.[17] Lin graduated from the

National Taiwan University in 1964. He subsequently received a master's degree in plant physiology. Lin received a doctorate in plant physiology from the University of Illinois at Urbana-Champaign in 1971. Lin had served in several academic positions in Taiwan before joining the firm that was to become Amgen in August 1981.

The paper described the identification of the human erythropoietin gene. Using information from the amino acid sequence of purified erythropoietin, the researchers created oligonucleotide sequences of DNA to use in screening libraries. The paper also depicted the structure of the human erythropoietin gene. The gene encoded a protein composed of 193 amino acids. The gene, inserted into a Chinese hamster ovary cell system, produced a molecule the team demonstrated, through bioassays in cultured bone marrow cells and in studies using mice, acted biologically similarly to erythropoietin. The authors acknowledged the paper of Jacobs and colleagues and stated that the techniques used in both studies were similar. They noted that the proteins produced in each study had identical amino acid sequences. They abbreviated the protein they synthesized as "Epo." The report came from Amgen (which employed twelve of the thirteen authors) and the Department of Biochemistry and Molecular Biology at the University of Chicago. The acknowledgment stated that part of the work done in the University of Chicago laboratory of Dr. Eugene Goldwasser, the senior author, had been supported by funds from the National Heart, Lung, and Blood Institute (NHLBI) of NIH.

These two studies, using amino acid fragments derived from purified human erythropoietin to create nucleic acid sequences that could be used to identify the gene responsible for coding the hormone, and subsequently using the gene to manufacture perfect copies of the native human hormone, represented a tour de force use of molecular technologies at the time. The research, creating a means for synthesizing what was imagined to be an important drug, as well as developing a lucrative pharmaceutical product, succeeded in achieving both goals. The work revolutionized molecular biology as well as the pharmaceutical industry.

Goldwasser and colleagues from Amgen published the structure of human erythropoietin a little later, in March 1986,[18] after the biotech company had gotten the necessary manufacturing and publishing head starts.

Clinical Studies of Erythropoietin

Dr. Christopher Winearls of the Royal Postgraduate Medical School, in London, and colleagues published the first report of the treatment of anemia in ESRD patients maintained on chronic hemodialysis with recombinant erythropoietin in the *Lancet* in November 1986.[19] They studied eight men and two women, treated with hemodialysis for ESRD. Their ages ranged from twenty-six to sixty-five years. The patients received recombinant human erythropoietin in a nonrandomized fashion, intravenously three times weekly, at the end of dialysis. Doses of erythropoietin ranged from 3 to 192 units/kg body weight, which were increased as tolerated from lower to higher levels. The ten patients all showed an increase in hemoglobin concentration. Nine of the ten patients reported an "improved sense of well-being" and eight of the ten described "increased exercise tolerance." In one patient, blood pressure increased precipitously, affecting brain function, and two patients had clotting of their fistulas. The authors noted the improvements in patients' subjective evaluations of their health and the potential benefits that would be associated with eliminating blood transfusions in this population. They suggested attention would have to be paid to blood pressure control and clotting disorders in ESRD hemodialysis patients treated with erythropoietin. They concluded that "the long-term effects of near-normal hemoglobin concentrations from maintenance therapy remain to be evaluated." They were prescient.

This British team had scooped Eschbach and Adamson. The acknowledgments section of Winearls's paper noted "Ortho-Cilag Pharmaceutical Ltd provided the rHuEpo, which was manufactured by Amgen and is being jointly developed by Amgen, Thousand Oaks, California, USA, by Cilag Schaffhausen, Switzerland, by Kirin, Tokyo, Japan, and by Ortho Pharmaceutical, Raritan, New Jersey, USA." At this time, the companies were all in it together.

In January 1987 in the *NEJM*, Eschbach, Adamson, and colleagues reported on phase 1 and 2 studies of therapy with recombinant erythropoietin in twenty-five anemic ESRD hemodialysis patients (the study Eschbach had presented in Capri several months earlier).[20] Patients were twenty-one to sixty-nine years old. Seven were treated with home hemodialysis. Twelve were dependent on frequent regular blood transfusions. The average patient's hematocrit (percent of the blood that was red blood cells) before treatment was frighteningly low at 19.4%. (Normal hematocrits range from 37.5% to 51.0%, depending on the laboratory. Normal hemoglobin concentrations range from 12.6 to 17.7 g/dL.) Six doses of erythropoietin given three times a week intravenously after dialysis were tested, from 1.5 to 500 units per kg of body weight. Some patients responded to doses as low as 15 U/kg. At doses over 50 U/kg, consistent, dose-dependent increases in hematocrit and improvement in iron use were noted. The rate of rise of hematocrit was dose-dependent. At 500 U/kg, the average increase of hematocrit was 10% over three weeks. The authors noted no "cardiac, pulmonary, hepatic, or other organ dysfunction that could be attributed to the treatment.... No changes, at any dose, in the white-cell count, white-cell differential count, or platelet count ... in serial studies of liver function, lipids, or uric acid, chest films or electrocardiograms." Iron deficiency could occur as red cell production increased, especially if supplemental iron was not administered. The authors pointed out that the iron deficiency could be easily treated. A figure in the paper showed average dose response curves for the different administered erythropoietin levels over time in the patients. At 500 U/kg the response approached a right angle, almost completely pitched toward the vertical. (Such a response is almost never seen in biologic systems.)

When the hematocrit increased above 30%, four patients developed new or worsening hypertension. In one of these patients, on the highest dose of erythropoietin, the increased blood pressure was accompanied by a seizure. One patient "who did not adhere to dietary potassium restrictions and who refused to prolong the duration of dialysis went on to have recurrent, severe hyperkalemia" and died. No anti-erythropoietin antibodies were found in the patients. No patient receiving recombinant erythropoietin during the trial required transfusions. The authors suggested that blood pressure control in patients receiving erythropoietin treatment would be "an important aspect" of care. Because of the increase in hematocrit, and as a consequence of improved diet and appetite with better well-being, provision of dialysis would probably have to increase. The article noted that recombinant erythropoietin was "being developed jointly" by AMGen, Cilag, Kirin Brewery, and Ortho Pharmaceutical. The article came from authors at the University of Washington, the Northwest Kidney Centers, and AMGen Corporation. Grant support from the

Arthritis Metabolism Institute of NIH and a Center Grant from NIH were cited. The *Journal*, as part of its policy, noted that four of the five authors were stockholders in AMGen Corporation and three were company employees, signifying a crucial role of industry in the structure of the clinical research. The paper had a profound effect on the treatment of patients with kidney disease.

In July 1989, Eschbach and Adamson, and colleagues from the Northwest Kidney Center as well as the Ortho Pharmaceutical Corporation of Raritan, New Jersey, published another paper in the *NEJM*.[21] This time, they studied the effect of erythropoietin treatment in anemic patients with chronic kidney disease before the illness became so advanced that ESRD therapy with dialysis or kidney transplantation was necessary. The goal of the study was to assess the response of hematocrit to drug therapy, as well as evaluating whether kidney function would deteriorate with treatment. Seven women and ten men participated in the studies. They ranged from twenty-four to seventy-two years old and had a variety of kidney diseases. The patients had S[Cr]s between 4 and 11 mg/dL (signifying roughly between 25% and less than 9% of normal kidney function) and had anemia, with hematocrits less than 30%. All patients were treated with doses of erythropoietin of 50 to 150 U/kg body weight. Intravenous doses were given to the participants three times a week for eight weeks or until goal hematocrits (37% for women and 40% for men) were reached. Subcutaneous injections were given on a slightly different schedule with slightly different goals for hematocrit in the participants. Erythropoietin was "provided as recombinant human erythropoietin manufactured by Amgen and supplied by Ortho Pharmaceutical Corporation." A double-blind, placebo-controlled first phase, during which neither patients nor investigators knew who was getting the active drug, was followed by a maintenance phase in which the response of patients to different doses was monitored but the investigators were aware of the assignments.

All seventeen patients had an increase of hematocrit (from an average of 28% to 37%, in a clearly statistically significant manner) in a dose-dependent fashion. Hypertension developed and worsened in many of the patients, who needed additional modifications of antihypertensive drugs. The S[Cr] increased in the participants from an average of 6.5 mg/dL to 8.6 mg/dL, a change of almost one-third. This magnitude of increase would usually signify a clinically important decrease in kidney function, but because the levels of S[Cr] do not change in a linear fashion with kidney function, changes at high S[Cr]s translate into less extensive differences compared to changes of similar proportions or magnitudes at lower ranges of S[Cr]. In the study, because of the variation in S[Cr] levels in the individual patients before and after the trial of erythropoietin, as well as the small number of participants, the investigators could not detect statistically significant differences in kidney function attributed to treatment. But the measurements only indirectly assessed this parameter. The investigators also could not link deterioration of kidney function in the patient participants to increases in the value of their hematocrits or the presence or extent of high blood pressure. The investigators reported that all participants experienced improvement in "appetite, activity level, and sense of well-being." They acknowledged that although the results on renal function were "encouraging, this issue should be studied in larger groups of patients with the use of more precise measurement of renal function, such as iothalamate clearance, before and after correction of the anemia with erythropoietin." They concluded therapy with erythropoietin was "effective in correcting the anemia of patients with progressive renal failure without affecting renal function, although it may be associated with an increase in blood pressure." The study had been funded by NIH grants and by the Ortho Pharmaceutical Corporation (not Amgen). The *Journal* noted that of the authors, only Dr. Abels of Ortho Pharmaceutical Corporation was a stockholder in Johnson and Johnson.

That same year, with a group of distinguished clinical nephrology colleagues, Eschbach and Adamson published the results of a phase III multicenter trial of erythropoietin treatment in 333 anemic hemodialysis patients.[22] Besides assessing the response of red blood cells, and potential adverse effects on organ system function and dialysis efficiency, the study evaluated the effect of therapy with erythropoietin on the perception of quality of life of the participants before, during, and after the study. The investigators used questionnaires derived from an earlier seminal study of quality of life in ESRD patients, published by Roger W. Evans, Diane L. Manninen, and colleagues in the *NEJM* in 1985,[23] before the advent of erythropoietin, to evaluate perception of quality of life in a subgroup of 130 patients participating in the study. The authors reported "the rHuEpo was provided as Epogen by Amgen Inc., Thousand Oaks, California, and was purified from the growth medium of Chinese hamster ovary cells into which the human erythropoietin gene had been transfected and expressed." The study was "supported in part by Amgen, Inc., Thousand Oaks, California."

Study participants were 174 women and 159 men treated with dialysis for ESRD. Their average age was fifty-one years old. They had a variety of kidney diseases, including those caused by high blood pressure and diabetes, as well as glomerulonephritis, urinary tract obstruction, polycystic kidney disease, and a few others. The patients were recruited from major U.S. academic medical centers. Average hematocrits increased dramatically, from 22.3% to 35% after treatment with erythropoietin. Initial high doses of erythropoietin had to be decreased in maintenance phases in order not to overshoot hematocrit goals. Blood transfusions were eliminated in the participants after two months of therapy. A set of coexistent illnesses and conditions that might limit the response to erythropoietin were identified. Scores on a crude index of physical function, the Karnofsky Performance Status Scale, dramatically improved from baseline, during and at the end of treatment, as patients' hematocrits increased from 23.7 to 33.9%. Patients' reports of their activity, exercise tolerance, appetite, and energy levels improved as well. Average scores on the Nottingham Health Profile, a subjective measure of patients' perceptions of their health status, improved when values before and after treatment with erythropoietin were compared. Seizures, development of iron deficiency, and worsening of high blood pressure were noted to be major side effects of therapy. The authors concluded anemia in hemodialysis patients corrected by therapy with recombinant human erythropoietin (rHuEpo) resulted "in the elimination of transfusions, reduction in iron overload, and improved quality of life. Iron stores and blood pressure must be monitored and treated to maintain the effectiveness of rHuEpo and to minimize the threat of hypertensive encephalopathy."

The War between Amgen and Ortho

Amgen faced a crisis as erythropoietin was being tested and approval for marketing was sought. After originally obtaining venture capital backing in the early 1980s, Fu-Kuen Lin applied for a patent for the synthesis of recombinant erythropoietin in 1984. Amgen was a neophyte biotech powerhouse but lacked expertise in clinical trials science and experience with navigating the long and arduous FDA approval process. Amgen needed the financial and scientific resources to complete the hurdles involved in obtaining drug approval. The Japanese rights to recombinant erythropoietin were sold to Kirin Brewery for $24 million. Johnson and Johnson offered to buy Amgen, as the fledgling company attempted to complete an FDA application for a new drug. The financial future for Amgen, however, appeared bleak. Amgen later agreed to sell Johnson and Johnson rights to the marketing of erythropoietin for all indications in Europe and elsewhere (except China and Japan), as well as the rights to the U.S. market, excluding dialysis patients, in 1985.

Ortho Pharmaceutical, a subsidiary of Johnson and Johnson, would market the very same drug in the U.S., for anemic patients with chronic kidney disease who had not yet reached the stage where they needed dialysis under a licensing agreement with Amgen. People undergoing chronic maintenance dialysis for ESRD seemed to be the biggest patient group to need therapy with erythropoietin. Since their treatment was reimbursed by Medicare, a source of revenue to cover what was going to be an expensive drug had been identified. Johnson and Johnson would help obtain the regulatory approvals from the FDA for Amgen as well as Ortho. The deal was outlined in a "product license agreement," or PLA.

However, warfare broke out among these two companies almost immediately. (The early battles over markets and market shares are described by Kathleen Sharp in *Blood Feud*.[24]) The battle continued over the years, as the partnership quickly soured. The facts of the mess are perhaps best described in an unbiased fashion in the opinion rendered in one of several lawsuits between the companies.[25]

The companies differed over the strategies for submissions to the FDA. Amgen submitted its FDA application for dialysis patients in October 1987, without including Ortho's data on the predialysis population. Ortho sought an injunction to prohibit Amgen from marketing EPO unless Amgen made the filings that would allow Ortho to obtain FDA marketing approval for patients with kidney disease not treated with dialysis. Amgen was successful and received FDA approval for Epogen on June 1, 1989. Amgen wouldn't sell EPO to Ortho, and Ortho could not market or sell EPO. In the meantime, Ortho, realizing the problem, had filed suit claiming millions of dollars of damages for lost income since June 1989. Suits and countersuits ensued in what seemed like an endless legal battle between the companies. (There was a lot of money involved, since Amgen had $287 million in sales over eighteen months). In one of the cases, the Appeals Court noted "inconsistent claims and counterclaims by both sides." The whole complicated back and forth was an indication of bad faith and questionable practices between two companies competing for a huge market.

Ortho finally won approval to market erythropoietin as Procrit, a drug that was identical to Epogen, for the international and U.S. applications other than dialysis patients on December 31, 1990. These markets included patients with anemia and HIV infection treated with azidothymidine and those with CKD not requiring dialysis. The price of Epogen and Procrit was supposed to be identical, ten dollars for one thousand units. And Amgen survived as a commercial entity.

How Can a Pharmaceutical Company Maximize Profits?

In June 1991, Amgen was fined $164 million, to be paid to Ortho for violating terms of the PLA. In 1993, Ortho received FDA approval for the use of Procrit in patients with anemia and cancer. In all types of anemic patients, and for both marketing plans, it was critical that more units of erythropoietin per patient be sold. Since the response of hematocrit and hemoglobin was largely dose-dependent, how the companies could make sure high doses were used and high hematocrits were achieved was the critical question. Patients with "resistance" to the actions of erythropoietin (because of bone marrow disease or failure, iron deficiency, or other coexisting illnesses) could be a lucrative segment of the market because they needed high doses of the drug to get to target hematocrits. The pharmaceutical companies doggedly tagged this condition for special education for nephrologists and research for many years. And most importantly, it was clear that the medication costs had to be reimbursed by the government or insurance companies. The reimbursement rules at the time stipulated a maximum goal hematocrit of 35%. Another answer to the corporate need for higher doses and higher hematocrits was presumed to be quality of life.

Roger W. Evans, Ph.D., a sociologist at the Batelle Human Affairs Research Center, in Seattle, Washington, had worked with a colleague, Diane L. Manninen, Ph.D., since at least 1983. They had studied the responses of early heart and kidney transplant recipients, and rehabilitation of patients with chronic kidney disease. Evans and Manninen then led a seminal study on the quality of life of ESRD patients, published in the *NEJM* in 1985.[26] Their colleagues were leaders in dialysis research, involved with the foremost large dialysis organizations at that time, including Drs. Christopher R. Blagg of the Northwest Kidney Center in Seattle, Edmund G. Lowrie of National Medical Care Inc. in Boston, Alan R. Hull of Southwestern Dialysis Centers in Dallas, Texas, and Robert A. Gutman of Duke University. (Gutman and colleagues had written an influential article in the *NEJM* in 1981 characterizing the decreased physical activity and inadequate employment status of dialysis patients when *rehabilitation* rather than *quality of life* was the buzzword on the patient experience.[27]) They reported on the quality of life of ESRD patients, in a landmark paper, comparing several groups of patients with kidney disease. They demonstrated that patients who had lost a kidney transplant had poorer quality of life than that experienced by patients treated with dialysis or any other group of patients with kidney disease in the study. They showed the devastating effects on patients of the loss of a kidney transplant.

Evans, Manninen, and a colleague, Barbara Rader, next set their sights on the question of whether quality of life in ESRD patients treated with erythropoietin could be improved. Randomized controlled trials could yield data on interventions that could be linked more easily to drug effects than information from "observational" studies. They published another key paper in *JAMA* in 1990, with their colleagues listed as the "Cooperative Multicenter EPO Clinical Trial Group" on the changes in perception of quality of life experienced by chronic hemodialysis patients with anemia who had been treated with Epogen.[28] The study included 329 of the 333 patients in the Eschbach trial who were followed for changes in their clinical status related to the increase in hematocrit caused by erythropoietin. The participating sites were all first-class academic medical centers. The average age of patients in the study was about fifty-one, and they were split almost equally between men and women; 33.9% of the patients in the study were Black, reflecting the demographics of the national ESRD program. The most common diseases causing ESRD in the patients were chronic glomerulonephritis (23%), high blood pressure (23%), and diabetes mellitus (18%), accounting for about two-thirds of the cases. The patients had been treated with dialysis for an average of approximately six years, so they were "survivors." The target hematocrit for those treated with erythropoietin was 32 to 38%. The quality of life of the participants was compared before the start of erythropoietin therapy and at the end of the trial. The employment status of the participants was assessed, as was their functional status, using the Karnofsky scale. "Health" was assessed using a disease symptom checklist and "health status" by the Nottingham Health Profile questionnaire.

The investigators showed statistically significant improvements in the Karnofsky scale score. The average Karnofsky score decreased from 3.3 to 2.75 (out of 10—where 1 is normal and 10 is "moribund"). Participants' reports of "tires easily, no energy," "weakness," "fainting spells, dizziness," "nervousness, tension, anxiety," "shortness of breath, trouble breathing," "muscle weakness," and "leg cramps" also diminished while they were treated with erythropoietin. No changes could be detected in patients' perceptions of pain, depression, or tremors. Patients perceived improvement in energy, emotional reactions and social isolation, and sex life but not in sleep, mobility, job or work status, home or social life, or personal relationships. Participants reported improvement in measures of "well-being, psychological affect and life satisfaction." Their perception of happiness increased, to the point where the proportion of patients who were "very happy" at the end of the trial exceeded that of the American general population. The investigators could not demonstrate a change in patients' employment status or ability to work as a result of the treatment of anemia with erythropoietin.

The paper concluded with a key set of acknowledgments. The authors noted that "rHuEPO (EPOGEN) was provided by Amgen, Inc, Thousand Oaks, Calif." They reported at the end of the paper that the "study was funded by Amgen, Inc, through a contract to the Battelle Seattle (Wash) Research Center.

Many of the authors and coauthors have corporate affiliations or contractual agreements with, or own stock in, Amgen, Inc. The editors have been informed of these potential conflicts of interest." It was expected that these improvements in perception of quality of life would be a strong argument for physicians and payers regarding the benefits to hemodialysis patients of treatment of anemia and achieving high hematocrits with erythropoietin.

Dr. Dennis Cotter, who had trained as an engineer, worked with the esteemed health technology assessment expert Dr. Seymour Perry at Georgetown University before branching out to work for a congressional committee focused on diagnostic related groups (DRGs). In these positions, Cotter had become adept at health-care systems data analysis, concentrating on insurance claims information to assess practice patterns and costs of care. Cotter left Georgetown in 1986 to found the Medical Technologies and Practice Patterns Institute (MTPPI). The institute's mission was to understand and evaluate the development and dissemination of U.S. health-care technology and to quantify costs, benefits, utility, and harms as science advanced to create better therapies. Such knowledge would be critical for government policymakers, as well as insurance companies, pharmacies, and health maintenance organizations. But such data might be important for pharmaceutical manufacturers as well. Cotter was soon approached by Nick Ruggieri, the Washington representative for Johnson and Johnson. Ruggieri needed analyses of Medicare data to understand use of erythropoietin across the U.S., in part to monitor Amgen's sales. By 1991, Dennis Cotter had met Dennis Longstreet of Ortho Biotech in his office in Raritan, New Jersey. Cotter portrayed the ethos at Ortho as "the more product you sell, the more you advance." Cotter described Longstreet as a "product salesman, who didn't know any of the science behind erythropoietin." Cotter remembers 1989 as "an era of optimism. There was enormous enthusiasm about biotechnology. It could provide 'miracle cures.' The approval and successful use of recombinant insulin and tissue plasminogen activator for the treatment of strokes in progress provided support for the subsequent acceptance of biotechnology products. Amgen engaged in a lot of lobbying."

The FDA "unit" in charge of Amgen's application for Epogen was the Bureau of Biologics, which Cotter noted was "concerned primarily with the purity of the blood supply." The review was directed by Dr. Joseph Fratantoni.

The proposal was not treated as a new drug application, and therefore, Epogen was evaluated under a different set of criteria. (Epogen was approved in this manner by the FDA in June 1989.)

Ortho Biotech wanted information regarding the use of Epogen in the U.S. Cotter obtained data from the HCFA (the predecessor of Centers for Medicare and Medicaid Services [CMS]) on the doses of erythropoietin administered to dialysis patients covered by Medicare, and the patients' hematocrits at that time, to do precisely such analyses, in cooperation with faculty members at Johns Hopkins. The team could link initial situations with the amount of drug administered, clinical outcomes, and costs. These data were needed, as Cotter put it, "to solve a commercial dispute."

MTPPI went on to counter the scientific validity of treatment with erythropoietin by simultaneously evaluating clinical effectiveness and costs and consult on projects for Ortho Biotech.

Dr. Allan J. Erslev (1919–2003), a pioneer in the study of erythropoietin biology, in a review article published in the *NEJM* in 1991,[29] shortly after the beginning of the molecular biologic revolution in erythropoietin, summarized the new state of scientific knowledge regarding this hormone produced by the kidneys, largely enhanced by the molecular biologic work of Amgen. Erythropoietin is a glycoprotein, meaning a molecule composed of a chain of amino acids linked to carbohydrates. EPO functions as a growth factor, increasing the production or synthesis of a biomolecule, in this case the red blood cell or erythrocyte. Erslev posited EPO is produced by fibroblasts (a specific type of cell in the interstitium, the supporting structure of the kidneys, close to the proximal tubule and peritubular capillaries). EPO binds to bits of proteins (receptors) on the surface of so-called erythrocyte progenitor cells, stimulating the production of red blood cells by the bone marrow. In patients with anemia, the kidney senses a decrease in oxygen-carrying capacity, and the renal interstitial fibroblasts synthesize more EPO, which is released into the bloodstream to engender its effects. In this manner, the body responds to a physiologic stress, loss of blood for example, by eliciting the synthesis and release of erythropoietin and the increased manufacture and release of RBCs in response to the lowered oxygen-carrying capacity of the blood, which, in the presence of adequate iron, results in the restoration of blood concentrations of hemoglobin and red cell mass, improvement in anemia, and restoration of the oxygen-carrying capacity of the blood. Erslev speculated that alterations in the carbohydrate chains of EPO might change its pharmacologic properties, a notion that was not surprising to scientists or the captains of the pharmaceutical industry.

Dr. Juan P. Bosch arrived as the new director of the division of Renal Diseases and Hypertension at George Washington University, in 1985, from Mount Sinai Hospital in New York, after the previous GW director resigned. Several well-known senior and some junior nephrologists came to look the place over—as Washington, D.C., might be an attractive place to treat patients with kidney disease and do research in ESRD. The city was famous around the country at the time—not only as the capital, but as a majority African American enclave, whose government was directed mostly by native Washingtonians (although the federal government exerted tight control over the town). Perhaps as a consequence of the demographics, or the poverty of the inhabitants, the city had the highest incidence of ESRD in the nation. Bosch, although relatively young, had quickly become quite prominent in academic circles for spearheading three areas of research in kidney disease. In the field of dialytic treatment for ESRD, Bosch pioneered the technique of hemofiltration, popular in Europe but almost unknown in the U.S., as a safer and improved alternative to classic hemodialysis. Bosch had also investigated the old concept of "renal reserve," by showing that a high-protein meal could increase the level of renal function, measured by the glomerular filtration rate, or GFR, in normal people.[30] In contrast, patients with kidney disease had a relatively fixed level of renal function, and their GFR did not respond to a protein load. Therefore, the protein load became a meaningful test to evaluate whether a patient had renal disease. Finally, in the field of acute renal failure, Bosch pioneered the use of continuous arterial venous hemofiltration (CAVH) treatment to provide a low-cost but efficient type of well-tolerated, gentle dialysis that could nevertheless be employed around the clock to treat severely ill patients, despite perilously low blood pressures and massive fluid overload.[31] Bosch's achievement was to characterize the dynamics of blood flow and fluid removal through the system using the analogy of glomerular pressures and flows. In this manner, he established himself as a member of both of the two warring camps of nephrology—the dialyzers and the physiologists—as well as positioning himself as an expert in acute renal failure. In one fell swoop, Bosch confidently set out to establish the George Washington University School of Medicine as a center of excellence in renal disease, challenging the hegemony of Georgetown's George Schreiner in his own backyard. After the publication of Eschbach's paper, Bosch was invited to join a "guideline" group, convened by Amgen, to consider what the level of hematocrit should be in patients with anemia who had ESRD treated with hemodialysis. His recollection is that

> the company representatives pushed for hematocrits greater than 35% for dialysis patients treated with Epogen. We were manipulated. We were pushed to recommend the highest hematocrit we could achieve, not the lowest that would support health, and be less costly to the government or the taxpayer if the treatment was supported by Medicare. I pointed out that the higher the hematocrit was, the more dialysis the patient would need to provide the same clearance of blood. Treatment times would have to be increased. The process seduced us into supporting "group-think." If I didn't see therapy this way, how come all these smart people were advocating higher hemoglobin values? I was unprepared for this commercial set of recommendations. Now I am against guidelines. They support the hidden agenda of the company, to maximize profits by use of therapeutics. Corporations are putting profits ahead of patients.

Bosch had given interviews to John Iglehart, the national *NEJM* correspondent. During the early 1980s, in a series of conversations, Bosch explained to Iglehart that dialysis in the U.S. was inefficient and that the treatment and payment system lacked quality controls. The ESRD program in that regard was not run like a business. Shortly after those conversations, Representative Pete Stark (1931–2020), Democratic congressman from California, called Bosch in his office. In his capacity as chairman of the Ways and Means Health Subcommittee, Representative Stark was directly concerned with Medicare coverage and costs. The approval of Epogen by the FDA necessitated decision-making on the part of Medicare. Should Medicare pay for Epogen treatment for ESRD patients with anemia? What should the goals of therapy be? How much should the drug cost ESRD patients? How much would the government be prepared to pay for a patient? Should there be a cap in outlays per patient per year? Stark wanted to know what hematocrit Bosch would recommend as a cap for a goal, so, if the government decided to pay for erythropoietin treatments through the Medicare system, there would be clear targets and payment limits. Bosch recalls that after a wide-ranging conversation covering ESRD patients, dialysis techniques, and anemia, he recommended a goal hematocrit of 35% to the congressman. Of course, Bosch was not the only source of opinion available to the government regarding the goal of therapy with erythropoietin.

Medicare began coverage of costs for Epogen in July 1989 after its approval by the FDA for the treatment of anemia in ESRD dialysis patients in June. Reimbursement rates were set at forty dollars per administration of fewer than 10,000 units (U) and seventy dollars per administration of 10,000 U or more.

Dr. Neil Powe, an internist and public health scientist then at Johns Hopkins, had been interested in the care of patients with kidney disease for some time. Powe graduated from Princeton and then Harvard Medical School and pursued postgraduate studies, obtaining a master's degree in business administration to help understand the complicated tangle of health-care costs in a regulated system. In 1992, along with colleagues in academia and HCFA,[32] Powe published a study in *JAMA* of the use of erythropoietin in ESRD patients after its approval. One year after the approval of Amgen's Epogen by the FDA, 52% of all Medicare dialysis patients received the drug. The yearly cost paid by Medicare for treatment of dialysis patients with Epogen was approximately $228 million. This represented almost one-fifth of the payments for the outpatient (nonhospital) treatment of ESRD patients and about 6% of all ESRD program payments. The study showed Black patients were less likely to receive Epogen, as were home hemodialysis and peritoneal dialysis patients. Men were less likely to receive Epogen then women. Younger and older patients were more likely to be treated than patients between thirty-five and sixty-four years of age. Geographical variations in the use of Epogen were noted. Powe's study showed you were less likely to be treated with Epogen if your dialysis took place in Tennessee, Mississippi, or Alabama than if you lived in Montana, Oregon, Idaho, or Washington State. Patients receiving dialysis in for-profit units were more likely to be treated with Epogen.

By the mid-1990s, it had to be acknowledged that there were disparities in access to EPO for hemodialysis patients (despite government financial support for its prescription) and that provision of the recombinant hormone was costly. But scientific, medical evidence demonstrated that the quality of life of hemodialysis patients improved with treatment of anemia with the drug. So even if there were some side effects associated with the treatment of dialysis patients with Epogen, one could argue that the concomitant improvement in quality of life made it worthwhile. And the investigators and the companies that supported their research did. Dr. Peter DeOreo, a respected dialysis physician in Cleveland, Ohio, told me that "it was obvious that normalization of hematocrit in dialysis patients would improve their quality of life." Perhaps in selected ESRD patients treatment of anemia with EPO could save lives.

Could EPO Increase Quantity as Well as Quality of Life?

Dr. Anatole Besarab began the early part of his career in academic internal medicine and nephrology in Philadelphia, at Jefferson Medical College, after receiving his M.D. from the University of Pennsylvania, training in medicine at the old and distinguished Pennsylvania Hospital. He finished fellowship studies in nephrology at Harvard. Besarab had been trained as a basic physiologist. He had described the effects of potent catecholamines, such as epinephrine, on the function of kidney tubules, using a system known as the isolated perfused kidney. At Jefferson, Besarab met Drs. Jaime Caro and Allan Erslev, of the Cardeza Foundation for Hematologic Research. Besarab brought his physiologic skills to bear using the isolated perfused kidney model to show how changes in blood ion composition or changes in acid-base or hormonal status could modify kidney function. Besarab became skilled in clinical trials science while at Jefferson. He later moved to Henry Ford Hospital in Detroit, Michigan.

In 1998, Besarab, with colleagues Drs. Kline Bolton of the University of Virginia, Allen Nisenson of UCLA, and Steve Schwab at Duke, as well as a group of Amgen scientists, published a study in the *NEJM* evaluating the results of treating anemic ESRD hemodialysis patients with congestive heart failure or ischemic heart disease with erythropoietin.[33] The study had a formidable

212 + THE BODY'S KEEPERS

premise. Erythropoietin therapy, by alleviating anemia, would increase the oxygen-carrying capacity of the blood of hemodialysis patients, providing sustenance to the heart muscle, which was starved for oxygen by anemia and its compromised coronary arteries. It was well known that coronary artery disease was common in ESRD hemodialysis patients. The investigators thought restoring the hematocrits of these sick people, with combined advanced heart and kidney disease, to normal levels would ameliorate several outcomes, since the vital oxygen-carrying capacity of the blood would be regained as patients' hematocrits improved. The authors maintained that in previous studies of patients with anemia and kidney disease, normal hematocrit values were associated with improved quality of life, decreased length of hospitalizations, and increased ability to exercise. The authors extrapolated these findings to hypothesize that normalization of hematocrits in hemodialysis patients with heart disease would improve their survival.

The goal of the study was to create two experimental clinical groups, equal in all ways except for the way erythropoietin was used to treat anemia. One group of patients would receive enough erythropoietin to achieve and maintain a hematocrit of 42%, a normal laboratory result. The second group would receive just enough erythropoietin to maintain an average hematocrit of 30%, more typical of contemporary treated hemodialysis patients. (This was in part a consequence of the Medicare payment system, which would only reimburse for achievement of goals for patients' hematocrits set by the regulators.) Which arm of the trial patients participated in would be determined by the toss of a coin. This design is called a randomized controlled trial, or RCT for short.

While the main outcome of the study was survival, the investigators and the company assumed restoration of normal levels of hematocrit to such patients would also improve their ability to think, and experience an improved quality of life. The study would show which was the best and safest strategy.

The investigators recruited an impressive team of well-known clinical nephrologists, specializing in the care of dialysis patients, from across the country to enroll and treat patients, and monitor outcomes. The ongoing results and patients' safety during the study were overseen by an independent Data Monitoring Committee composed of a group of national and international experts in kidney disease, clinical trials science, and statistics. All patients enrolled in the trial had been treated with erythropoietin, with hematocrits between 27% and 33%. The study enrolled 1,233 patients, who were followed for an average of fourteen months.

The study blew up in the investigators' faces. The research was stopped by its Data Monitoring Committee, because statistical analysis of the trends showed that the patients in the "normal" hematocrit group had roughly a 30% greater chance of dying or sustaining a heart attack, compared with the group treated to a conservative hematocrit goal. In the paper, the survival curves showed that the "normal" hematocrit group always had poorer survival than those treated conservatively. The conclusion of the study was that "in patients with clinically evident heart failure or ischemic heart disease receiving hemodialysis, administration of erythropoietin to raise the hematocrit to 42% is not recommended." While the investigators acknowledged the bad news, they could not explain why the patients in the "normal" group had been more likely to die. Analysis of the hematocrits of those who died compared to those who survived and of the doses of erythropoietin administered to the different patients did not explain the survival differences.

Dr. David A. Goodkin was the senior author of the study. He had trained in nephrology at Temple University under the tutelage of the charismatic Dr. Robert Narins. After his fellowship at Temple, Goodkin entered private practice in Southern California but in 1992 was recruited by Amgen, which needed a clinical nephrologist to coordinate studies of Epogen in patients with kidney disease. He told me, "I was not so savvy about business at that time, but it was a 'heady' environment. I was excited about being on a steep new learning curve. Amgen was not a bureaucratic institution then. The best science and the best ideas won."

Goodkin noted that "an interim analysis of the independent Data Monitoring Committee revealed more access clotting in the high hematocrit group, and showing its superiority was futile. It was quite a disappointment, quite a shock." The investigators and Amgen were promptly informed of the results. Amgen immediately issued a press release, announcing that the study had been stopped. Goodkin wrote the paper that was sent to the *NEJM*. In the original version, using a log rank test, the investigators reported an increased risk of death in the high hematocrit group. The *Journal's* statistical consultant opined that accounting for an interim analysis, mortality rates between the two groups at the time the study was stopped were not significantly different. The final published paper reflected that review. In addition, Goodkin noted that the *Journal* removed a sentence stating, "There was no difference between groups in quality of life" in the final published report but retained a phrase suggesting differences in "physical function" could be detected. He was later able to clarify these and other issues in an invited review in *Seminars in Dialysis*, in 2009.[34] Goodkin has wondered whether the investigators selected a population that was too sick, with advanced heart and kidney disease, to show beneficial results. Perhaps, he surmised, "we should have chosen a younger population."

The study was difficult for clinicians to understand, not only because of the counterintuitive results and the revisions to the final paper by the *Journal*, but also because the science of clinical trials had not advanced enough at the time to allow physicians to understand the implications of a "stopping rule." There had been no statistically significant increase in death rates in the high hematocrit group, in part because the study was stopped prematurely to prevent such a result. Therefore, the researchers did not have to state that therapy with erythropoietin in the high doses needed to achieve a normal hematocrit in dialysis patients caused death. They were able to get away with a summary that stated that such a clinical goal could not be "recommended." The overarching message, however, was quite clear. There was no advantage to trying to achieve normalization of hematocrit in dialysis patients. Put more bluntly, erythropoietin, administered in the high doses needed to achieve normal hematocrits, killed dialysis patients. Had such results been apparent, they could not be used to sell more units of erythropoietin.

Adamson and Eschbach wrote the editorial in the *Journal* accompanying Besarab's paper.[35] They noted that almost ten years after the approval of erythropoietin for the treatment of anemia in ESRD hemodialysis patients, the number of patients treated had greatly increased and yearly costs of anemia treatment had increased by nearly fivefold since the first year it was available, to almost a billion dollars. They pointed out that many physicians were enthusiastic about the improvements erythropoietin had effected in their patients, and although the 36% hematocrit cap limited therapy, the average hematocrit of ESRD patients (at the time, in 1995) was 31%. They focused on the unknown relationship between iron administration, goal hematocrits, and outcomes that the study presented. However, they endorsed hematocrit goals of 33% to 36% and the use of intravenous iron supplements for the treatment of anemic ESRD hemodialysis patients. It was not revealed in the editorial whether the scientists had a financial interest in the companies supplying erythropoietin.

Cotter, Mae Thamer, John H. Sadler, and I reported, in a paper in *Kidney International* in 1998,[36] that between 1990 and 1996, the mean recombinant human erythropoietin dose increased between 7% and 39% (depending on initial hematocrit) in adult U.S. hemodialysis patients, achieving only relatively modest increases in the overall average hematocrit for the entire population. We could not show dosing was related to patient or provider characteristics in this study but noted that "African-Americans, the elderly, non-diabetics and persons receiving dialysis in a non-profit facility had a larger percent change in hematocrit compared to their counterparts." We concluded that the "results of the clinical use of rHuEPO seven years after FDA approval found in the general ESRD hemodialysis population have not equaled the results obtained in the initial clinical trials. Overall, our findings suggest that substantial increases in rHuEPO dose provided to anemic patients have resulted in only modest increases in hematocrit in the seven years since rHuEPO's introduction. Resistance to rHuEPO, prior rHuEPO treatment, inadequate use of supplemental iron, and policy and financial incentives may explain this finding." The use of erythropoietin had been widespread and was paid for by the government but had made little overall change in the hematocrits of the entire population of HD patients.

In summary, Cotter and colleagues showed although average erythropoietin doses per patient had steadily gone up, as the number of people treated for ESRD with dialysis increased, the patients' average hematocrit remained stubbornly unresponsive to the increase in drug administration, suggesting inefficiencies in the treatment system. These glitches could include giving high doses of erythropoietin to patients who had untreated iron deficiency or some other condition that made their bone marrows unresponsive. That inefficiency was a failure of physician diagnosis and a waste of taxpayer dollars.

A further setback to the industry came after a report from France in the *NEJM* in 2002 of pure red cell aplasia in patients with kidney disease treated with erythropoietin.[37] One of the concerns of the original Amgen investigators regarding recombinant human erythropoietin was whether the production of antibodies reacting with the drug would be stimulated by the treatment. Because the recombinant product was thought to be identical to the human hormone, it was anticipated that there would not be a discernible antibody response in patients. The early investigators were gratified to report in their first several papers that there was no important antibody response. Several cases of patients treated with erythropoietin who continued to have anemia were reported by the end of the 20th century, including two patients with red cell aplasia, where bone marrow disease prevents red cell production in the presence or absence of erythropoietin. The French investigators reported thirteen cases of patients with anemia treated with erythropoietin, who, after initially responding, developed antibodies to erythropoietin and worsening of anemia. Most of the patients had ESRD and were treated with dialysis. They had been treated with subcutaneous erythropoietin and had developed resistant anemia from three months to more than five years after starting drug therapy. Erythropoietin therapy was stopped in all these patients, who had antibodies directed against the drug that were documented in a series of elegant experiments performed by the investigators. The antibodies of all the patients prevented red blood cell formation in Petri dish experiments. Six of the thirteen patients recovered some ability to produce RBCs after various treatments, including immunosuppressive medications, were used to halt patients' antibody production. Several of the patients remained dependent on blood transfusions to survive.

Like Erslev in 1991, the French investigators pointed out that recombinant erythropoietin had a slightly different carbohydrate side chain structure compared with the native molecule and that these structures differed between various erythropoietin compounds (epoetin alfa and epoetin beta, marketed by different companies [Johnson and Johnson in Puerto Rico and Roche in Germany]). The investigators could not prove that the antibody response was engendered by the carbohydrate side chains. Although the side effect of red cell aplasia was rare, it was potentially devastating to the affected patients, who might need lifelong transfusions. The investigators concluded that antibodies against erythropoietin that may develop during treatment of patients with kidney disease and anemia can result in the development of pure red cell aplasia as a complication of therapy. The study was supported in part by funds from Amgen.

A key part of the licensing agreement between Amgen and Ortho Biotech was the provision that allowed Ortho to market erythropoietin for the treatment of nondialysis patients in the U.S. and across the globe, with the exception of Japan and China. This turned out to be a much larger market than the one Amgen had reserved for itself, U.S. dialysis patents, since ESRD is merely the "tip of the iceberg" of patients with CKD. Could Ortho show Procrit was just as effective at improving hematocrits, and perhaps quality of life, in CKD patients as Epogen was in dialysis patients, without the pesky side effects? While they were the same molecule, potentially, Procrit might be a safer and more effective drug in the larger CKD population. Although Besarab's paper had raised safety concerns, Ortho Biotech set out to show that its premise was sound for the larger and healthier population of CKD patients.

Could Higher Doses of EPO Increase Patients' Lifespans as Well as Corporate Profits?

No one knew what the optimum goal was for treatment of anemia in patients with kidney disease not needing dialysis. Kidney guideline groups, including those sponsored by the National Kidney Foundation, made suggestions of hemoglobin concentration goals between 11.0 and 12.0 or 13.0 g/dL, but these were not usually based on the hard evidence provided by randomized clinical trials. Hemoglobin concentration is often estimated as one-third of the hematocrit. For instance, a hemoglobin concentration of 13 g/dL roughly corresponds to a hematocrit of about 39%. Guidelines, especially in this field, were based primarily on conjectures regarding quality of life and mostly derived from observational studies rather than the gold standard of randomized controlled clinical trials. The relationships between hemoglobin levels and quality of life assessments were really uncertain because of differences in methods used to assess patients' perceptions, different characteristics of the populations studied, and the different scientific study designs used in different research projects. And none of the previous studies could systematically evaluate adverse effects, including importantly, death.

The Correction of Hemoglobin and Outcomes in Renal Insufficiency
(CHOIR) study was designed to test the results of treatment of anemia in CKD
patients not treated with dialysis with two hemoglobin goals: one close to that
of normal people and one closer to the guidelines put forth by various kidney
disease advocacy groups. The CHOIR study would assess all pertinent CKD
patient outcomes related to the treatment of anemia, including survival. Dr
William F. Owen Jr., a young nephrologist at the Brigham and Women's Hospital, had participated in key observational research studies while at Harvard. He
had published an important paper in the *NEJM* in 1993, showing survival of
dialysis patients was related to their nutritional status as well as the dose of
dialysis provided to them.[38] Owen contributed to the initial planning and development of a protocol for a study of erythropoietin treatment of anemic CKD
patients supported by Ortho Biotech. Dr. Ajay Singh was a nephrologist at the
Brigham and Women's Hospital in Boston, who took charge of the CHOIR study
after Bill Owen left Harvard to assume leadership positions at the University of
Medicine and Dentistry of New Jersey. Singh trained in medicine at University
College London School of Medicine, and undertook fellowship training in
nephrology at the Tufts–New England Medical Center in 1987, joining the faculty thereafter. In 1998, he joined the faculty of the Brigham and Women's Hospital as clinical director of the Renal Division and director of Dialysis Services.
He was appointed associate professor of medicine at Harvard Medical School.

The world had changed. Instead of hematocrit, hemoglobin concentration
was now the gold standard for the assessment of treatment of anemia trials.
The CHOIR study set out to show cardiovascular complications and death rates
would be lower in CKD patients treated with recombinant erythropoietin to
achieve a hemoglobin level of 13.5 g/dL (corresponding to a hematocrit of about
40.5%) than those treated to a goal hemoglobin concentration of 11.3 g/dL. For
the study, 1,432 patients were enrolled at 130 sites, with many of the U.S.'s most
well-known clinical nephrologists collaborating with colleagues in private
practices. Enrolled patients had to have anemia, with hemoglobin concentrations below 11.0 g/dL, and estimated glomerular filtration rates (eGFR) ranging
from 15 to 50 mL/min/1.73m^2.

The study started swimmingly, with recruitment on target, and the
prompt achievement of a separation between the average hemoglobin levels of

the two groups. Average hemoglobin levels increased about 2.5 g/dL in the high goal group, about 25%, compared with 1.2 g/dL in the comparison group, or about 12%, a highly statistically significant difference, just as planned. The high hemoglobin group needed an average of about twice as much erythropoietin a week compared to the comparison group, a difference that was also significant. The study, however, was ended early by its Data and Safety Monitoring Board, because there was little chance the high hemoglobin group would have better outcomes than the less aggressively treated patients. The results were reported at the American Society of Nephrology meeting in November 2006 and in the *NEJM* in the December 16, 2006, issue.[39] At the time the study was stopped, patients in the high hemoglobin group were 34% more likely to have experienced one of the adverse events, death or a cardiovascular disease, that were the study outcomes. There were practically no differences between the perceptions of quality of life at the end of the study between patients in the high and low hemoglobin groups. The patients in the low hemoglobin group, contrary to expectations, had improvement in only one of the many quality of life measures assessed. That finding was one of the only significant results of the study, but there were no comparable beneficial effects in the high hemoglobin group. This result, a study stopped early by its oversight group, because of ill effects in the high goal group, was startlingly similar to the outcome of the Besarab study of hemodialysis patients almost a decade earlier. And you couldn't say that although the risk might be greater, patients treated to higher hemoglobin goals had better quality of life. The quality of life figures in the low and high groups were almost identical. So, insurers would be paying more for more hospitalizations and deaths for an equal quality of life if they endorsed more intensive treatment of anemia in patients with kidney disease. The study was supported "by Ortho Biotech Clinical Affairs, and Johnson and Johnson Pharmaceutical Research and Development, both subsidiaries of Johnson and Johnson." The paper noted that Dr. Singh and other investigators had received consulting fees and other support from the sponsors, but in the case of a study that did not support more extensive drug treatment, that might be forgiven.

Meanwhile, the Europeans had an equal say in the matter. Dr. Tilman Drüeke, a respected nephrologist from Paris, France, based at the famous Necker Hospital, a center for research on the kidney for decades with a long-standing interest in the bone disease and anemia of kidney failure, led the Cardiovascular Risk Reduction by Early Anemia Treatment with Epoetin Beta (CREATE) study, a European trial quite similar to the CHOIR study. The results of CREATE were published in the same *NEJM* issue as the CHOIR study results.[40] CREATE was designed to see if a high hemoglobin goal (13.0 to 15.0 g/dL) in CKD patients not dependent on dialysis would lower the incidence of cardiovascular disease compared to similar patients treated to more modest targets (hemoglobin concentrations of 10.5 to 11.5 g/dL). For the study, 650 patients were enrolled, and 226 patients completed the trial in the high dose arm, while 250 finished the study assigned to the lower doses. Erythropoietin was supplied as epoetin beta (NeoRecormon) by F. Hoffman–La Roche. The initial estimated GFR of patients was about 24.5 mL/min (using the Cockcroft Gault formula) and the average baseline hemoglobin concentration was 11.6 g/dL. There was no difference in the incidence of cardiovascular events or mortality between the two groups. The decrement of renal function was similar in the groups as well, although more patients randomized to the high hemoglobin group needed to start dialysis. Perception of quality of life improved in the high hemoglobin group compared with those treated to lower goals, but the high group experienced more hypertension and headaches. The authors concluded, "Thus, the CREATE study adds direct evidence to confirm the current best practice guidelines, which recommend partial correction of anemia and not routine normalization of hemoglobin levels." They reported the study was supported by F. Hoffmann–La Roche and that several of the lead authors had accepted grant support and consulting and lecture fees from the sponsor.

An editorial regarding these two large, important studies by esteemed nephrologists Giuseppe Remuzzi and Julie Ingelfinger was published in the same *NEJM* issue.[41] Dr. Remuzzi, an Italian nephrologist, was famous for studies of clotting in patients with renal failure and for the intensive study of kidney diseases associated with blood disorders. He was on the *Journal*'s editorial board. Dr. Ingelfinger was a pediatric nephrologist at the Massachusetts General Hospital, and a deputy editor of the *Journal*. The editorial pulled no punches.

Taken together, these two studies suggest caution in the full correction of anemia in patients with chronic kidney disease. Currently, there are several additional multicenter trials of complete as compared with partial correction of anemia in patients with chronic kidney disease; Dr. Remuzzi is participating in one of them. Although we need more information about the ideal target level and should consider the present guidelines incomplete, it seems wisest to refrain from complete correction of anemia in persons with chronic kidney disease.

The *Journal* noted, "Dr. Remuzzi reports receiving lecture fees from Abbott, Sanofi-Aventis, and AstraZeneca. No other potential conflict of interest relevant to this article was reported." The editorial sounded the death knell for high doses of erythropoietin, high levels of iron repletion, and normalization of hemoglobin in CKD patients with anemia. The next year would be a busy year for industry, for researchers in the field of treatment of anemia with erythropoietin in patients with kidney disease, for Congress, and for the FDA. Consideration of the Medicare payment structures for erythropoietin would be at the forefront of discussions.

Patients, Payments, and Profits

In 2006 the typical reimbursement rate for a hemodialysis treatment was about $130, and administration of 1,000 units of erythropoietin was paid at $9.45.

In January 2007, *NEJM* national correspondent Dr. Robert Steinbrook reviewed the complex interactions between the Medicare payment system for dialysis and erythropoietin treatments, and patient outcomes.[42] He highlighted that in

2005, the ESRD program covered about 390,000 beneficiaries and spent $7.9 billion for dialysis services, including $2.9 billion for medications that are reimbursed separately. Epoetin alfa accounted for $2 billion of this spending and was the highest-expenditure drug in all of Medicare Part B.

Dialysis facilities can make more money from administering epoetin than from dialysis and related routine services, which Medicare has reimbursed at a composite rate since 1983. Monthly spending per patient for epoetin has soared to about half that for dialysis, which has remained relatively flat.

Steinbrook noted that Congress might reconsider the Medicare payment schemes for dialysis and associated administered drugs to reduce costs and discourage excessive use of erythropoietin, consistent with medical recommendations for patient safety. Steinbrook quoted a letter from Representatives Bill Thomas and Pete Stark to the Centers for Medicare and Medicaid Services (CMS) stating, "We are deeply concerned that the current CMS policy is not aggressive enough to stem the systemic abuse of [epoetin alfa], resulting in costs to taxpayers and potential health dangers to patients." Steinbrook pointed out that on "November 16, 2006, the day the CHOIR study was published, the FDA issued a public health advisory to 'underscore the importance of following the currently approved prescribing information' by raising hemoglobin levels no higher than 12 g per deciliter." Steinbrook reported

> Medicare's spending on epoetin reflects the reimbursement rate, the frequency of administration, the dose, and the monitoring policy for epoetin use, which the CMS revised in 2006. Also in 2006, the CMS set payment levels for drugs that are billable separately under Medicare Part B, which covers physician services and hospital outpatient services, at the average sales price plus 6%. In October 2006, the reimbursement rate for epoetin was $9.45 per 1000 units. Patients undergoing dialysis typically receive injections at nearly every treatment; Medicare beneficiaries who required dialysis averaged about 10.5 administrations per month in the first half of 2006, and the average dose was about 7500 units.

Steinbrook quoted testimony suggesting that as long as dialysis facilities "receive a separate payment for each administration of each [separately billable] drug and the payment exceeds the costs of acquiring the drug, an incentive remains to use more of these drugs than necessary." Steinbrook explained contemporary Medicare monitoring policy required dialysis providers and others to reduce the erythropoietin dose by 25% if the hematocrit of the patient was greater than 39% (roughly corresponding to a hemoglobin concentration of 13.0 g/dL), in addition to reducing the payment. Steinbrook reported that Ways and Means Committee members objected to the CMS policy because the outlined targets exceeded those recommended by the FDA. Steinbrook noted that the Government Accounting Office recommended extending bundled payments to include the costs of the administration of commonly prescribed drugs, to limit overprescription of erythropoietin, both to promote patient safety as well as to control costs. Steinbrook wrote that creation of a new payment bundle would be challenging, and that reimbursements would have to acknowledge that the costs of caring for sicker ESRD patients treated with dialysis had to be considered. He ended the article by pointing out that a new bundled system for dialysis payments had been required of CMS in 2006 by legislation but that such a plan had not yet been released.

On March 9, 2007, in response to the release of the CHOIR and CREATE studies, the FDA issued a "black box" alert, a warning regarding the treatment of patients with chronic kidney disease with erythropoiesis-stimulating agents, such as Epogen, Procrit, and Aranesp.

WARNINGS: INCREASED MORTALITY, SERIOUS
CARDIOVASCULAR and THROMBOEMBOLIC EVENTS, and
TUMOR PROGRESSION
Renal failure: Patients experienced greater risks for death and serious cardiovascular events when administered erythropoiesis-stimulating agents (ESAs) to target higher versus lower hemoglobin levels (13.5 vs. 11.3 g/dL; 14 vs. 10 g/dL) in two clinical studies. Individualize dosing to achieve and maintain hemoglobin levels within the range of 10 to 12 g/dL.

Mae Thamer, Yi Zhang, James Kaufman, Dennis Cotter, Fan Dong, and Miguel Hernán published a paper in *JAMA* in April 2007,[43] continuing the investigations previously made by Cotter's MTPPI, into the relationship of profit status of dialysis units and prescription of erythropoietin. They noted that since "1991, epoetin payment has been based on the amount of drug administered, creating a financial incentive for increased use of this therapy."

They pointed out that Medicare payments for erythropoietin for dialysis patients amounted to $1.8 billion and that this sum accounted for 11% of all ESRD costs. They summarized their findings at the end of the paper.

> Our results indicate that facility ownership and chain status have a strong effect on epoetin dosing practice patterns. Compared with other facility types, we found that large for-profit chains administered higher epoetin doses, used higher dose increases, and had higher achieved hematocrit levels, as well as a larger proportion of patients above the upper limit of hematocrit level (target of 36% was recommended by the National Kidney Foundation and the US Food and Drug Administration during the time of our study). Our adjusted analyses suggest that the differences in epoetin dose levels among dialysis chains are not explained by differences in patient characteristics or responsiveness to epoetin therapy....
>
> ... These findings suggest that reimbursement policy and clinical performance measures may provide incentives for dialysis facilities, in particular for-profit facilities, to target hematocrit levels exceeding those recommended by the clinical guidelines. As existing guidelines are reevaluated, it will be important for policy makers to design an epoetin reimbursement policy that provides an incentive to achieve desired clinical outcomes while optimizing epoetin usage.

The authors concluded, "Dialysis facility organizational status and ownership are associated with variation in epoetin dosing in the United States. Different epoetin dosing patterns suggest that large for-profit chain facilities used larger dose adjustments and targeted higher hematocrit levels." Besides the profit motive, the investigators implicated policy incentives that promoted practice patterns perhaps not in the best interests of patients or taxpayers. In search of higher profits with higher EPO prescriptions, were dialysis corporations putting their patients at risk, while costing the federal government more money?

In the same April 2007 issue of *JAMA*, Dr. Daniel W. Coyne, a well-known nephrologist at the School of Medicine of Washington University in St. Louis, provided editorial comment on the Thamer paper.[44] Coyne had received a bachelor's degree in chemistry from St. Louis University and then graduated from the medical school at Case Western Reserve University. He finished his residency in internal medicine at Emory University and completed his fellowship training in nephrology at Washington University in St. Louis. Thereafter, he remained on the faculty of the university's medical school. Coyne had become a critic of guideline-driven practices in nephrology and industry conflicts of interest in patient care. (Coyne's focus on conflict of interest between researchers, clinicians, and commercial entities brings up memories of Bud Relman and his indictment of the medical-industrial complex.) Coyne noted that the MTPPI paper was timely in light of the recent "US Food and Drug Administration (FDA) advisory warning that epoetin and darbepoetin (erythropoiesis stimulating agents [ESAs]) result in 'an increased number of deaths and of non-fatal heart attacks, strokes, heart failure, and blood clots when ESAs were adjusted to maintain ... hemoglobin more than 12 g/dL.' The FDA recommends using just enough ESA to maintain the lowest hemoglobin level necessary to avoid the need for transfusions and ensure hemoglobin level does not exceed 12 g/dL." Coyne reviewed the RCTs that could not show survival benefits associated with higher erythropoietin doses or hemoglobin targets as well as observational studies suggesting benefits of therapy for ESRD patients that were not borne out by national treatment or mortality statistics. Coyne pointed out that nephrologists might, perhaps unwittingly, sign standard orders crafted by dialysis organizations designed to maximize EPO doses. Coyne noted the potential profit that might accrue to dialysis organizations associated with prescription of higher doses of erythropoietin. His assessment of the situation and the pertinent economics was blunt.

Epoetin is profitable for dialysis facilities. The 2 largest dialysis chains in the United States reported in their 2006 annual reports filed with the Securities and Exchange Commission that 21% to 25% of their revenue was from epoetin. Epoetin is reimbursed by Medicare at 6% above the average sales price. In addition, contractual agreements with Amgen provide rebates to facilities and chains for growth in epoetin purchases and in patient outcomes, which could potentially include achieving a high percentage of patients at hemoglobin levels higher than 11 g/dL. Chief medical officers have clear conflicts of interest because they generally own stock in the company and directly or indirectly influence anemia management policies. Dialysis chains also may provide to their employees bonuses or other payments tied to certain employee-specific "outcome" performance, and generally tied to the financial performance of the corporation. The significant dependence of dialysis providers on epoetin for income, and the ease at which a higher hemoglobin target affords greater epoetin use, creates a tempting situation for all involved.

Coyne also raised the issue of potential conflict of interest on the part of medical organizations making treatment recommendations. He implicated advocacy groups that produced clinical practice guidelines, such as the National Kidney Foundation, as having accepted contributions from pharmaceutical companies and large dialysis organizations, perhaps preventing them from being unbiased. Coyne ended his editorial stating physicians "need to challenge industries that appear to be using patients as profit centers based on bad science." Interestingly Coyne's financial disclosures included "being or has been a consultant/advisor to Abbott, Amgen, Roche, and Watson; a speaker for Abbott, Amgen, Merck, Watson, and the National Kidney Foundation; and a research investigator funded by Abbott, Advanced Magnetics, Amgen, Genentech, Roche, and Watson." And Coyne continued to be a participant in industry-supported studies of the treatment of anemia in patients with CKD and ESRD. Coyne was functioning as a kind of whistleblower. The editorial dialogue illustrates how difficult it is to find completely unbiased umpires in this field where medicine and industry are so intertwined. Interactions between medical researchers, industry, and policymakers could potentially become a problem for both science and industry. Resolution of conflict of interest in evaluation of new drugs is a key issue for the Food and Drug Administration. An old adage is "where there's no conflict, there's no interest." And vice versa.

Two articles published in the *NEJM* on June 14, 2007, added to the feeding frenzy regarding the possible dangers of treating sick patients with erythropoietin. Fadlo R. Khuri, M.D., of the Emory Winship Cancer Institute in

Atlanta, Georgia, wrote in a Perspectives article that appeared shortly after the black box warning regarding erythropoietin treatment of patients with kidney disease was released that the Oncology Drug Advisory Committee of the FDA had met to consider the possible adverse effects of erythropoietin in cancer patients with anemia, including blood clots, tumor growth, and patient mortality.[45] The author noted that several RCTs of treatment with erythropoietin in such patients showed reduced survival in the erythropoietin groups. The FDA had released a black box warning regarding the treatment of patients with cancer with erythropoietin in March 2007. Dr. Robert Steinbrook, national correspondent for the *Journal*, reported on the FDA "alert" issued on March 9, 2007, regarding treatment with erythropoietin.[46] He noted that in 2004, epoetin ranked first in Medicare Part B expenditures for drugs (with darbepoetin coming in second), but that in 2005 darbepoetin was placed first and epoetin second. Steinbrook emphasized that the Medicare reimbursement for these drugs was 106% of the average sales price rather than taking advantage of the widely available discounts offered to providers. An article entitled "Doctors Reaping Millions for Use of Anemia Drugs" by Alex Berenson and Andrew Pollack in the *New York Times* on May 9, 2007, had made the issue clear to the nonscientific reader just shortly before the articles appeared in the *NEJM*.

Putting Profits Ahead of Patients?

The controversy regarding target hematocrit, patient safety, and financial incentives continued in other venues. On June 26, 2007, a hearing took place in Congress, under the auspices of the House of Representatives Subcommittee on Health of the Committee on Ways and Means to address "ensuring kidney patients receive safe and appropriate anemia management care." Amgen, Kidney Care Partners, the National Renal Administrators Association, the Renal Support Network, and the Research Utilization Project Proposal all submitted statements to the subcommittee. In printed comments, Chairman Stark stated,

> My priority for Medicare ESRD policy is to ensure patient safety while also protecting taxpayers from unnecessary expenditures. . . . Health risks associated with higher doses and well-documented flaws in a

payment system that encourages higher dosing highlights that this issue is ripe for reexamination. We must do better for our ESRD beneficiaries and for the taxpayers.

At the hearing Stark noted:

First, we must put patient safety first. We'll hear from the FDA that when anti-anemia drugs are used to raise red blood cell levels above a certain threshold there's a risk of death, blood clots, strokes, heart failure and heart attacks. We need to keep this in mind as we're dealing with populations that are more vulnerable to these conditions.

Second, we're stewards of taxpayers' dollars. The current Medicare reimbursement system creates incentives for higher dosing of ESAs, which lead not only to the aforementioned health risks, but also come at a higher cost to taxpayers and beneficiaries.

The Office of the Inspector General will present their new report, released today, documenting that large dialysis organizations make a profit on each and every dose of Epogen. Recent research published in *JAMA* shows that for-profit dialysis centers dose Epogen at higher levels than not-for-profit centers. The payment system leads to perverse incentives that we cannot ignore. . . .

. . . This announcement proves however that there are additional efficiencies that can be gained by reducing Epogen doses. Clearly what I've been saying all along is true. The industry only responds when we threaten to do the right thing and remove their incentive to inflate doses as a way to reap profits. Medicare can be a better purchaser of care for dialysis beneficiaries and can do so in a way that ensures more efficient use of ESAs and better health outcomes for beneficiaries.

A report from the Government Accounting Office, entitled "Medicare Should Pay a Bundled Rate for all ESRD Items and Services," was appended to the documentation of the hearing, as well as a report from the NIDDK, using information from the USRDS documenting that the use of erythropoietin in dialysis patients had increased over the years. Testimony from John K. Jenkins,

M.D., director of the Office of New Drugs at the Center for Drug Evaluation and Research at the FDA, suggested that clinical guidelines for administration of erythropoietin used by DaVita, a large dialysis organization, were not consistent with FDA recommendations.

Ajay K. Singh, M.D., the director of dialysis services at the Brigham and Women's Hospital who had led the CHOIR study, addressed three issues in his testimony at the hearings: the target hemoglobin in kidney disease patients, the "extensive off-label use and over utilization" of erythropoietin, and bundling payments for ESRD services. Singh full-throatedly supported the FDA alert "that a hemoglobin level should be maintained to less than 12 grams per deciliter." Singh quoted Cotter's recently published *JAMA* paper, which documented "overuse of Epoetin in for-profit dialysis chains as compared to not-for-profit chains." Singh offered explanations for this finding, including "flaws in the current CMS reimbursement system" that encouraged overuse, and "use of standing orders that are based on corporate guidelines in dialysis facilities." Singh stated,

> I believe bundling of drugs such as ESAs will remove incentives for overtreatment. It will reduce the escalating cost for injectable drugs. It will encourage the use of subcutaneous administration of Epoetin, a practice which is widely utilized in the Veteran Administration system [and] in Kaiser, and is certainly the case in Canada and other European countries.
>
> . . . . And, finally, I believe that if bundling takes some time, CMS should modify its reimbursement policy so that the current over utilization that has accrued since and higher hemoglobin levels above 39 that have occurred since April 2006 gets corrected.

Singh had gone from being a researcher supported by biotech companies, to a public health advocate, presumably as a result of his own research endeavors. Alan S. Kliger, M.D., a clinical professor of medicine at Yale University School of Medicine, and chairman of the Department of Medicine at the Hospital of St. Raphael in New Haven, Connecticut, emphasized that "I'm an employee of a not-for-profit hospital, and for the record, I'm not in the employ of any drug companies or other commercial enterprises. I'm also President of the Renal Physicians Association, the professional organization of nephrologists, whose goals are to ensure that patients suffering from kidney disease receive the best care delivered under the highest standards of medical practice." Kliger pointed out, as did the executive director of the American Association of Kidney Patients (AAKP), that individual patients might need higher hematocrits to feel well or to function adequately and that such situations should be resolved by communication within the doctor/patient relationship. He noted that profits from erythropoietin prescriptions did not accrue to the physicians who worked in dialysis units. During later testimony, Dr. Kliger generally agreed with the positions taken by Dr. Singh.

Leslie V. Norwalk, the acting administrator of the Centers for Medicare and Medicaid Services, who had spoken before the physicians, testified:

> Shortly we will release a report to Congress on the elements and features of such a payment system for ESRD. Today I want to highlight some of the major design issues in an ESRD bundled payment system and also talk about the use of ESAs. In contrast to our current system, which pays separately for drugs and encourages their use, a bundled PPS [prospective payment system] would focus on appropriate delivery of the full range of ESRD services. Such a PPS would change the incentives for ESA use, potentially eliminating their overpromotion and overdosing and could obviate the need for a specific monitoring policy targeting ESA utilization, and with a collection of measures facilitate a broader focus on quality. An ESRD bundled PPS would establish a fixed payment amount for a set of services furnished to a patient in an ESRD facility. The PPS would give facilities flexibility of managing ESRD patient care and eliminate incentives that have led to the overutilization of some medications.

Really, Can't We Give CKD Patients Higher Doses of Erythropoietin-Stimulating Agents?

But the industry couldn't take this lying down. In a last hurrah, about three years after the publication of the results from the CHOIR and CREATE studies, in November 2009, results of the Trial to Reduce Cardiovascular Events with Aranesp Therapy (TREAT) trial, sponsored by Amgen, were published in the *NEJM*.[47] The rationale for TREAT was to demonstrate that in patients with type 2 diabetes mellitus and CKD who had anemia, increasing hemoglobin levels would lower rates of death, cardiovascular events, and progression of disease to ESRD. This was despite findings from the CREATE and CHOIR trials, which did not show such salutary outcomes.

Erslev had pointed out in his 1991 review that the erythropoietin molecule had carbohydrate (glycosyl) side chains attached to its main amino acid structure.[48] Scientists speculated that the number and type of glycosyl side chains might affect the body's metabolism of erythropoietin. Perhaps extra glycosyl side chains would impede erythropoietin's metabolism and breakdown, allowing an erythropoietin molecule to have a longer half-life in a patient's body. A longer drug half-life (due to the extra side chains) could be associated with longer times between administration of medicines, perhaps once a week rather than three times a week. Patients might really appreciate a schedule of less-frequent drug-dosing, especially if the medication was administered by inconvenient injections under the skin. For a drug company with a patent on an erythropoietin drug, such a modification might lead to a new drug, a new patent, and FDA approval for a new but similar agent, allowing the period of sales exclusivity to be extended and profits to be maximized. Amgen had produced just such a drug, darbepoetin. If Amgen developed a new, effective, erythropoietin agent, perhaps with a better dosing profile, which was more acceptable to patients, it could recapture the market that it had ceded to Ortho Biotech more than a decade before. Amgen could market such a drug to the nondialysis-dependent CKD population, and to other patients with anemia as well, such as those with cancer or HIV infection. Aranesp, a novel erythropoiesis-stimulating protein (NESP), was approved by the FDA in September 2001, for use in patients with chronic renal failure and for those with ESRD treated with dialysis. In March 2006, Aranesp, the trade name for darbepoetin, was approved for the treatment of anemia in patients with cancer who experienced anemia while receiving chemotherapy. Its clinical utility in CKD patients was tested in the TREAT study.

Once again, TREAT was a large, international trial, in which many leading kidney and cardiovascular disease experts participated as investigators. The authors maintained a key limitation of previous erythropoietin therapy trials in patients with kidney disease was the lack of placebo-treated patients, hampering the ability of investigators to discern true drug effects. TREAT was a well-designed, randomized, placebo-controlled double-blind study, the gold standard for clinical trials, in an important, vulnerable population, patients with both diabetes and chronic kidney disease. TREAT randomized more than 4,000 patients with diabetes and chronic kidney disease, not treated with dialysis, half to darbepoetin to achieve hemoglobin concentrations of 13 g/dL and half to placebo, with some drug administration allowed if hemoglobin concentrations fell below 9 g/dL in the placebo group. The investigators determined rates of death, heart attacks, congestive heart failure, development of ESRD, strokes, or hospitalizations for acute lack of blood flow to the heart in the two groups.

The investigators achieved rapid and sustained differences in the hemoglobin levels between the two groups, which overall had similar clinical characteristics at baseline. There was a modest effect to improve fatigue and to decrease transfusion rates in patients treated with darbepoetin. Most of the quality of life indicators assessed in the study were not different between the two groups at the end of the trial. Although there were no differences in rates of death, heart attacks, congestive heart failure, or ESRD, strokes were almost twice as likely in the patients treated with darbepoetin. The authors concluded that treatment of moderate anemia in patients with CKD with darbepoetin did not reduce the risk of death, cardiovascular disease, or development of ESRD, and there was an associated "increased risk of stroke. For many persons involved in clinical decision making, this risk will outweigh the potential benefits."

In 2010, the *NEJM* published a new analysis of the TREAT study.[49] The investigators, supported by Amgen, evaluated adverse events in the participants in the trial according to their ability to respond to darbepoetin. They noted that a poor initial response to the drug was associated with a higher rate of subsequent death or development of new cardiovascular complications during the trial. The investigators admitted that they could not establish the mechanisms underlying the findings. It was unclear if poor outcomes were related to patient factors or dose of Aranesp. The authors couldn't determine if the sickest patients were less likely to respond to the drug or if the higher doses of darbepoetin used in these patients caused bad outcomes. The investigators, however, raised important questions regarding the whole notion of hemoglobin targets for patients with kidney disease and anemia that unfortunately could not be answered by the information generated by the trial. They concluded the "findings raise concern about current target-based strategies for treating anemia in patients with chronic kidney disease."

The Government Revises the Rules

In January 2010, the *NEJM* published a paper by Drs. Ellis Unger, Aliza Thompson, Melanie Blank, and Robert Temple, all physicians employed by the FDA, entitled "Erythropoiesis-Stimulating Agents—Time for a Reevaluation."[50] Such a paper, by federal officials, usually has the imprimatur of policy. The authors reviewed the history of the original studies of erythropoietin treatment in patients with anemia and renal disease, as well as the Normal Hematocrit Trial and the CHOIR, CREATE, and TREAT trials. The FDA was concerned about two main possible pathways through which high-dose ESA treatments and high hemoglobin goals might be associated with poor patient outcomes. Healthier patients may have had a better response to ESAs, needing lower drug doses, leaving the sicker, or more-EPO resistant patients to treatment with higher doses. Also, rapid increases in hemoglobin levels may have led to blood vessel and organ injury. The officials also outlined a third possibility in their critical analysis of the results from the Besarab and CHOIR studies.

> During a review of the marketing application for darbepoetin alfa, an association was found between rates of increase in the hemoglobin level exceeding 1 g per deciliter per 2-week period and the risk of cardiovascular and thromboembolic events. This observation provided the basis for a warning on the label for darbepoetin alfa (and eventually a stronger warning on the label for epoetin alfa) regarding excessive rates of increase in hemoglobin concentrations. Subsequently, the FDA found a similar relationship between such excessive rates of increase and the risk of adverse cardiovascular events in analyses of data from the

Normal Hematocrit Study and the CHOIR trial. A third possibility is that the adverse cardiovascular events are not related to hemoglobin concentrations at all but are instead due to some off-target effect of ESAs—for example, trophic effects on vascular endothelial or smooth muscle cells, or conditions precipitated by higher exposure to ESAs (e.g., iron deficiency). We have already found one such effect—the ability of ESAs to enhance tumor progression and shorten survival in patients with some types of cancer.

The FDA physicians reviewed that the agency had to modify the original hemoglobin goals of the TREAT study in 2004 (before the publication of the results of CHOIR) since they were too high. "The FDA allowed the trial to proceed only after working with Amgen to develop conservative dosing and monitoring schemes to limit overshoots of the hemoglobin target, oscillations in the concentration, and rapid rates of increase and only after ensuring that there would be oversight by an independent data and safety monitoring committee.... Despite these measures, the TREAT investigators documented adverse consequences of using an ESA to raise hemoglobin levels." The FDA officials noted, "Clearly, the trials did not yield convincing evidence of any consistent quality-of-life benefit that would appear to outweigh the increased risks of nonfatal myocardial infarction, nonfatal stroke, and death. What the Normal Hematocrit Study, the CHOIR trial, and TREAT do show, however, is that hemoglobin-concentration targets of 14.0, 13.5, and 13.0 g per deciliter—and the ESA regimens used to achieve them—are harmful." The FDA officials concluded by acknowledging that "modest" increases in hemoglobin concentrations in anemic kidney diseases patients might be "beneficial," and called for randomized controlled trials that would establish optimal, presumably lower hemoglobin targets "well below 12 g per deciliter."

In addition, EPO-resistant patients were a cash cow. Payment policies paradoxically encouraged physicians and dialysis organizations to give higher and higher doses of ESAs to patients who were not going to respond to the treatments. The government, at many different loci, appeared to be fed up with the marketing and prescription of drugs that led to the achievement of higher hemoglobin levels in patients than were indicated by guidelines, than were necessary, that could not be shown to improve quality of life in correlation with hemoglobin levels, that were harmful, and that cost taxpayers inordinate amounts of money. It would be neither cynical nor uncharitable to wonder whether the government, because of its remuneration policies, had perhaps been paying biotech companies and dialysis organizations to encourage harmful outcomes in ESRD patients to achieve higher profits. CMS went on with a clear goal to eliminate incentives to higher ESA dosing and to establish a new approach to paying for dialysis therapy and erythropoiesis-stimulating agents.

On July 26, 2010, CMS released a "fact sheet" entitled "New Bundled Prospective Payment System for End-stage Renal Disease Facilities Designed to Promote Efficient Care and Improve Patient Outcomes," describing the final rule that had been issued by the agency on July 23. It took CMS more than three years after Ms. Norwalk's testimony to Representative Stark's committee to release its new policy. The fact sheet reviewed previous CMS reimbursement practices, noting 38% of dialysis payments were for injectable drugs, nonroutine laboratory tests, and other supplies and services. The fact sheet also outlined that the Medicare Improvements for Patients and Providers Act of 2008 (MIPPA) required CMS to develop a "bundled prospective payment system" in place of the "composite rate payment methodology." The fact sheet announced that a new bundled Prospective Payment System (PPS) for facilities that provided "renal dialysis services and home dialysis" to Medicare beneficiaries with ESRD had been created. CMS would make a single payment to facilities for each dialysis, which included the treatment as well as the administration of ESAs, iron, and vitamin D analogues. Adjustments in payment would be made for patient characteristics such as age, body surface area, and body mass index, as well as some coexisting conditions, but not for the sex or race of the patient. Adjustments were provided for pediatric ESRD patients, as well as for dialysis facilities providing fewer treatments and in certain geographic locations and for facilities caring for patients with certain clinical characteristics. The base rate for a dialysis treatment would now be $229.63. The payment included "non-routine laboratory services and all ESRD-related part B drugs and their equivalent forms covered under Part D." The fact sheet justified the amount of the new reimbursement in detail. The base rate would be updated annually. The rule also created a Quality Incentive Program (QIP) that would link payments to a facility's performance standards. Performance measures would include measurement of the dose of dialysis provided to each patient and parameters related to each patient's anemia management, assessed by hemoglobin concentrations. The QIP was lauded in the fact sheet as "the first pay-for-performance program in a Medicare fee-for-service payment system." The new system would become effective January 1, 2011. Succinctly, CMS had converted the treatment of dialysis patients with ESAs from profit centers to cost centers. The bundle payment for 2023 was $265.57.

Rise of the ESAs—Medical Advances or Me Too Drugs?

Were erythropoietin congeners the only drugs that could stimulate erythropoiesis (RBC synthesis) in patients with kidney disease? New, effective drugs that enhanced erythropoiesis (the newly termed erythropoiesis-stimulating agents, or ESAs) could result in new patents and indications for treatment in target populations that could benefit the bottom line of pharmaceutical and biotech companies. Hoffman–La Roche produced methoxy-polyethylene glycol-epoetin beta (Mircera), called a continuous erythropoietin receptor activator (CERA), and obtained approval for its use in patients in Europe, and then in the U.S., in 2007. By adding methoxy polyethylene glycol butanoic acid side chains to an erythropoietin backbone (as Erslev had anticipated), the drug lasted longer and could be sold as a new, perhaps more expensive product, if patents on epoetin alfa expired.

Affymaz and Takeda Pharmaceutical developed another, new substance to perform the job erythropoietin and its modified descendants had accomplished over approximately the previous decade and a half. In another triumph of biology, using "phage display technology," small peptides (short strings of amino acids) could be identified that bound to the erythropoietin receptor. In other words, small protein fragments, not related to erythropoietin, using specialized scientific techniques, were found that could mimic the action of the natural hormone. A peptide was identified that did not have the same amino acid sequences as natural erythropoietin, but bound to the EPO receptor in a manner similar to human EPO. In a secondary step, making a synthetic peptide in an industrial laboratory and artificially adding polyethylene glycol side chains to the amino acid structure resulted in a compound that stimulated RBC production in cellular systems just as erythropoietin did. And that compound could be marketed as a new drug.

Peginesatide was a peptide (rather than a natural protein) that had an amino acid sequence unrelated to erythropoietin. A key feature of this manufactured molecule was the extra side chains (made of many units of polyethylene glycol [PEG]), which were added to its amino acid backbone. This technique is used fairly frequently by the biotech industry to increase the biologic half-life of drugs. If longer half-lives are achieved, they allow dosing to be relatively infrequent. In some cases such altered drugs may need to be administered only once a month.

In March 2012 peginesatide was approved by the FDA for treatment of anemia due to chronic kidney disease in adult patients treated with dialysis. As Omontys, it could be prescribed once a month to dialysis patients. In January 2013 the results of studies of peginesatide in anemic patients with ESRD treated with hemodialysis and in patients with CKD and anemia before the onset of ESRD were published in the *NEJM*.[51] Drs. Steven Fishbane, Anatole Besarab, and a group of distinguished international dialysis doctors reported that peginesatide taken once a month was "non-inferior" (technical clinical trials language for "about the same") to erythropoietin in maintaining hemoglobin concentrations in hemodialysis patients. In a companion article in the same issue of the *Journal*, Dr. Iain Macdougall, as first author (who was a coauthor on the dialysis paper) reported, in the PEARL study, similar increases in hemoglobin in 983 CKD patients achieved by once-a-month peginesatide or darbepoetin administered twice a month, with a goal hemoglobin concentration between 11 and 12 g/dL. Again, the effects of peginesatide on hemoglobin concentration were "non-inferior" to those in the darbepoetin group. However, patients treated with peginesatide were 32% more likely to experience death, unstable angina, or irregular heartbeats than the patients treated with darbepoetin in the studies. The authors concluded in the abstract that "cardiovascular events and mortality were increased with peginesatide in patients with chronic kidney disease who were not undergoing dialysis."

Tilman Drüeke, who led the CREATE trial, questioned in an accompanying editorial:

Is there any advantage of using peginesatide rather than the existing ESAs? Less frequent dosing may be an advantage under certain circumstances. . . . As with any new class of drugs, prolonged experience and monitoring are necessary. Another important issue is cost. At a time when the prescription of much cheaper, biologically similar ESAs is steadily growing outside the United States, expensive new drugs will be competitive only if proven to result in better patient outcomes. Such outcomes remain to be demonstrated for peginesatide and other new types of ESAs that are in development.[52]

Drüeke bluntly hit the nail on the head for readers of the *Journal* as well as physicians, regulators, policymakers, and perhaps patients. Cheaper and the same is better. The same and more expensive is not. In a population where drug administration is highly regulated, "me too" drugs must outperform their competitors and be of value to patients and insurers providing reimbursements.

Less than one year after the approval of peginesatide, a report of anaphylaxis (a severe allergic reaction culminating in shock and occasionally death) in dialysis patients treated with the drug was published in the *NEJM*.[53] Anaphylaxis had occurred in approximately 1.4 out of 1,000 patient treatments. On February 23, 2013, Affymax and Takeda announced that all lots of peginesatide on the market would be recalled. In June 2014 the manufacturers announced they would work with the FDA to withdraw the medication's New Drug Application.

Is There a New, Safe Way to Increase Hemoglobins and Profits in CKD Patients?

Another approach to increasing erythrocyte production in patients with kidney disease was to modify the cellular biologic systems that enhance erythropoietin synthesis or action. Drug companies had been working on these pathways for decades. Scientists knew, since at least the 1970s, that low levels of oxygen in the blood, known as hypoxia, were sensed by the kidney and induced the synthesis and release of erythropoietin. That's why people who live at high altitudes have high hematocrits, and why athletes train in places like Mexico City or Colorado Springs, to build up endurance and performance by increasing their RBC mass. A key question for corporations, scientists, physicians, and patients was, could a drug be fashioned that would mimic the effects of erythropoietin on the production of erythrocytes that would not raise the safety concerns intertwined with the use of ESAs?

As the system was explored, hypoxia-inducible factors (HIFs) appeared on the to-do lists of scientists and biotech companies. The initial basic studies of HIFs were reported in papers published as early as in the beginning of the 1990s and over the next decade.[54] William G. Kaelin Jr., Sir Peter J. Ratcliffe, and Gregg L. Semenza won the Nobel Prize in Physiology or Medicine in 2019 for their discovery of

> how cells can sense and adapt to changing oxygen availability. They identified molecular machinery that regulates the activity of genes in response to varying levels of oxygen.
>
> The seminal discoveries by this year's Nobel Laureates revealed the mechanism for one of life's most essential adaptive processes. They established the basis for our understanding of how oxygen levels affect cellular metabolism and physiological function. Their discoveries have also paved the way for promising new strategies to fight anemia, cancer and many other diseases.[55]

Hypoxia-inducible factors, and drugs that cause their production and release (activators) increase synthesis of erythropoietin but also facilitate the use of iron in biologic systems. Improving iron use could obviate the need for patients to receive intravenous iron supplements, which were being increasingly assessed for their own safety risks. Therefore, if a drug company could safely harness the twin benefits of erythropoietin production and improved iron availability, a useful medication with a better safety profile for patients with kidney disease and anemia could be marketed, engendering huge profits. One such set of substances, prolyl hydroxylase inhibitors, as HIF stabilizers, seemed to be attractive as drug candidates. The fact that they could be administered orally was also a great potential benefit.

From 2015 to 2016, Drs. Robert Provenzano, Anatole Besarab, and colleagues published a series of papers in *Nephrology Dialysis Transplantation*, *AJKD*, and *CJASN* on the treatment of anemic patients with CKD before the onset of ESRD, as well as dialysis patients, demonstrating the safety and efficacy of roxadustat.[56] The studies were supported by a biotech company, FibroGen Inc., of San Francisco, California.

In July 2019, the *NEJM* published online the results of a trial of roxadustat in dialysis patients with anemia who had previously been treated with erythropoietin.[57] Roxadustat is a hypoxia-inducible prolyl hydroxylase inhibitor that can be administered orally. For the study, 305 dialysis patients in China were randomized to be treated with either roxadustat or epoetin alfa for twenty-six weeks. The goal of the study was to see if the treatments were equivalent in achieving hemoglobin concentrations of 10 to 12 g/dL. To test this, researchers treated 204 patients with roxadustat and 101 with epoetin alfa. The increases in hemoglobin were similar in both groups. Patients treated with roxadustat had better indices of iron metabolism, while hypertension was more common in patients treated with epoetin. Patients in the roxadustat group had more episodes of abnormally high blood potassium levels and more respiratory infections. The study was funded by FibroGen and FibroGen (China) Medical Technology Development. A companion article on the treatment of anemic nondialysis-dependent CKD patients with roxadustat was published in the same issue of the *Journal*.[58]

In February 2020, FibroGen announced the FDA had accepted a new drug application for the use of roxadustat to treat anemia in nondialysis- and dialysis-dependent CKD patients. The company's partners worldwide were Astra-Zeneca and Astellas. The drug had already been approved for clinical use in Japan and China.

Concern, however, had been raised about the class of drugs and the design of the trials to assess the safety and effectiveness of the HIF stabilizers. The trials used "non-inferiority" designs, where the drug only had to demonstrate equivalence to the comparison group, not superiority. Disturbing safety signals were noted in some of the trials of roxadustat, and other HIF stablizers, related to the incidence of cardiovascular and blood clotting (or thrombotic) events in patients treated with the novel drugs. These drugs did not seem to convey a clear safety advantage compared to the older ESAs. In addition, although there may have been advantages of the HIF stabilizers, especially in peritoneal dialysis and home dialysis patients, now a focus because of the President's Executive Order of 2019, clinicians and scientists worried about the wisdom of fundamentally changing the biology of cellular systems of patients. Should the cells of patients be fooled, on an ongoing basis, into thinking that they have been deprived of oxygen? Is it possible that cellular systems, hoodwinked into believing that they are starved of oxygen, may initiate "death star" protocols, perhaps delayed in time, that will result in other, unknown adverse effects in patients? Long-term studies, such as the randomized controlled trials that showed high erythropoietin doses causing high hemoglobin concentrations were associated with mortality, would ultimately be required to evaluate the HIF stabilizers.

Finally, the admonition of Tilman Drüeke regarding the costs of equivalent therapies had to be considered. Of course, if any of the HIF stabilizers were to be approved for use in ESRD or CKD patients in the U.S., the price would be a key issue, to be balanced by patients, providers, and payers.

The FDA Considers a New Drug Class for Treatment of Anemia in CKD Patients

On July 15, 2021, the FDA Center for Drug Evaluation and Research (CDER) Cardiovascular and Renal Drugs Advisory Committee (with the unfortunate acronym of CRDAC) met to consider the new drug application for approval of roxadustat for the treatment of anemia in patients with chronic kidney disease.

The Roster of Advisors included cardiologists and clinical trialists, a biostatistician, and nephrologists.[59]

Julia B. Lewis, M.D., a nephrologist and professor of medicine in the Division of Nephrology at Vanderbilt Medical Center in Nashville, Tennessee, served as chairperson. She served in leadership positions in kidney disease scientific societies as well as participated in NIDDK-supported clinical trials in patients with kidney disease, and industry supported studies.

Paul T. Conway, of Falls Church, Virginia, a leader of the American Association of Kidney Patients, representing the community of people with kidney disease, served as a temporary voting member.

FDA Opening Remarks were delivered by Dr. Ellis Unger, a cardiologist.[60] Unger reviewed the history of the involvement of the FDA in the approvals of ESAs, and highlighted the salient issues related to the review of the roxadustat application. Unger revealed that he had been the FDA officer in charge of the application for approval of darbepoetin twenty years before. He made the point that the committee was there to evaluate the safety of the new drug. He noted that the studies were complex and that in nondialysis CKD patients, there had been more dropouts in the placebo arm, which made valid comparisons difficult. Unger noted, "With respect to the standard analyses of safety, there were greater rates of some important adverse events with roxadustat than even epoetin alfa, thrombotic events in particular."

Applicant presentations on behalf of FibroGen Inc. as well as its partner AstraZeneca were made by R. Wayne Frost, Pharm.D., J.D., senior vice president of regulatory affairs at FibroGen. Frost had had several successes in drug development. Frost called roxadustat "a novel, oral therapy to treat patients with anemia of CKD and the first major innovation in the management of this condition in 30 years. Patients with anemia of CKD need options beyond existing therapies." Frost emphasized the need for treatments for patients who were resistant to erythropoietin and who were on home dialysis therapies and needed oral medications to treat anemia to counteract the "unacceptable risk of red blood cell transfusion." Frost cited the Nobel Prize awarded about two years before to the investigators of hypoxia inducible factors and reviewed physiologic and pharmacologic aspects of the system. He stated the "CV safety profile of roxadustat was comparable to placebo in NDD (non-dialysis dependent CKD patients) and epoetin alfa in DD (dialysis dependent) and the general safety profile appears to be acceptable." Frost affirmed: "All external experts have been compensated for their time."

Roberto Pecoits-Filho, M.D., Ph.D., F.A.S.N., F.A.C.P., led off with a brief presentation on behalf of FibroGen on "Unmet Needs." He held leadership roles in the International Society of Nephrology and the Kidney Disease Improving Global Outcomes (KDIGO) group. Pecoits-Filho was a senior research scientist at Arbor Research Collaborative for Health in Ann Arbor, Michigan, and a professor at the School of Medicine, Pontifícia Universidade Católica do Paraná, in Brazil. Pecoits-Filho had studied and written papers on inflammation in patients with kidney disease as well as anemia in patients with CKD.

His presentation focused on the burden of anemia in patients with kidney disease, the current lack of therapeutic options for anemia, the need for new drugs to treat anemia, and the innovative, first-in-class nature of the drug to be considered in the day's proceedings. He reviewed the drug's beneficial effects on iron metabolism and the special benefits that might accrue to patients with erythropoietin resistance who were on home dialysis therapies and might prefer an oral medication. He noted that he had participated in some of the trials on CKD and anemia. He summarized—perhaps overdramatically—"my options to care for patients with CKD anemia, or CKD, are clearly insufficient, and sometimes non-existent. Physicians and patients would benefit from an oral therapy for anemia that promotes endogenous erythropoiesis, improves iron utilization, and offers a choice for ESA hyporesponders."

Lynda Szczech, M.D., M.S.C.E, presented the efficacy data on roxadustat for FibroGen. Szczech was the vice president for clinical development and medical affairs at FibroGen Inc. Szczech had held faculty positions at New York Medical College and Duke University School of Medicine and had served as the president of the National Kidney Foundation. Her research included seminal studies of the treatment of anemia in patients with kidney disease and in HIV infection and kidney disease.

Szczech described the results of the six trials considered by the committee, focusing on the ability of roxadustat to increase hemoglobin levels in the participants. She stated the "prespecified primary efficacy endpoints were met in each individual study." She noted that the drug was effective in patients with high levels of inflammation and improved the status of patients with disordered iron metabolism. Szczech summarized the clinical results of FibroGen's trials as suggesting roxadustat was comparable to epoetin alfa.

Szczech did not comment on safety. Dr. Dustin Little, who presented the safety data, had an uphill battle on his hands. Little was a nephrologist and the roxadustat global clinical head at AstraZeneca. The key endpoints for the roxadustat studies he presented included major adverse cardiovascular events (MACE), consisting of all-cause mortality, myocardial infarctions, and strokes. In addition, the studies evaluated hospitalizations for heart failure or unstable angina in the participants. In some of the studies, different rates of discontinuation in participants treated with placebo compared with the drug made interpretation of these adverse events difficult. Little had to spend quite a bit of time explaining these complicated concepts to the committee as well as the implications of different analytic approaches, especially since there were more adverse events in people treated with roxadustat in the studies. He concluded the first part of his presentation by highlighting that the cardiovascular outcomes with the drug had been safe.

Little went on to review the results of outcomes related to seizures, infections, vascular access thrombosis, and deep vein thrombosis, noting there were more of these adverse events in the patients treated with roxadustat. But Little, on behalf of the sponsors, had a solution.

> In light of these findings, we are proposing changes to roxadustat dosing to mitigate thrombosis risk. First, we plan to lower the hemoglobin target from 10.5 to 12 grams per deciliter to 10 to 11 grams per deciliter. As I will show you, this allows for us to use lower roxadustat doses throughout the treatment period and it also allows us to minimize hemoglobin overshoots with roxadustat treatment. Additionally, we plan to lower roxadustat starting doses both in ESA untreated and ESA conversion patients.

In effect, the sponsors proposed a whole new set of studies, under the rubric of "mitigation," to be undertaken later, provided roxadustat achieved approval.

> In conclusion, our large database allowed for a comprehensive evaluation of the roxadustat safety profile. We observed comparable cardiovascular risk for roxadustat versus placebo and versus ESA in non-dialysis patients compared to ESA in dialysis patients. Patients treated with roxadustat had an increased incidence of vascular access thrombosis, deep vein thrombosis, and seizures, and we saw a higher

incidence of fatal infections versus placebo in NDD patients, but not compared to ESA in DD patients.

We are proposing several strategies to manage these risks. First, product labeling will communicate warnings and precautions to physicians and a medication guide will communicate these risks to patients.

We're also proposing changes to dosing that will decrease the risk of thrombosis with roxadustat treatment, and we're proposing a post-marketing, real-world study of 10,000 patients to confirm that risk of VAT is similar for roxadustat and ESA with the proposed changes to roxadustat dosing. We will continuously evaluate, communicate, and mitigate risks, and we are committed to working with the FDA to further characterize the roxadustat safety profile in the post-approval setting.

Finally, Dr. Steven Fishbane gave his clinical perspective. He was a professor of medicine at the Donald and Barbara Zucker School of Medicine at Hofstra/Northwell and chief of nephrology for the Northwell Health System. Fishbane was a well-known clinical trialist with long experience in studies of patients with CKD and anemia, with many ties to industry. Fishbane emphasized the length of time he had spent in the field and his membership in the KDIGO Global Anemia and Kidney Disease Guideline Group. He noted, perhaps somewhat pessimistically, the "approval of ESAs in 1989 was an important advance for patients, but there's not been much innovation in anemia treatment since the first ESA approval. I believe roxadustat now represents an important advance."

Fishbane concluded a long presentation with a perhaps lopsided encomium to the virtues of roxadustat and despair regarding the current state of treatment of patients with kidney disease with erythropoietin, with its multitude of logistical challenges, while deemphasizing safety issues. He contributed his "strong belief" regarding the favorable benefit/risk ratio of roxadustat, noting he had "carefully reviewed the sponsor's plan to adjust recommended roxadustat dosing to limit hemoglobin rate of rise to mitigate thrombosis risk . . . and the sponsor's new dosing plan should be highly effective for reducing risk."

Fishbane, however, did not add much to the material Pecoits-Filho had presented earlier, aside from including his personal opinions. Fishbane did ringingly endorse the sponsors' proposal to reduce doses and proceed with new pertinent studies only after drug approval. After Fishbane's presentation the sponsors briefly took questions. Ravi I. Thadhani, M.D., M.P.H., professor of medicine and dean for academic programs at Harvard Medical School in Boston, Massachusetts, a nephrologist, asked a question regarding the rationale of the mitigation plans to reduce the dose of roxadustat in order to decrease the occurrence of side effects such as thromboses. Little answered that the mitigation strategy was focused on reducing thrombotic events but not other adverse events that had been noted in the presented studies. The sponsor perhaps could be characterized as being focused on the benefits of the new drug, while minimizing its risks. After lunch, the FDA scientists had the chance to present their interpretation of the studies.

The FDA presenters were skeptical. Dr. Saleh Ayache focused on the safety of roxadustat as illustrated in the clinical trials. He outlined the four ESAs that had been approved for use in the U.S. by the FDA, noted that none of those drugs could be administered orally, and reviewed the studies that led to their approval. Ayache reviewed the design and the endpoints of the roxadustat studies, and their safety evaluations. The FDA agreed with the sponsors' assessment of the efficacy of the drug, but one concern was that "hemoglobin concentration in the roxadustat groups in these studies tended to overshoot its target." In the dialysis population, Ayache agreed that roxadustat had shown a comparable effect on change in hemoglobin levels to that of epoetin alfa. Ayache acknowledged the differences in dropout rates in the nondialysis CKD patient studies that the sponsor had outlined in earlier presentations. In contrast to the sponsors' analyses, the FDA found a clear difference in safety in the studies, with worse outcomes in the patients treated with roxadustat. In the nondialysis population, the FDA found that roxadustat "shows a clear signal for serious thrombotic events." In the pooled dialysis population, the FDA pointed out the "the rate of early discontinuation was higher in the roxadustat group than the epoetin alfa group. . . . The reasons for discontinuation were adverse events and subject or physician decision to leave the study." In unequivocal terms Ayache emphasized the presence of serious thrombotic events and seizures in the patients treated with roxadustat.

Although the sponsors had denigrated the older, noninnovative erythropoietin, which was not available in oral preparations, treatment of patients with roxadustat in dialysis was associated with a higher rate of important adverse events. Dr. Song, the FDA statistical reviewer, continued the FDA analyses of cardiovascular events in the studies, noting that the "FDA does not agree on the interpretation of the results using strictly a noninferiority hypothesis testing approach. Rather, our interpretation of the trial findings focuses on the estimation of MACE risk and the uncertainty around it."

Song presented data showing that in nondialysis-dependent CKD patients, there were no significant differences in the major adverse cardiovascular events (MACEs) between the two groups in the primary analyses. However, FDA analyses evaluating only patients who had been treated suggested that up to 38% more patients treated with roxadustat might have had a MACE outcome. In dialysis patients, similar findings were evident. When Song presented comparisons of death in the dialysis patient studies, the conclusion was that in primary analyses, patients treated with roxadustat were at a 17% higher risk of death. In contrast, in secondary analyses there was no difference in mortality between the groups.

Ayache then presented findings in nondialysis CKD patients suggesting "a fairly strong association between the roxadustat dose and thrombotic events, but no association in the placebo-treated patients," with similar, but not identical results in the dialysis patients in the studies. Ayache concluded that the risks of cardiovascular events and mortality were difficult to interpret but that the results of the administration's sensitivity analyses were "unfavorable for Roxadustat."

Clearly the roxadustat study findings were complex, open to different interpretations using different analytic tools, and subject to radically different interpretations by the FDA scientists and the sponsors. When the FDA presentation was opened to questions from committee members, several presented queries to the speakers. Among those, Ms. Alikhaani asked about the erythropoietin "hyporesponsive" (or resistant) patients in the study, and Dr. O'Connor asked about the boundaries for risks used in the studies. Susan T. Crowley, M.D., M.B.A., F.A.S.N., professor of medicine at Yale University and director of the National Kidney Disease and Dialysis Program at the Veterans Health

Administration, asked about the strategies involved in decreasing the proposed dose of roxadustat.

The FDA had changed over the years. Representatives of the patient community, who would be affected by the agency's decisions, were now invited to participate in meetings regarding approval of drugs. In an "open public session," people were invited to comment on roxadustat. The ground rules put forth by Dr. Lewis stated:

> FDA encourages you, the open public hearing speaker, at the beginning of your written or oral statement to advise the committee of any financial relationship that you may have with the sponsor, its product, and if known, its direct competitors. One of our goals for today is for this open public hearing to be conducted in a fair and open way, where every participant is listened to carefully and treated with dignity, courtesy, and respect.

Sixteen speakers contributed. There was a mix of physicians (most of whom had participated in anemia studies, some of whom had conflicts of interest) and patients or relatives of CKD patients. A representative of the American Kidney Fund spoke. Some speakers did not address financial conflicts of interest. All endorsed the use of roxadustat, citing different reasons but typically focusing on the convenience of oral administration or absence of need for transportation to a health-care facility. Thereafter, the committee returned to questions addressed to the sponsor. Among them, Mr. Conway's question may have been the most critical.

> In plain language, can you tell the patient community that's listening why you should move forward on this if you're relying on a model to show safety and efficacy by reducing dosing and mitigation measures as opposed to waiting and seeing what that actually looks like if you do some other type of study on that? Why should this move forward into a patient population relying on modeling? That I think is a fair question.

Questions from the FDA were then presented to the committee members for discussion. In some cases, key questions for committee members included their public votes on aspects of approval of roxadustat. For example, committee members were asked to comment on plans for "mitigation" or changing the dosing of roxadustat and, by extension, if another clinical trial was necessary before approval. Lewis opined, "I think the trial needs to be prior to approval, and the hypothesis that the dose adjustments and different algorithms will mitigate those safety signals needs to be tested. Further, I would actually think there's enough of a safety signal that there may need to be a formal dedicated cardiovascular study." Conway remarked,

I'm very concerned about this idea of taking the data that we have and try and extrapolate from that, through a model or through some other kind of tangential effort, in my opinion, to show that there is safety. So the frustrating thing in listening to this, for me, is that the patient burden is well documented, in my opinion, but the burden is on the sponsor to show why this should move forward before it's tested out as opposed to waiting and doing that postmarket. I think we should get it checked out before it goes into patients. I really do.

The third question was the first that required committee member votes. They were asked, "Should roxadustat be approved for the treatment of anemia due to chronic kidney disease in adult patients not on dialysis?" The vote was one yes, thirteen no, without any abstentions. Concerns were raised about safety and about the untested nature of the proposed mitigation strategies.

Lewis summarized the arguments underlying the first vote:

I think that the consensus is that the safety signal is concerning to the panel members, concerning enough that they feel that a mitigation study needs to be done prior to approval. I think that many people, including Dr. Crowley who voted yes, but many other people—and I really appreciate our consumer and patient reps here—are very empathetic to the patient's voice of wanting an oral or an easier therapy, but not at the expense of unknown or perhaps negative safety profile. I think it's also important to note that there is concern about effects that will not in any way be related to the hemoglobin rise or to the mitigation study that's being proposed to be done at the recommendation of this committee prior to approval. I think the points were well made that there should be a very careful consideration for what will most efficiently and effectively answer this question in a study, and I applaud us being reminded that we should include patients' and families' voices in feedback on that design as well.

The second question requiring voting was "Should roxadustat be approved for the treatment of anemia due to CKD in adult patients on dialysis?" The vote was two yes, twelve no, and no abstentions. Dr. Thadhani joined Dr. Crowley in the affirmative position.

Once again, Dr. Lewis clearly and succinctly summarized the view of the committee:

I think the two people who voted yes did so because they felt that there was an unmet need, particularly for home dialysis patients, and there was more control over this population of patients, and the patients and physicians involved would understand the risks. There also was an interest in having a very careful label perhaps for only hyporesponsive patients and maybe home patients, and that would give a doorway to a risk mitigation and post-approval process as well. I think the majority who had voted no are still concerned about the adverse safety signal, particularly the on-study mortality. I don't think people are convinced that modeling supported by a phase 2 study can replace a clinical trial for safety. . . . I think we all felt challenged by the unmet need for alternatives in this population, but the safety concerns outweighed the desire to help meet that unmet need.

Dr. Unger addressed all the participants and noted,

I'd like to thank all of you for your thoughtfulness, for your objectivity, and I thank the people who have tried to follow the data and the science. Those are our guiding stars at the FDA and I really appreciate that. I know this wasn't the vote that the applicant had hoped for, but I would like to credit the applicant for running I think a very impressive development program here. There wasn't always agreement with the FDA, apparently, but nevertheless, it was an impressive program. It's the largest body of data we may ever see for a drug like this, so I think a shout-out to them is in order as well.

Dr. Lewis concluded her remarks by reiterating the importance of the inclusion of patients on the committee and during the open public session. And so, after a full day's work, the meeting was adjourned.

A sense of high drama emerges in the transcript of what was after all an administrative meeting. The FDA and the sponsor did not interpret the clinical data in the same manner. The decisions made from the results of the meeting involved the potential profit or loss of hundreds of millions of dollars for the sponsors. Roxadustat was not approved by the FDA. But the meeting had never been about the ability of the HIF stabilizers to increase hemoglobin levels in patients with CKD. Rather, after more than thirty years' experience with the effects of a molecular biologic breakthrough used in patients—the ESAs, which had risks and benefits—committee members focused on the safety and the unknown, potential off-target effects of unleashing a new molecule that might undermine the biology of every cell in the body. Would this new class of drugs perform better for patients with CKD than the erythropoietin analogues or drugs that interacted with the erythropoietin receptor—known entities? Perhaps Tilman Drüeke's question lingered in the minds of committee members. The committee was not buying what FibroGen had to sell. The committee opted for safety first. It could be argued that the sponsors deemphasized the safety issues brought up by the studies and focused on the potential benefits of this new drug. The committee, however, did not believe that a dose reduction, chosen without the rigorous clinical trial testing provided by a randomized controlled study, could ensure the safety of the many people in the U.S. with CKD and anemia. Presentations and analyses were delivered by disinterested public servants, and a multidisciplinary panel of experts, consumers, and patients did the right thing—almost unanimously.

Several trials of other HIF stabilizers in patients with CKD and anemia have since been published in the medical literature, including in high-impact journals. In general, the studies show similar efficacy to the older ESAs, but many raise the same kind of questions about safety that were brought up at the FDA committee meeting in July 2021. At least six HIF stabilizers have been developed. By the end of 2021, four HIF stabilizers had been licensed in Japan, and roxadusat was licensed in China and Chile.

On December 16, 2021, the *NEJM* published two papers, "Daprodustat for the Treatment of Anemia in Patients Undergoing Dialysis" and "Daprodustat for the Treatment of Anemia in Patients Not Undergoing Dialysis," with Ajay Singh as the first author and an international team of nephrology collaborators.[61] The study in nondialysis patients randomized 1,937 to treatment with daprodustat and 1,935 to treatment with darbepoetin alfa, evaluating changes in hemoglobin concentrations, and the first occurrence of a major adverse cardiovascular event in the two groups. The authors concluded that in "patients with CKD and anemia who were not undergoing dialysis, daprodustat was noninferior to darbepoetin alfa with respect to the change in the hemoglobin level from baseline and with respect to cardiovascular outcomes." The design of the study in dialysis patients was similar. Patients were randomized to treatment with daprodustat (three times a week) or epoetin alfa or darbepoetin alfa (for hemodialysis and peritoneal dialysis patients, respectively). The two primary outcomes were the mean change in the hemoglobin level and the first occurrence of a major adverse cardiovascular event. In the study, 1,487 patients were randomized to daprodustat and 1,477 to an ESA. During the follow-up period, a major adverse cardiovascular event occurred in 25.2% in the daprodustat group and in 26.7% of the ESA group. The authors concluded in "patients with CKD undergoing dialysis, daprodustat was noninferior to ESAs regarding the change in the hemoglobin level from baseline and cardiovascular outcomes." The CRDAC met on October 26, 2022, to consider an application from GlaxoSmithKline, regarding the risks and benefits of the use of daprodustat, for the treatment of anemia in CKD patients.

The format was similar to that of the meeting on roxadustat. This time Dr. Ann Farrell was the director who gave the opening remarks to the group.[62] Farrell reviewed the pathophysiology of anemia of kidney disease and previous

FDA actions on ESAs. She noted prespecified analyses of drug safety that were critical for the meeting. She reviewed several potential adverse events associated with the use of daprodustat in CKD patients who had not yet started dialysis, and a more limited set of complications in dialysis patients treated with the drug. The advisory committee was composed of many of the same members who had participated in the meeting on roxadustat. The course of the meeting was similar to the earlier one, but the consequences were different.

Dr. Kirsten Johansen, professor of medicine at the University of Minnesota and principal investigator of the contract for the United States Renal Data System, an investigator in both studies, presented on "Unmet Needs." She noted that anemia was associated with diminished quality of life, hospitalizations, and other complications. Johansen, like Pecoits-Filho, emphasized that oral medications could provide a great advantage for patients with CKD not yet on dialysis and for people who lived far from medical centers. Alexander R. Cobitz, M.D., Ph.D., of GlaxoSmithKline presented data showing that daprodustat was as effective as ESAs in causing hemoglobin concentrations to increase in patients with chronic kidney disease. Dr. Khavandi presented safety data, noting "both studies met the primary safety endpoints of MACE, demonstrating that daprodustat is non-inferior to the standard of care ESA comparators." There was further discussion of the increased stroke rate and hospitalization for heart failure in nondialysis patients treated with daprodustat as well as complications of stomach lesions and gastrointestinal bleeding in patients treated with the novel drug. In general, risks with daprodustat therapy appeared to be greater in the population of CKD patients not yet on dialysis, for unclear reasons. Dr. Ajay Singh summarized the GSK presentations by noting his experience in the field of ESAs in patients with CKD and suggested the novel drug could ameliorate disparities in the treatment of anemia in racial and socioeconomic groups, improve perception of quality of life, and decrease transfusion rates. Singh challenged some of the FDA analyses on statistical grounds. He concluded by "respectfully" submitting "that the committee should also consider the views of the well-informed patient who may want to have the ability to choose their preferred option to treat their anemia. These patients may select the convenience and flexibility of dosing from an oral treatment."

The FDA staff noted there had been no disparities in discontinuation rates in the daprodustat studies (which had plagued the roduxastat presentations) and pointed out higher rates of heart failure hospitalizations, AKI, and gastrointestinal and other complications, particularly in patients not on dialysis treated with daprodustat. A lively discussion ensued regarding the potential for bias in evaluating secondary outcomes in clinical trials and using various analytic techniques. Once again, patients, physicians, and advocacy organizations lent support for the approval of daprodustat, with the notable exception of Public Citizen. The organization felt there were no additional benefits but increased risks associated with the novel therapy.

The FDA asked committee members to discuss the risks and benefits of treatment with daprodustat in CKD patients treated and not treated by dialysis. Some committee members agreed with the Public Citizen position, while others did not consider the safety analyses to be cut-and-dried and could not come to the conclusion that there was clear evidence of increased harm with the drug. Committee members noted that for in-center hemodialysis patients, receiving an ESA intravenously, oral medications had little benefit. Several committee members agreed with Singh's position regarding patient choice and convenience, including Mr. Conway. There was consensus that for unknown reasons, risks were higher in the CKD patients not treated with dialysis. There were also questions regarding whether there was a "class effect" of the HIF-prolyl hydroxylase inhibitors (HIF-PHIs), suggesting the side effects of the drug were intrinsically linked with the action of the drugs. Clinician scientists offered counterarguments that different molecular configurations in the class of HIF-prolyl hydroxylase inhibitors might be associated with different drug effects and varying safety profiles.

In many ways, the committee had an easier task than with the evaluation of roxadustat, which had logistic issues in the clinical studies and a poorer safety record. It is impossible to determine what were the contributions of different drug effects, dosages and dosing schedules, population differences between the studies, and other unknown confounders to the different outcomes of the trials using the different HIF-prolyl hydroxylase inhibitors, as is often the case with RCTs. Such knowledge will have to await the coming of true precision medicine evidence, which may be relatively far off in the future.

Committee members were asked to vote on whether benefits of treatment with daprodustat for nondialysis patients outweighed risks. Five voted yes, and eleven no. Regarding whether benefits of treatment with daprodustat for dialysis patients outweighed risks, thirteen voted yes, and three voted no. On February 1, 2023, the FDA approved the use of daprodustat for the treatment of anemia in adult CKD patients treated with dialysis but not for those not yet on dialysis.

What Is the Current Situation?

Contemporary studies do not suggest bias in the provision of ESAs to patients according to race. However, studies do show differences in various parameters related to the treatment of anemia in patients with kidney disease. Janet K. Freburger and colleagues showed in 2012, that between 2002 and 2008, the average doses of ESAs and iron were higher for Black patients than White, Asian, or "other" ESRD patients.[63] During the same period, hemoglobin levels were higher in the "other" group of patients but not statistically different between Black and White patients. Interestingly, the average dose of ESAs administered to patients in this sample decreased after 2006. The study was supported by Amgen Inc., and two of the authors were Amgen employees, suggesting a corporate interest in the findings. In 2015, Marc N. Turrene and colleagues studied whether changes to the payment system in 2011 had affected practice patterns in U.S. hemodialysis patients.[64] In their sample, studied from August 2010 to December 2011, the average patient hemoglobin concentration decreased from 11.5 to 11.0 g/dL. The average dose of erythropoietin decreased from 20,506 to 14,777 units a week. These findings suggested government policies were indeed having an effect on clinical practice as well as patient outcomes. The authors reported that no "meaningful differences by race were observed regarding the rates of change of management practices or laboratory measures." However, as in the study by Freburger and colleagues, the average dose of erythropoietin was higher in Black patients. The authors concluded that despite "evidence that anemia and mineral metabolism management practices have changed significantly over time, there was no immediate indication of racial disparities resulting from implementation of the PPS or ESA label change." The study was

supported by NIH's National Institute on Minority Health and Health Disparities, and individual authors received support from the NIDDK and Fresenius.
The corresponding author was from Arbor Research Collaborative for Health,
which received support from "Amgen, Inc., Kyowa Hakko Kirin, AbbVie Inc.,
Sanofi Renal, Baxter Healthcare, Vifor Fresenius Medical Care Renal Pharma
Ltd., and Fresenius Medical Care, without restrictions on publications," so it is
difficult to evaluate possible conflicts of interest in this report.

More recently, John Danziger, M.D., and Kenneth J. Mukamal, M.D., M.P.H.,
of the Beth Deaconess Hospital and Harvard Medical School, and Eric Weinhandl, Ph.D., M.S., of the Chronic Disease Research Group, Hennepin Health-
care Research Institute, Minneapolis, Minnesota (now with the USRDS),
showed higher lead levels in local drinking water were associated with lower
hemoglobin levels and higher prescription of ESAs in almost 600,000 patients
initiating dialysis across the U.S. between 2005 and 2017.[65] The investigators
also found significantly higher water lead levels among Black patients' resi-
dences compared to those of White patients. The authors concluded that "even
low levels of lead that are commonly encountered in community water systems throughout the United States are associated with lower hemoglobin levels and higher ESA use among patients with advanced kidney disease." If one
believes higher doses of ESAs are associated with adverse events, these findings, from several studies, show Black dialysis patients in the U.S. incur higher
risks from treatment of anemia. These results implicate the social determinants of health in affecting life and death outcomes in African American
patients with kidney disease in the U.S. As Dr. Rudolph Rodriguez and colleagues put it in a seminal paper on residential associations with outcomes of
dialysis patients in 2007, Geography Matters.[66]

———— ✦ ————

What paths have the kidney community traveled over the last approximately
one-third of a century? The landscape has changed. I remember hemodialysis
patients with hematocrits of less than 10% receiving weekly transfusions who
were too weak to walk and who could barely engage in the activities of daily
life. Molecular biologic tools were brought forth in the 1980s that resulted in
wonder drugs that changed the lives of patients. The contribution of Fu-Kuen

Lin's and Joe Eschbach's teams cannot be understated or dismissed. Over the next three decades, controversies emerged regarding the goals of the treatment of anemia in patients with kidney disease, the safety of CKD patients, and the place of the profit motive in the medical industrial complex, affecting patient care and well-being. The policy controversies after the publication of the CRE-ATE and CHOIR studies, although concerned about patient survival, focused on the profits that the dialysis organizations and pharmaceutical companies would net, and the costs the government would provide. Eschbach and Adamson were just as correct in 1985 as they would be today when they wrote, "Only through careful physiologic studies will it be possible to determine the optimal red cell mass in such individuals." And only through rigorous, well-designed, and well-performed randomized clinical trials can the efficacy and safety of new drugs be evaluated.

The FDA, which emerges as a hero in this story, addressed the thorny issue of approval of a new class of drugs that could increase the hemoglobin of patients with CKD and anemia with pluralistic inputs, including listening to the voices of patients, and made the right decisions in the eyes of the public. Its task, to ensure the safety and effectiveness of drugs prescribed in the U.S., is critical to the health of the nation. The decisions of the agency, usually informed by the discussions of experts with differing points of view, have profound consequences for both patients and corporations.

Drug companies have conflicts of interest in marketing and promoting drugs whose powerful short-term (surrogate) benefits have side effects and whose long-term results may not be salutary for patients. Adverse effects on survival may only be noted when carefully designed trials are performed after a drug is first released, as has been the case with certain nonsteroidal anti-inflammatory drugs (such as Vioxx). It is difficult to know whether the pursuit of normalization of anemia in patients with CKD not on dialysis was ethical after the publication of the Normal Hematocrit Study of hemodialysis patients in 1998, and controversial views exist on this point. It can be questioned whether the TREAT study was ethical after the negative results of the CHOIR and CREATE trials were published in 2006. However, scientific and ethical counterarguments were indeed made at the time, and government regulatory agencies approved the research. Studies took place in different populations, where outcomes may have differed. Whether the biotech companies manufacturing and selling erythropoietin and its biosimilars pursued profits at the expense of putting patients first is a question each physician and patient must confront.

It is often repeated that Albert Einstein stated "the definition of insanity is doing the same thing over and over again, but expecting a different result." The pharmaceutical houses, however, spent more than two decades repeating the same experiment with different drugs and different populations and achieving the same distressing results, while marketing drugs in high doses to millions of patients and making profits at the same time. The truth was evident in Eschbach's original presentation at the Capri Conference in 1986 and in the landmark papers published in the *Lancet* in 1986 and in the *NEJM* in 1987. High doses of erythropoietin, rapid increases in hematocrit, and attempts to restore hematocrits to normal levels in patients with ESRD (and, later, CKD patients) result in unacceptable complications such as high blood pressure, blood clots, seizures, strokes, brain dysfunction, and death. Patients, drug companies, and physicians just had to see it.

Physician investigators accept emoluments from drug companies for participating in clinical trials or recommending their products. Academic physicians working in the clinical arena are often embedded in relations with industry. Physicians supervising dialysis units for dialysis organizations may have interests in the finances of the parent companies, and practicing physicians invest in stocks, without disclosures.

A sea change has occurred from 1989 to the present at several levels of American society that is reflected also in federal regulatory approaches. The time from the approval of erythropoietin for the treatment of anemia in dialysis patients to the consideration of roxadustat and daprodustat for patients with CKD and anemia has represented a new era in medical care, molecular biologic achievements, as well as regulatory oversight. In evaluating safety and efficacy, regulatory agencies have given safety greater prominence. Patients now have input into the regulatory process. We can appreciate the advances while remaining wary about pitfalls that may not have changed. Risk/benefit balances considered by regulatory agencies as well as in the patient/physician relationship have become more nuanced, and patient choice may have gained a firmer foothold. It is important for physicians and other health-care providers to collaborate with patients in an uphill battle to decrease the role of profit in health care.

Over the last forty years, medicine and medical care have undergone profound transformations as well. Relman decried the medical industrial complex in an article in the *NEJM* in 1980.[67] Since then, medical providers as well as dialysis chains have undergone a process described by Dr. John Geyman as "corporatization."[68] This includes a substantial shift in medical entities from nonprofit to for-profit status around the nation over the years. The challenge is to continue to provide care for patients in this relatively new but all-pervasive corporate environment, largely driven by financial considerations.

Corporate goals to sell as much product as possible may not always be compatible with patient welfare. It is the duty of corporations as well as physicians to maintain the balance in favor of patients' safety at all times. Corporate greed must be kept in check by employees of regulatory agencies such as the FDA and the European Medicines Agency who remain free of conflicts of interest and by physicians who closely monitor the responses of the patients they care for after they prescribe drugs. Reviewers must not be seduced by the beauty of molecular biologic triumphs or the unraveling of heretofore unknown physiologic pathways but, rather, put the consequences of treating patients with the drug in question at the forefront. In addition, it is a moral imperative that drugs that may improve quality of life be available equitably to patients without regard to gender or race.

8

---·✳·---

APOL1

Genetics of Kidney Disease, Race, and Equity

In an era when epidemiologists did not have access to supercomputers and there were few large databases collecting information on the health of individuals, physicians had been taught that kidney disease was different in White and Black Americans. In the 1970s, clinicians and pathologists informed medical students that the outcomes related to high blood pressure were different in different ethnic and racial populations. Conventional wisdom suggested that hypertension was common and the result of a variety of aberrations in human organ systems. The stiffening of blood vessels (atherosclerosis) with age, excessive salt intake, the abnormal production and release of hormones from the adrenal glands or the kidneys (or, rarely, other glands), the use of certain medications, the narrowing of the renal artery connecting the aorta to the kidney (thereby providing its blood supply), and disease of the kidney tissue itself could all result in increased blood pressure.

Two Types of High Blood Pressure

At the time, hypertension was classified into groups. "Essential hypertension" was the most common condition, where no underlying cause could be

ascertained. Essential hypertension could just be treated. "Secondary hypertension" was caused by the aforementioned conditions. The task of the clinician was
to identify any possible underlying cause and relieve it, resulting in the improvement or normalization of blood pressure. Patients with high blood pressure
underwent a variety of chemical tests, including analyses of twenty-four-hour
urine collections, to ensure that there was no endocrine disease present. The vast
majority of these tests were negative. The most feared entity, "malignant hypertension," was characterized by extremely high blood pressure occurring in association with new or worsened disease of the brain, heart, and kidneys.[1] The
presentation of malignant hypertension often involved a dramatic, sudden
increase of blood pressure with rapid deterioration of kidney function, heart failure, and evidence of involvement of the central nervous system, such as visual
disturbances or blindness, disorientation, delirium, or stroke. People with essential hypertension rarely went on to develop kidney disease, while those with
malignant hypertension had kidney disease by definition. Most people with
essential hypertension were White and did not have kidney disease caused by
hypertension. A disproportionate number of patients with malignant hypertension were Black, and their condition often progressed to renal failure after one or
more acute episodes. These differences were not lost on public health experts,
pathologists, or nephrologists. By the early 1980s, it was apparent that the ESRD
dialysis program had up to three times as many Black Medicare beneficiaries
compared with other racial groups in the U.S. population.[2] These facts led to consideration of the age-old environment versus genetics controversy regarding this
epidemiologic disparity. Although socioeconomic status, living conditions, poor
dietary habits, and risky behaviors might affect the prevalence of kidney disease,
it was widely believed by medical scientists that there must be a genetic difference between the populations accounting for the radically different incidence of
kidney disease in Black and White Americans.

Were Genetic Differences Associated with the Presence of Kidney Disease?

Genetic science had advanced dramatically over the decades since the original studies of Watson and Crick on the structure of DNA in 1953. By the 1990s,

several studies showed a "clustering" of kidney disease in families of patients with diabetes, suggesting underlying genetic mechanisms for the initiation of kidney disease. In 1989, Drs. Elizabeth Seaquist, Frederick C. Goetz, Stephen Rich, and Jose Barbarosa from the University of Minnesota published an article in the *NEJM*, showing kidney disease clustered in families with diabetes.[3] The authors noted this pattern was consistent with a heritable cause of kidney disease in the families, but they could not exclude shared environmental influences, such as diet, playing key roles in generating the results, especially in the absence of the identification of a specific gene associated with the findings.

These and other studies suggested that the kidney disease of diabetes, a common cause of ESRD, "ran" in families. If a genetic basis for kidney disease could be found, evaluation of these families might well provide the answer.

Dr. Josephine Briggs was recruited to lead the Division of Kidney Urologic and Hematologic Disease at the NIDDK in 1997 from the University of Michigan, where she had attained the rank of professor of medicine and had established a reputation for distinguished research in kidney disease and the function of the renin system. Briggs realized that the genetic investigation of kidney disease was timely and feasible and represented a burgeoning research opportunity that policymakers, physicians, scientists, and patients could all support. Advocacy from multiple entities and stakeholders is often key to initiating large research projects funded by the government. In addition, the study of the kidney disease of diabetes united two of the divisions within the institute.

In 1998, NIDDK was poised to take action. The leadership of the institute convened a workshop that summer to explore the genetic underpinnings of kidney disease in patients with diabetes. The workshop included scientists from many disciplines, including geneticists, diabetologists and endocrinologists, biostatisticians, nephrologists, epidemiologists, public health experts, and public policymakers. Presentations focused on evaluating current evidence for the genetic background of common kidney diseases, proposing solutions to identifying specific genes associated with the risks of developing kidney disease, and estimating the number of patients required to participate in a meaningful, definitive study. At the time of the workshop, Briggs knew she needed a new recruit to direct a program in the genetics of kidney disease. The ideal candidate would be a nephrologist with expertise in medical genetics. Most successful clinical and basic science researchers in genetics, however, could not be lured to take a job in the government, which barred many forms of independent research and usually paid much less than private practice, academic, or industry positions. There was a person who wanted the job, however unqualified he might be. Josie Briggs chose me to lead the study from NIDDK.

At that time, two different approaches to identifying gene sequences associated with disease were widely used. Family studies used "linkage analyses," while comparisons between groups with and without a particular disease could be used to power "association" studies. In 1998, researchers thought linkage studies could provide answers related to the genetic basis of kidney disease with superior power, taking advantage of the strong genetic relationships seen in close family members with the same disease. Workshop participants suggested linkage studies would yield the answer to the scientific question in part because of the evidence of clustering of kidney disease in certain diabetic families. If a gene was tightly linked to a disease or a complication of a disease, a researcher might only need a small number of families with two affected patients to detect the culprit.

RFA DK 99–005, Diabetic and Non-diabetic Nephropathy Susceptibility Genes, appeared in the NIH Guide for Grants and Contracts in January 1999. The Request for Applications (RFA) called for scientifically justified proposals from the research community for a genetic analysis and data coordinating center (GADCC) to lead the study and participating centers to recruit patients to donate their medical histories and DNA for research purposes. The NIDDK allocated $4 million a year for five years to this effort. Case Western Reserve University was the successful applicant for the GADCC, led by the eminent geneticist Dr. Robert Elston. Dr. Elston had developed statistical tools for analyzing genetic data in large populations of people. The successful participating centers that joined the consortium were a diverse group, including Wake Forest University, the University of California, Los Angeles, Case Western Reserve University, the University of New Mexico, the University of Texas at San Antonio, and Johns Hopkins. The consortium would study White, African

American, Hispanic, and Native American families, accounting for ethnicity in their analyses, a relatively novel approach at the time. NIDDK scientists interested in the genetics of diabetic kidney disease who had worked with the Pima Indians in Arizona joined the consortium, led by the renowned diabetologist Dr. William Knowler. Dr. Elston was assisted by a young geneticist, Dr. Sudha Iyengar. Dr. Barry Freedman of Wake Forest emerged as the leader of the consortium.

Freedman's overriding interest was the genetics of kidney disease. In early, small studies, he noticed kidney disease ran in families and that at times, certain families had several members with similar as well as different kidney diseases. Freedman gave lectures across the country positing that a "renal failure gene" must exist. His case was strengthened when just such a gene was identified in rodents by Dr. Howard Jacobs, then of the Medical University of Wisconsin, in Milwaukee. Jacobs called the rodent gene *Rf-1*.[4]

The FIND Study

Most of the successful sites, including the GADCC, proposed using family linkage studies as the basis for the genetic research. However, the Johns Hopkins group, led by Dr. Michael Klag, proposed a radically different approach. Building on work that had been done by a career NIH staff geneticist, Dr. Stephen O'Brien, the Hopkins group proposed an approach that used "mapping by admixture linkage disequilibrium" (MALD). The MALD technique assumed there would be great power if a clinical characteristic, such as kidney disease, differed markedly between groups with different ancestries. Genetic markers associated with different ancestries in different groups could be "linked" to genetic sequences associated with the disease. The Hopkins group recruited Dr. Mike Smith from the O'Brien laboratory to spearhead the genetic part of the grant work, in cooperation with Klag, a physician/epidemiologist who had worked on studies of patients with kidney disease for many years.

The consortium first met in the autumn of 1999. As the consortium developed its research plan, it became clear that two approaches would be taken, using the information from many of the same participants. The consortium members would recruit family members with diabetes and kidney disease as well as, in "Plan B," analyzing data from dialysis patients with diabetes and a control group of dialysis patients without diabetes. Typically, NIDDK recruits a group of distinguished scientists to provide oversight for large, consortial studies, giving direct advice to the institute. The oversight group, at that time termed an External Advisory Committee, or EAC, was headed by Dr. David Warnock, a well-known nephrologist from the University of Alabama at Birmingham who had worked on studies focusing on the physiology of the proximal tubule as well as genetic research and studies involving large groups of patients. The NIDDK also recruited a geneticist from Howard University in Washington, D.C., Dr. Georgia M. Dunston, to provide perspectives on genetic studies and the ethnic groups being evaluated. In addition, the NIDDK, concerned about availability of the genetic samples, both for the investigators and eventually for the entire research community, wished to set up a facility for maintaining the precious DNA donated by study participants. NIDDK contracted with Dr. Cheryl Winkler of the O'Brien laboratory to provide facilities for immortalizing cells as a renewable DNA source, preserving the DNA and ensuring its quality. The consortium named itself the Family Investigation of Nephropathy and Diabetes, or FIND, among friends. A nice catchy study title might enhance recruitment, the investigators thought.

Early meetings between the research consortium and its EAC focused on tracking samples, recruiting participants, and ensuring DNA quality. As recruitment reached critical levels, Dr. Dunston would frequently ask the investigators, "What are you going to do if you find a gene that confers a high risk of developing kidney disease in African Americans?" She was interested in how the investigators would consider the information and how it would be reported in the scientific literature as well as to the study participants and, perhaps most importantly, to the public. Dunston was concerned that such a finding, while widely expected in the kidney and genetic research circles, could end up conferring stigma in the African American community. In addition, she wondered whether uncovering a genetic cause of kidney disease in African Americans, without identifying a cure—or at least an intervention strategy—could lead to despair in a vulnerable population. Or, even worse, would such findings lead to racist interpretations and undesirable clinical outcomes?

A Parallel Research Approach

Dr. Jeffrey Kopp, who was not involved in the FIND study, had worked on the problem of a specific kidney diagnosis, focal segmental glomerulosclerosis (FSGS), for many years. This disease was associated with striking loss of protein in the urine and, in many cases, with relatively rapid progression to ESRD. FSGS was clearly more common in African Americans in the U.S. than in people of other backgrounds. Kopp attended the University of Pennsylvania School of Medicine after graduation from Harvard College and pursued residency training and a fellowship in nephrology at the University of Washington in Seattle. Originally, he had been interested in the bone disease associated with kidney disease, which was one of the strengths of the UW program. After joining the National Institute of Dental Research at NIH, he concentrated on the study of laminin, a structural protein intrinsically associated with the pathophysiology of FSGS. Kopp transferred to NIDDK to focus his studies on kidney disease, including FSGS and HIV-associated nephropathy, which was diagnosed almost exclusively in individuals of African ancestry. Recognizing the power of assembling groups of patients with a single disease who are followed over time, Kopp put together a consortium of academic nephrologists, whose practices included patients from New Orleans, Philadelphia, Chicago, Baltimore, Washington, D.C., New York City, Marshfield, Wisconsin, Galveston, Texas, and Morgantown, West Virginia. These clinicians were interested in FSGS and had information over time on the outcome of many patients with the disease. The investigative group enrolled FSGS patients into a study where they donated their DNA for research, and their clinical course was followed.[5] One of Kopp's key laboratory collaborators was Dr. Cherie Winkler.

Dr. Winkler received her Ph.D. in immunogenetics from the University of Maryland and worked at the National Cancer Institute studying genetic variations in patients with infectious and noncommunicable diseases. Her laboratory developed expertise in growing immortalized cells from immunosuppressed individuals. Winkler applied this expertise to immortalizing cells from FIND participants with ESRD. Previous attempts to immortalize blood cells from dialysis patients had failed repeatedly.

Kopp and Winkler hypothesized that the gene variant predisposing African Americans to progressive kidney disease would be more prevalent on African-origin chromosome segments and less prevalent on chromosome segments derived from Europeans. They studied 190 patients with two kidney diseases that are much more prevalent in African Americans, FSGS, and HIV-associated nephropathy (HIVAN, a form of FSGS that rapidly progresses to ESRD) and compared findings with 222 control participants. Using a set of genetic variants that differed in frequency between Africans and Europeans, Winkler and her genetics team were able to identify blocks of chromosomes of either European or African ancestry. This method, called mapping by admixture disequilibrium, identified a region of excess African ancestry on chromosome 22 in the patients with FSGS and HIVAN but not in the control group. Compared to either the rest of the genomes of the cases only or to the controls, the chromosome 22 region of the patients with FSGS was greatly enriched in African-origin chromosome blocks. The probability of this happening by chance was only about one out of a billion, or fewer, experiments. Kopp and Winkler speculated that the gene of interest in this region was MYH9 (myosin heavy chain 9), which coded a protein found in the podocytes of the kidneys known to cause FSGS-like renal damage in patients with MYH9 mutations. They validated the chromosome 22 association with FSGS in this study in another group of patients treated with dialysis because of nondiabetic ESRD. They summarized their findings in a manuscript that they intended to submit to a first-rate medical journal.

Smith and Winkler were also associated with the FIND study, which was nearing completion of patient recruitment. They met with the FIND MALD investigators who were working on a similar study involving diabetic and nondiabetic dialysis patients. After sharing these dramatic results with the Johns Hopkins group, working as part of the FIND consortium, the FIND investigators confirmed the same region Kopp and Winkler had identified with nondiabetic ESRD (but not with the smaller group of patients with diabetic ESRD), validating the remarkable association of chromosome 22 with nondiabetic ESKD.

Publication Issues

Kopp, Winkler, and their consortium colleagues sent the manuscript describing the research results to the *NEJM*. After initial favorable reviews, the paper was rejected. One reviewer thought it was impossible to show such strong genetic associations in a small study that recruited a few hundred rather than the more customary thousands of participants seen in major genetic studies. At this point, the FIND team and the Kopp-Winkler group decided to submit their papers for publication to another high-impact journal, *Nature Genetics*.

In contrast to the *NEJM*, *Nature Genetics* was interested in the work of the FSGS consortium, in addition to the results of the FIND study, and published both papers as companion pieces in the same issue in 2008, solidifying, in a respected scientific forum, the notion that there was a genetic basis to common kidney diseases.[6] Interestingly, considering the initial hypothesis, as well as the NIH institute funding the research, NIDDK, the investigators could not show that the region they identified was associated with kidney disease in patients with diabetes.

A challenge in genetic discovery research projects in human populations is that they often show associations rather than establish causal relationships. Determining causality typically entails the deployment of an intervention. Scientists often decide to "knock out" a gene in an animal model, such as a mouse, to show the lack of a gene or gene product will result in a disease that mimics the human illness. Or they can "knock in" an abnormal gene and show the animal develops something akin to the human disease with the new gene mutation. The FIND and NIH investigators did not have animal data regarding the gene loci they identified on chromosome 22. They devoted a good deal of space in the *Nature Genetics* papers trying to link *MYH9* with kidney disease, but their arguments were not totally convincing. Myosin heavy chain was a muscle protein, and the push to connect this biologic product with kidney disease hinged on its association with some rare kidney diseases and platelet disorders. It was just difficult to construct a solid scientific story in which *MYH9* disturbances caused kidney disease on a widespread basis. But the strength of the association with a gene on chromosome 22 seemed incontrovertible. The FIND researchers hedged their bets in the paper, stating, "it is likely our results have simply identified genetic variants that are in strong linkage disequilibrium with the causal variant." They were right.

What Will We Do If We FIND a Gene?

Acting on Dr. Dunston's advice, the NIDDK convened a workshop in April 2010 to address the implications of finding a gene linked to high susceptibility to developing kidney disease in a minority population. The workshop was named "MYH9 and Kidney Disease: Clinical and Public Health Implications of Recent Genetic Findings in Populations." The conference brought together experts in kidney disease, genetics, public health, and testing and screening procedures. The conference participants divided into breakout groups to provide perspectives on clinical implications, to explore possible avenues for future research, and to make recommendations about possible screening and treatment strategies. A highlight of the meeting was a lecture by Dr. David Williams, the eminent sociologist from Harvard. Williams outlined the stark disparities between races in the U.S. in income and life expectancy across age groups. He did not think the election of President Obama would change these distressing realities, but held out some hope for the effects of improvements in education, health-care access, and fiscal policies, if they could be realized. Workshop participants felt screening for *MYH9* was not yet justified, because there was no intervention to offer if genetic abnormalities were detected. The workshop attendees thought research incorporating genetic analyses might be useful in patients at risk for the development of kidney disease because of traditional factors, such as race, or the presence of diabetes or hypertension, but such studies might be costly, because of the number of patients required and the length of follow-up time necessary to detect the beginning signs of disease. The attendees, however, felt that the study of genetics in patients who had received a kidney transplant might be valuable. They conjectured that fewer kidney transplant patients might be needed for shorter follow-up times in order to make meaningful conclusions.

A Way Forward

Besides the overarching goal of translating the findings into clinical practice, which could improve the quality and quantity of the lives of those affected by this genetic variant, a big challenge was demonstrating how changes in *MYH9* biology might cause and/or worsen kidney disease. This issue was put to rest by findings of a multidisciplinary research team of nephrologists and geneticists led by Dr. Martin Pollak from Harvard. They had invited Barry Freedman and Cherie Winkler from the FIND study, as well as Jeffrey Kopp, to collaborate on the project. They recruited Dr. Etienne Pays, an expert in parasitology from Belgium, to help in crucial analyses.

Reports of studies that include NIH scientists must go through a clearance process before being prepared for submissions to scientific journals. A scientist without a direct connection to the research is asked to review the findings to point out flaws or make suggestions before the paper is permitted to be submitted for publication. Jeffrey Kopp asked me to review the paper in February 2010. He sent me the manuscript on a Wednesday and asked me Thursday if I had read it. I laughed because reviewing a paper is a bit of a chore, requiring a great deal of concentration. Jeffrey was eager to have the paper reviewed and sent out for publication as soon as possible. I promised him I would review it over the weekend. I had spent the weekend in New York at the opera and finally took the paper out to read on the air shuttle trip back to Washington, D.C. I almost fell out of my seat. The results were clearly a major finding, indeed a paradigm shift. I quickly gave my consent for clearance, as, subsequently, did the NIDDK.

The paper was published in that most prestigious journal, *Science*, in August 2010.[7] The investigators noted the association of *MYH9* with kidney disease in the FIND and Kopp papers previously published in *Nature Genetics* but pointed out that the causal variants underlying the disease had not been identified. They also highlighted that genes in the region in question on chromosome 22 had probably been subject to changes engendered by natural selection. The investigators pointed out that genes encoding apolipoproteins were in the same region on chromosome 22 identified by the FIND and Kopp groups, quite close to *MYH9*, and that their protein products had many variations and several precise functions in humans and other primates. These apolipoprotein gene products also varied in different populations. The investigators hypothesized that variants in an *APOL* gene might be more tightly linked to kidney disease than the *MYH9* gene. They used data from the 1000 Genomes Project, funded by the National Human Genome Research Institute (NHGRI) of the

NIH and the Wellcome Trust, to "identify polymorphisms within this expanded risk interval that showed large frequency differences between Africans and Europeans . . . to test for association with renal disease." (In other words, the investigators used previously identified areas on chromosomes that had already been determined to be different in populations of White and Black people.) The investigators first compared genes from 205 patients with FSGS determined by the gold standard, a kidney biopsy, with those of 180 African Americans without kidney disease. The majority of these patients came from Kopp's consortium, but the investigators from Harvard's Brigham and Women's Hospital contributed the rest. The strongest signal was in the gene encoding apolipoprotein L-1 (*APOL1*) at a variant site they termed G1. The G1 allele was present in 52% of those with FSGS, but in only 18% of the controls, a finding that could be explained by chance only about once in a trillion trillion times. (That's 1 in 10^{23} times.) They also identified another allele, G2, associated with kidney disease in that population. In analyses where G1 and G2 were considered together, the G1 and G2 variants accounted for practically all the kidney disease in the study participants. Indeed, when the G1 and G2 variants were considered, there was no association of kidney disease with the *MYH9* locus. The link had been with *APOL1* all the time, but the *APOL1* gene was on the same ancestry block as the *MYH9* gene, and the two genes tended to be inherited together. In another group of ESRD patients, the study findings were replicated, with even stronger statistical relationships between the G1 and G2 alleles and kidney disease. (The statistical significance and the strength of the association for the *APOL1* variants were much greater than those seen with *MYH9*.)

Furthermore, the investigators showed that the presence of one variant allele in a person was not enough to result in the development of kidney disease. The presence of two variant alleles was associated with a high probability of the presence of kidney disease, but not all people with two variant alleles developed kidney disease. These findings were consistent with what is known in genetic circles as a "recessive model of inheritance with incomplete penetrance." The findings suggested the presence of another source of risk, such as another culprit gene or an environmental factor, like a viral infection, might be involved in the pathogenesis of expression of kidney disease. Their findings suggested the gene variants associated with disease might be present in about 20% to 40% of African American ESRD patients and 23% to 52% of African Americans who had FSGS but in only 13% to 21% of African Americans without kidney disease. In retrospect, the FIND and NIH investigators simply chose the wrong locus. This was understandable because the peak of association centered on *MYH9*, but there were thirty-two other genes closely packed under that peak.

Perhaps the most exciting part of this dramatic, landmark, paper was the explanation of why *APOL1* variants might be linked to kidney disease. (This had been the key element lacking in the *MYH9* story.) The investigators cited work from the 1000 Genomes Project that showed the variants were relatively common in Nigerian populations but were not found in people of European, Japanese, or Chinese ancestry. These findings suggested that the gene variants associated with disease might have arisen relatively recently in African populations because of some environmental factor or event (sometimes termed "pressure") associated with natural selection. In other words, gene variants associated with the development of kidney disease might have appeared over time in selected populations if they conferred a health advantage related to another deadly illness.

There was precedent for this analogy in a disease that was known to be common in African Americans—namely, sickle cell disease. Sickle cell disease was also a recessive genetic disease. It had been established that the presence of at least one sickle cell variant gene protected people from severe malaria, an infectious disease caused by parasites invading red blood cells. The abnormal hemoglobin gene products in RBCs prevented the parasites from engaging with the erythrocytes. In those people with two variant hemoglobin genes, however, the adaptation went awry. Sickled RBCs clogged blood vessels, resulting in pain and, over the long-term, the development of bone and kidney disease as the vessels supplying blood to the organs died. Anemia, as a consequence of the abnormal RBC hemoglobin, was a prominent feature of the disease as well. Therefore, the price paid for protection from malaria in a large population was that some unlucky people who inherited two variant genes would be afflicted with an awful illness that diminished quality of life and shortened life span. Could a similar process be at work with *APOL1* gene variants?

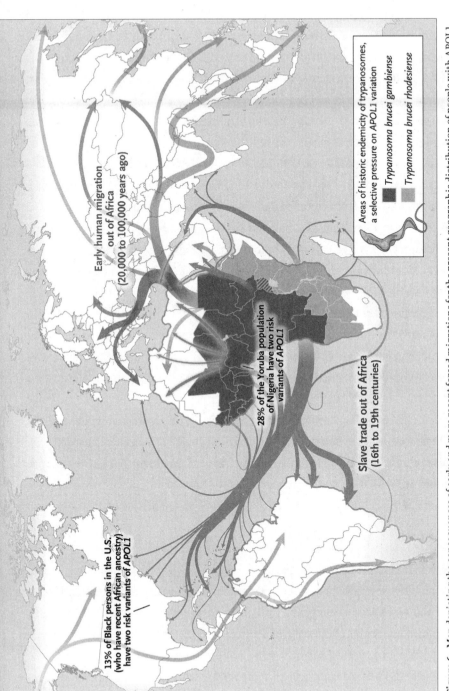

Figure 6. Map depicting the consequences of early and more recent forced migrations for the present geographic distribution of people with APOL1 gene variants across the globe. From the *New England Journal of Medicine*, Winfred W. Williams and Julie R. Ingelfinger, "Inhibiting APOL1 to Treat Kidney Disease," vol. 388, pages 1045–49, © 2023 Massachusetts Medical Society. Reprinted with permission from Massachusetts Medical Society.

The Winkler group was already working with Pays and his colleagues and introduced Dr. Pays to the Pollak investigative team. Pays and colleagues had shown as early as 2003 that ApoL1, the protein gene product of *APOL1*, in the human bloodstream is toxic to the parasite *Trypanasoma brucei brucei*, the agent responsible for African trypanosomiasis (sleeping sickness), but it is not toxic to the two strains of *T. brucei* that cause human African trypanosomiasis. This dread disease, spread by the tsetse fly, only exists in sub-Saharan Africa. The researchers designed a series of elegant experiments to show that the variants might have evolved from the natural (or ancestral) *APOL1* gene in order to provide protection from trypanosomiasis. The investigators demonstrated, in Petri dish studies, that plasma from patients with the G1 or G2 variant and laboratory-generated G1 and G2 proteins coded by the variant gene sequences were more likely to kill the parasites than plasma from patients not carrying the variant or proteins generated by the ancestral gene. The analogy to sickle cell disease was self-evident, and this, as well as the extremely high probabilities noted in the clinical studies and the difference in the prevalence of the variant genes in groups of people with recent African descent compared to other populations, made a strong case for invoking a causal relationship between the *APOL1* gene variants and kidney disease. The next challenge remained the formal demonstration of causality in an animal model and the elucidation of the mechanisms whereby abnormal *APOL1* genes caused kidney disease. When these mechanisms are identified, treatment for kidney disease could be devised. At least that was and is the hope.

Clinical Studies on *APOL1*

While investigators in different groups were showing that variant ApoL1 proteins adversely affected several kidney cellular functions, clinical studies moved forward at a rapid pace. Dr. Afshin Parsa did his fellowship training in nephrology at the University of California, San Francisco, where he gained expertise in genetics. Afterward, he joined the faculty at the University of Maryland. He had been eager to show relationships between *APOL1* variants and the course of kidney disease. He joined forces with the Chronic Renal Insufficiency Cohort (CRIC) study to determine if the presence of *APOL1* variants was associated with hard clinical outcomes. The CRIC study had been initiated by Josie Briggs and the NIDDK at the beginning of the millennium to recruit patients with kidney disease and follow them over a long period of time in order to assess the course and outcomes of patients with early stages of kidney disease. Dr. Briggs had often referred to the CRIC study as a "Kidney Framingham study," a research study that would establish important clinical risk factors to predict if specific groups of patients with chronic kidney disease did well, went on to need dialysis or kidney transplantation, developed heart disease, or died prematurely. Parsa thought this would be an ideal group to study. The work they did, published in the *NEJM* in 2013, galvanized the kidney research community.[8] The paper described the CRIC participant population as well as the population of participants in the African American Study of Kidney Disease and Hypertension (AASK), a study initiated by the NIDDK in the 1980s to determine the best treatment for hypertension in African Americans and to follow the course of their kidney disease. The AASK study was exclusively made up of African American participants, while the CRIC study intensively and preferentially recruited African Americans with kidney disease. The CRIC population included 2,955 White and Black people with various kinds of chronic kidney diseases. Almost half had diabetes mellitus. Participants were evaluated for the rate of loss of kidney function while they participated in the study as well as the end points of loss of half of their initial kidney function or development of ESRD. Almost 700 AASK participants were also evaluated for loss of half of kidney function from study entry or entry into ESRD. Therefore, information from the two groups could be easily combined. The presence of *APOL1* gene variants was evaluated in all participants. About 58% of patients with poor outcomes in the AASK study had two high-risk variants, while only a little more than a third of patients in the low genetic risk group had the undesirable outcomes. These findings indicated that the presence of two *APOL1* risk variants conveyed almost double the risk of losing kidney function or entering ESRD in this group compared to those without the genetic risk. In Black CRIC participants, those with two *APOL1* variants had a statistically significant more rapid decrease in kidney function and approximately twofold more common development of ESRD. The authors concluded, "Renal risk variants in *APOL1* were associated with the higher rates of end-stage renal disease and progression of chronic kidney disease that were observed in black patients as compared with white patients, regardless of diabetes status."

Barry Freedman, who was an author with Afshin Parsa on the *NEJM* paper, further concentrated on the kidney transplant population. In a series of studies, he and collaborators showed that kidney transplant recipients who received a kidney with two variants lost their grafts much faster than recipients who got a kidney from a donor with no abnormal variants or only one *APOL1* gene variant. These findings had implications for people waiting for kidney transplantation, as well as for the national system that determined kidney allocation among potential recipients. The algorithm for risk in kidney recipients focused on the race of the kidney donor. Genetic information, rather than using the construction of race, might provide far more accurate estimates of risk of loss of kidney function in kidney transplant recipients. (This might be an early type of "precision medicine.") Scientific, policy, and personal health considerations conjoined to make further research in this field, using prospective studies, imperative.

Meanwhile, over the previous several years, Drs. Ali Gharavi and colleagues at Columbia University and Friedhelm Hildebrandt and collaborators at Boston Children's Hospital, Harvard Medical School, and elsewhere, as well as others, had shown that many different genetic mutations are associated with unsuspected kidney disease in patients in populations distinct from those of recent African descent.[9] Paradoxically, their work showed that rare or private genetic variations are commonly linked to what were previously thought of as complex kidney and urologic diseases in the general population. Some of these diseases fall under the spectrum of CAKUT, or congenital abnormalities of the kidney and urinary tract. Both Hildebrandt and Gharavi were honored with the Homer Smith Award of the American Society of Nephrology.

The Birth of APOLLO

The NIDDK held a workshop in June 2015 and invited basic and clinical scientists to discuss fruitful areas of research for studies in *APOL1* genetics, apolipoprotein biology, and kidney physiology. The conference participants also highlighted ethical considerations in studies of *APOL1* genetics. Participants recommended further studies to delineate mechanisms underlying the toxic effects of *APOL1* variant gene products on the kidney and their possible roles in disease pathogenesis. Another key recommendation of attendees was to focus on the kidney transplantation population, where prospective studies, thought to have high power (needing relatively few participants to be followed for comparatively short periods of time), might provide clinically useful information more rapidly.

In November 2016, the NIH Guide published RFAs DK 16–024 and DK-16–025, initiating the *APOL1* Long-Term Kidney Transplantation Outcomes, or APOLLO, study. The funding for the APOLLO study was provided primarily from NIDDK, but the National Institute on Minority Health and Health Disparities (NIMHD) and the NIAID participated as well. The Requests for Applications called for proposals for a scientific data research center (SDRC) to lead the study and clinical centers to recruit living and deceased African American kidney donors to donate their DNA for research purposes while also recruiting the recipients of these kidneys. Recipients would be followed for several years to determine whether *APOL1* variants in the donors predicted recipients' outcomes. The study started in September 2017. The NIH allocated almost $4 million per year for five years to this effort. Wake Forest University, led by Barry Freedman, was the successful applicant for the SDRC. Thirteen successful clinical centers joined the consortium.[10] The consortium had the goal of recruiting every recipient of a kidney from every African American donor across the U.S., whether transplantation occurred at a large or small center. Dr. Marva Moxey-Mims of Children's Hospital in Washington, D.C., was chosen by NIH to lead the consortium. An innovative but key component of the study was the creation of the Community Advisory Council, a group of African American people who had kidney disease, had undergone kidney transplantation, or had served as a kidney donor or who were relatives of a person with kidney disease. The CAC advised the investigators on matters related to recruitment and retention of study participants and regarding all aspects of study procedures. A member of the group, Ms. Nichole Jefferson, was appointed to the steering committee, the governing body of the study. These innovations helped ensure that the patients' voices were heard as an important component of a large, federally funded study. Study results for APOLLO, expected by 2026, should have a major impact on counseling kidney donors and recipients on the effect of *APOL1* risk alleles on the kidney health of African American living donors and the recipients of kidney transplants.

New Hope for Interventions in *APOL1* Kidney Disease

The study of kidney disease has been revolutionized by advances that have occurred in genetic science since the 1980s. Genetic studies have shown that the disparities in kidney diseases in populations in the U.S. are not solely due to the social determinants of health. Powerful genetic forces, probably engendered by infectious diseases prevalent across the African continent, have resulted in a huge burden of kidney disease in African Americans. Several studies from investigators at Columbia and Harvard, as well as other research institutions, have demonstrated that much of the burden of kidney disease in children, as well as adults, is due to myriad genetic causes. The challenge for the 21st century is to translate these advances in science to clinically applicable treatments and perhaps cures for patients at risk for or with kidney disease.

It's always an issue in genetic studies if physicians can do anything about the findings that will favorably affect the health of patients. An answer for *APOL1* came in a series of exciting articles published in the *NEJM* in March 2023. Investigators at Vertex Pharmaceuticals had tested the ability of a small molecule, inaxaplin, to inhibit one of the functions of *APOL1* gene products in an animal transgenic mouse model of kidney disease and proteinuria.[11] They showed the experimental molecule reduced proteinuria in the mice. They then performed a small study, working with nephrologists in the research community, in a group of thirteen patients with focal segmental glomerulosclerosis, and proteinuria, with two *APOL1* variants, who were able to complete the study, giving them inaxaplin daily for thirteen weeks. The investigators showed inaxaplin reduced urinary protein excretion in the patients. Although a small research step, the study showed a drug could influence the effects of a genetic modification that could cause harm in humans. The investigators reported mild adverse events occurring during treatment, but noted that in most cases, they were not attributed to treatment with the novel molecule. The hope, of course, is that long-term and early treatment with such a drug could prevent the onset or ameliorate the course of focal segmental glomerular sclerosis in patients with two injurious *APOL1* gene variants. The investigators cited their study as an example of precision medicine, where genetic status might be more important than kidney biopsy results in determining who would qualify for, and respond to, treatment.

The *NEJM* published an accompanying paper, with beautiful explanatory illustrations, by editors Winfred W. Williams and Julie R. Ingelfinger that reviewed *APOL1* genetics and its epidemiology and relationship to kidney disease.[12] In addition, the *Journal* published an editorial in the issue by Dr. Neil Powe, entitled "A Step Forward for Precision Equity in Kidney Disease."[13] Powe, the leader of the University of California, San Francisco, Medicine Service at the Priscilla Chan and Mark Zuckerberg San Francisco General Hospital, reviewed the disproportionate burden of kidney disease in African Americans, and previous findings related to *APOL1*. He thought the research "appears to be a major scientific breakthrough with enormous implications, especially for persons of African ancestry." Powe outlined the more definitive studies that would be needed to demonstrate the efficacy of treatment and to bring the drug to market. However, Powe noted the significance of these proof-of-concept studies and the enormous potential of such research to address inequities in the prevalence, treatment, and outcomes of kidney disease. Industry-based research and collaborations with academic investigators could enhance equity for patients with kidney disease.

The Vertex investigators are currently engaged in another, larger placebo-controlled trial of inaxaplin.

Many physician researchers addressed the study of genetics of kidney disease over the decades from the 1980s to the third decade of the 21st century, making both incremental and dramatic discoveries that showed how often kidney disease is a result of genetic determinants in people of all racial groups. Dr. Martin Pollak won the prestigious Homer Smith Award in 2017 for his groundbreaking and ongoing work on the science of *APOL1* genetics related to kidney disease. In the next chapter, we see how genetics have interacted with a potent environmental factor, systemic racism, to magnify the effects of kidney disease for African Americans.

9

--- ✤ ---

MATURITY OF KIDNEY
TRANSPLANTATION

Clinical Success and Lingering Inequities

Is There Something Better Than Imuran?

By the late 1970s, the search for better immunosuppressive drugs was on. Jean Borel, born in 1933, received his doctorate in immunogenetics in 1964. After joining the international pharmaceutical giant Sandoz, based in Switzerland, Borel became interested in the chemical product of a fungus a botanist fellow employee had brought back to the company after travels in Norway. Cyclosporin A, as it then was called, was isolated by Sandoz in 1971. (The drug would undergo several name changes and was cited under different terms in different papers over the ensuing years.) Borel established that this ring-shaped biochemical made by the fungus had immunosuppressant properties. In 1976, Borel and colleagues published an article on the novel compound in the journal *Agents and Actions*.[1] They described cyclosporin A as a small protein that delayed rejection of skin grafts and graft versus host disease in mice and ameliorated arthritis and immune-mediated central nervous system inflammation in animal models of disease. In contrast to clinically available immunosuppressants, cyclosporin A had relatively minor effects on white blood cell counts in the animals they tested. In 1977, in the highly regarded journal *Immunology*,[2] Borel and colleagues described cyclosporin A as a "small cyclic peptide," with effects on immune cells that mediated delayed hypersensitivity and humoral (or antibody) responses. They suggested the effects might be selective for T-cells, a key part of the body's immune regulatory system. The investigators emphasized its relative lack of toxic effects, implying cyclosporin A might be a safer immunosuppressive drug than those currently used in clinical practice. In subsequent studies published in 1979[3] and 1980,[4] Borel and colleagues further elucidated the effects of cyclosporin A on the biology of lymphocytes and the outcome of skin grafting in mice and dogs.

In 1978, the *Lancet* reported a study of rabbits that received kidney transplants treated with cyclosporin.[5] Another *Lancet* article, published shortly thereafter by Roy Calne and colleagues, reported on seven ESRD patients maintained on dialysis who received cadaveric kidney transplants and were treated with cyclosporin as an immunosuppressant in combination with other therapies designed to blunt the immune response.[6] Although cyclosporin appeared to be a powerful immunosuppressant, adverse events included, paradoxically, kidney toxicity as well as side effects involving the liver. Starzl and colleagues reported in 1980 on twenty-two patients in Denver, Colorado, who received cadaveric renal transplants and were treated with cyclosporin.[7] Although the results were preliminary, in most cases the relatively short-term outcomes were satisfactory. Long-term results were needed to put the findings into proper clinical perspective. The patients reported by Starzl's team had only been evaluated for two to four and a half months. They emphasized that other supplementary immunosuppressive drugs or therapies were required in combination with cyclosporin. Several studies in humans and animals, many by Calne and colleagues, followed over the next several years, which suggested the drug might have kidney toxicity, but what was really needed to show clinical effectiveness was a randomized controlled trial of this new immunosuppressant drug, assessing long-term outcomes.

By 1982, clinical trials of the effectiveness of cyclosporin were being published. In 1982, preliminary results of a European Multicentre Trial, "Cyclosporin A as a Sole Immunosuppressive Agent in Recipients of Kidney Allografts from Cadaver Donors,"[8] showed that in 117 patients randomized to receive cyclosporin, kidney transplant survival was 73% compared to 53% in 115 patients randomized to treatment with the usual drug combination of azathioprine and steroids. Patients had been followed for up to eleven months. Approximately four-fifths of patients in the experimental group had been treated with cyclosporin alone. Kidney function in patients in both groups at six months was similar. The authors suggested cyclosporin was an effective and superior immunosuppressive agent, since the use of steroids could be curtailed in patients receiving this drug.

In 1982, Dr. John S. Najarian (1927–2020), with colleagues David E. Sutherland, Richard L. Simmons, and others at the University of Minnesota, published their findings on the use of cyclosporin in kidney transplantation in *Surgery*.[9] One hundred recipients of kidneys from cadaver donors were randomized to receive either cyclosporin A combined with prednisone or antilymphoblast globulin, azathioprine, and prednisone, the typical immunosuppressive regimen at Minnesota. One-year kidney transplant survival was 93% in those treated with cyclosporin compared with 81% in those who received usual therapy. Patients in the cyclosporin group had fewer rejection episodes as well as fewer infections than patients in the usual care group. They reported cyclosporin therapy impaired kidney function; however, the toxicity was reversible if the drug dose was decreased. The investigators admitted that studies evaluating the effects of longer treatment were needed.

Shortly afterward, in 1982, the final data from the European Multicentre Trial that had been previewed in the *Lancet* earlier that year were published.[10] Randomization of the 232 patients who received kidney transplants from cadaveric donors occurred at eight medical centers across the continent. The authors concluded these preliminary results suggested cyclosporine appeared "to be more effective than conventional immunosuppression and avoids the necessity of long-term steroid therapy."

In 1983, the advances that transplant physicians, surgeons, and their patients had been anxiously awaiting finally appeared.

Starzl and colleagues reported the results of a randomized trial in twenty-one kidney transplant recipients treated with cyclosporin and prednisone compared with twenty patients who received immunosuppression with azathioprine and prednisone.[11] One-year graft survival was 91% for those treated with cyclosporin and 56% for those treated with Imuran. The difference between the graft survival in the two groups was statistically significant, despite the small number of patients in the trial.

In 1983, the *NEJM* published "A Randomized Clinical Trial of Cyclosporine in Cadaveric Renal Transplantation," performed by the Canadian Multicentre Study Group.[12] Cadaveric kidney transplant recipients were randomly treated either with cyclosporine and prednisone or with the clinical standard of azathioprine and prednisone, using contemporary rigorous clinical science best practices. The study took place over five years. The authors subtly criticized the methodologies of some of the previously published randomized studies of the new immunosuppressant. A total of 103 patients received cyclosporine and 107 received azathioprine at twelve Canadian transplant centers. Some patients in the standard care group received antilymphocyte globulin as well. Patients were followed for one to seventeen months. The median follow-up was still a relatively short eight months. Predicted kidney transplant survival in those who received the renamed "cyclosporine" was estimated at 80.4%, while graft survival was estimated at 64.0% in those treated with more conventional forms of immunosuppression, a highly statistically significant difference. Patient survival was also significantly better in those who received cyclosporine. Kidney function, as assessed by S[Cr], three months after the procedure, however, was significantly worse in those who received cyclosporine. The study group carefully reported and characterized complications in the two treatment groups, including high blood pressure, infections, cancers, decreased white blood cell counts, and liver toxicity as well as deaths. In general, the investigators were not able to show differences in complications of transplantation between the two treatment groups, perhaps because of the relatively small number of patients randomized. The investigators acknowledged that the role of concomitant steroid therapy in patients undergoing kidney transplantation treated with cyclosporine was unclear and could not be addressed by their study. The authors concluded the "significant improvement in graft survival in this and other studies suggests that cyclosporine rather than azathioprine is the immunosuppressive agent of choice in cadaveric renal transplantation." The investigators noted that additional clinical studies needed to be performed to "determine the optimal regimen for the use of cyclosporine."

This clear, well-designed, and carefully analyzed study was received appreciatively by researchers and clinicians. The study put the nail in the coffin of the use of azathioprine, a drug that had been the state of the art in clinical practice for twenty years. The medical community and ESRD patients had eagerly awaited FDA approval of cyclosporine for clinical use in patients receiving kidney transplantation in the U.S. Approval came in the autumn of 1983.

In 1984, two critical papers related to cyclosporine and kidney transplantation were published in the *NEJM*. In one paper, Dr. Robert Merion, a young surgeon working with Calne and other colleagues, reported on a retrospective analysis comparing seventy-nine patients who received kidney transplants treated initially with cyclosporine alone as the immunosuppressive agent to twenty-nine patients who received conventional immunosuppression, simultaneously, using azathioprine and steroids.[13] Patients were followed from five to fifty-four months after transplantation. Those in the comparison group treated with conventional approaches had variations in the exact regimen used. None of the patients had diabetes mellitus. Patients treated with cyclosporine had higher four-year survival (86% vs. 76%) and better kidney graft survival (70% vs. 62%) than the comparison group. The differences in patient and kidney graft survival were not statistically significant. Acute transplant rejection occurred in 62.1% of those treated with cyclosporine and 65.5% of those treated conventionally. The authors noted that S[Cr]s were higher in the cyclosporine group (but the difference was not statistically significant throughout the course of treatment), suggesting, but not proving, that kidney function was poorer in the cyclosporine group. They attributed the difference primarily to nephrotoxicity associated with the use of the wonder drug, but acknowledged, without the use of renal biopsies consistently in both groups, that kidney rejection and nephrotoxicity could not be definitively differentiated. They stated, "Associated nephrotoxicity has not been satisfactorily explained or clinically resolved." They advocated for limiting kidney toxicity from the drug by monitoring cyclosporine levels in the recipients frequently and adjusting drug doses accordingly or switching to other forms of immunosuppression later in the course of therapy. They concluded that cyclosporine was a viable and effective form of immunosuppression for kidney transplant patients and that in many ways, it was superior to immunosuppressive strategies based on steroids and azathioprine. In some cases steroid treatment in such patients could be avoided when cyclosporine was used. They emphasized that longer and more controlled studies were needed to establish norms for practice in this field. Although the study was not randomized and had an unconventional design, it had a relatively long observation period and had been accepted by the *Journal*, granting it an important imprimatur in the medical community. The study was supported by the University of Michigan, the Medical Research Council of Great Britain, and the East Anglia Regional Health Authority.

More clarity was brought to the issue of nephrotoxicity when a paper on use of cyclosporine in patients undergoing transplants not involving kidneys, entitled "Cyclosporine-Associated Chronic Nephropathy," appeared in the *Journal*.[14] The study was led by Dr. Bryan Myers, a graduate of the University of Cape Town, who had worked in Israel and San Francisco before joining the Stanford faculty. Myers specialized in the field of glomerular pathophysiology. He was an expert measuring glomerular filtration by direct laboratory methods, using techniques with markers that were freely filtered by the kidneys but were not affected by the function of the tubules. His work had been extensively funded by various NIH institutes. The investigators took advantage of the heart transplant program at Stanford University, which had begun to use cyclosporine in their patients. They measured the glomerular filtration rate (GFR) in seventeen heart transplant recipients treated for a year or longer with cyclosporine compared with fifteen similar patients treated with azathioprine, using traditional and newer methods developed by Myers and colleagues.

The average S[Cr] was similar in both groups before transplantation, about 1.3 mg/dL. In patients treated with cyclosporine, S[Cr] levels had increased significantly from 1.3 ± 0.1 to 2.1 ± 0.2 mg/dL over a year, consistent with an important decrease in renal function. In contrast, in patients treated with azathioprine, the S[Cr] levels significantly decreased from 1.3 ± 0.1 to 1.0 ± 0.4 mg/dL, suggesting improvement in GFR. Differences in the S[Cr] levels were seen between the two groups as early as a month after heart transplantation and prescription of cyclosporine. Many of the patients in the cyclosporine group developed high blood pressure. Far fewer, only about 6%, developed hypertension if they had been treated with azathioprine. Although both groups of patients had similar cardiac function, after one year, those treated with cyclo-sporine had worse kidney function, with GFRs of 51 ± 4 (about half normal levels) compared with 93 ± 3 mL/min (a normal result) in patients treated with conventional immunosuppression. The patients treated with cyclosporine had higher mean arterial blood pressure. Two of the patients treated with cyclospo-rine developed end-stage kidney failure. The authors noted their results with S[Cr]s were consistent with the Canadian and European kidney allograft trials. Although the investigation was not randomized or controlled, the advantage of studying the effects of cyclosporine in patients who did not have kidney dis-ease and did not need renal transplantation was immediately obvious. The kid-neys were no longer a confounding factor, and the results of therapy with cyclosporine on their function was clear. The authors interpreted the findings as showing that cyclosporine had direct nephrotoxicity, affecting the tubules, resulting in decreased glomerular filtration and renal function. Myers and col-leagues bluntly concluded, "Long-term cyclosporine therapy may lead to irre-versible and potentially progressive nephropathy. We recommend that cyclosporine be used with restraint and caution until ways are found to miti-gate its nephrotoxicity." The wonder drug had problems and its use incurred consequences, notably an impairment in kidney function. Before this study the effects of cyclosporine on kidney function in transplanted patients had been particularly murky in the absence of routine evaluation by use of renal biopsies. Perhaps, even at the outset of the availability of cyclosporine, a better nonpurine analogue immunosuppressant drug was still needed.

Kidney Transplantation and the Revolution in Quality of Life

As nephrology developed as a subspecialty of internal medicine, because of advances in technology and increasing complexities of treatment, nephrology clinicians further divided into transplanters and dialyzers. Since the modali-ties of ESRD therapy were not determined randomly, it was difficult to pre-cisely compare outcomes of patients treated with transplantation and dialysis. By the 1980s, dialysis had expanded into accepting elderly, sicker patients, while the patients favored for transplantation were younger and often had dis-ease limited to the kidneys. In this new ESRD care era, supported by seemingly unlimited funds from the federal government, dialysis units had shifted to accepting many more patients with diabetes mellitus for treatment in contrast to their earlier, more restrictive policies. Patients, physicians, and researchers were interested in whether kidney transplantation truly provided improved quality and length of life to patients who successfully underwent the procedure. It would be hard to determine differences in the absence of well-designed randomized clinical trials. The issue was soon addressed by a distinguished multidisciplinary group.

In 1985, the *NEJM* published "The Quality of Life of Patients with End-Stage Renal Disease" by Roger W. Evans, Diane L. Manninen, Louis P. Garrison Jr., L. Gary Hart, Christopher R. Blagg, Alan R. Hull, and Edmund G. Lowrie.[15] Dr. Evans was a sociologist who worked at the Battelle Human Affairs Research Centers in Seattle, Washington. Drs. Manninen and Garrison were also social scientists at Battelle. Evans and Manninen had worked as a team since 1983, studying patients' responses to ESRD therapies. Dr. Blagg (1931–2022), a nephrologist, had become the director of the Northwest Kidney Center in Seattle in 1971, succeeding Dr. Belding Scribner. Blagg had moved from Leeds, England, to work with Scribner in the early days of dialysis. Blagg had always been interested in the human experience and long-term consequences of being treated with hemodialysis. Evans and Blagg had published together previously as well. Dr. Lowrie worked at National Medical Care, one of the oldest for-profit dialysis organizations, based in Boston. Dr. Gutman was a transplant nephrologist at Duke who had previously published a two-part review on kidney transplantation in the *NEJM* and had published early studies on rehabilitation in dialysis patients. Dr. Hull was a nephrologist specializing in dialytic care at the Southwestern Dialysis Center in Dallas, Texas.

The authors started their paper by reviewing the early findings related to the costs as well as the benefits patients experienced from enrollment in the ESRD program. At the time, the focus on patient outcomes was on "rehabilitation" and whether dialysis patients were able to return to work. The investigators acknowledged the ESRD program had changed over its first decade, admitting older patients with medical comorbidities, such as diabetes mellitus and heart disease, who were primarily treated with dialysis. Such patients were not deemed to be good transplant "candidates." The notion of "quality of life" was only beginning to be explored by researchers, and the tools to measure the concept were largely lacking. The authors quoted book chapters regarding the assessment of quality of life and a 1982 *Kidney International* paper by Johnson, McCauley, and Copley,[16] but the previous investigations largely focused on dialysis patients. Although it was generally thought self-evident that life and health were vastly improved for ESRD patients by kidney transplantation, information to prove this, especially if the cohorts of patients in each group were similar in age and had similar systemic illnesses, was not available.

Using multiple psychological measures to measure "quality of life," Johnson, McCauley, and Copley, in their very small study with only fifty-nine patients in four groups, suggested cadaveric transplantation might not convey advantages in mood and attitudes of ESRD patients. They did point out that transplantation seemed to confer some improved perceptions regarding quality of life for the patients, but perhaps more importantly, they showed that patients whose transplants had failed and who had returned to dialysis treatment had, even in such a small sample, diminished and dismal perceptions of their quality of life. The investigators used measures that Angus Campbell and colleagues had previously employed to evaluate the quality of life in a large U.S. population sample, published in 1976 in a book titled *The Quality of American Life*.[17] The investigators were therefore able to speculate about ESRD patients' quality of life compared to national norms. Studies comparing perceptions of quality of life between transplant and dialysis patients were hampered, however, for at least two reasons. A randomized study of the same patients eligible for either transplantation or dialysis was clearly impossible when the choices involved in making such decisions were so different and so grave. No one could imagine patients giving up their autonomy, allowing their treatment to be determined by the toss of a coin, for such an investigation. In addition, merely comparing patients treated with transplantation or dialysis, even prospectively, could not account for the fact that the populations were very different, a classic case of "comparing apples and oranges," a scientific anathema. Transplant patients were younger, healthier, and drawn from more privileged, wealthier communities than patients treated with dialysis. The quality of life investigators attempted to address these scientific design issues head on to answer whether kidney transplantation really conferred better quality of life for ESRD patients, all things being equal, using statistical techniques for nonrandomized, "observational" studies.

Evans, Manninen, and coauthors, to try to rectify the flaws of previous studies, evaluated a relatively large number of ESRD patients (859 people), treated with different therapeutic modalities (home hemodialysis, in-center hemodialysis, continuous ambulatory peritoneal dialysis, and transplantation), coming from different settings (rural and urban, for-profit and not-for-profit dialysis centers). Patients from eleven medical centers across the country participated. Interviewers, who had been centrally trained, directly obtained information from the patients, literally about how they were feeling. The investigators attempted to control for differences between the patients treated with the different modalities by statistical methods. The authors used "objective" quality of life indicators, such as self-reported work status and staff-reported Karnofsky scores. The Karnofsky score of functional status, conceived as "objective," starkly ranging from full function to "moribund" or "dead," had been used in studies of the response to treatment with erythropoietin. The "subjective" or "emotional" measures, linked to the patients' moods or the way they felt, were similar to those used by the Campbell and Johnson groups.

The investigators found that transplant patients were most able to work and had the highest scores on the "subjective" quality of life measures—well-being, psychological status, and satisfaction with life. The transplant patients were thought to have a more positive perception of quality of life than the dialysis patients, similar to that of average Americans. The study, supported by a grant from HCFA, was a ringing endorsement for the benefits of kidney transplantation. The authors quoted *Gift of Life: The Social and Psychological Impact of Organ Transplantation* by Roberta Simmons, Susan Klein, and Richard Simmons, Fox and Swazey's *The Courage to Fail*, and the work of Dr. Paul Eggers.[18]

Kidney Transplantation versus Dialysis: A Tale of Two Treatments

By 1988, Dr. Paul Eggers of HCFA put the results of the improved availability and outcomes of kidney transplantation after the introduction of cyclosporine in the ESRD program into perspective in an article entitled "Effect of Transplantation on the Medicare End-Stage Renal Disease Program" published in the

NEJM.[19] Eggers did his undergraduate and graduate work at and received a Ph.D. from Purdue University. His dissertation was "An Ecological Analysis of the Spatial Distribution of Pharmacists." Eggers had always been interested in social justice. After finishing his graduate work, he joined HCFA, which administered Medicare claims and payments, in its Office of Research. In 1985, he became the chief of the office's Program Evaluation Branch, which had purview over the U.S. ESRD program.

At that time, the growth and success of kidney transplantation resulted in the patient population with functioning grafts becoming "the fastest-growing group of beneficiaries of the Medicare end-stage renal disease program." By 1985, such transplant patients composed about 18% of ESRD patients and almost one-third of those less than fifty-five years old. The proportions of transplant patients in the ESRD program were higher than those reported by Henry Krakauer and colleagues only five years previously,[20] demonstrating that the procedure was effective, popular, and becoming relatively more common as well as conferring better survival. The rates of graft survival for transplanted kidneys improved markedly between 1983 and 1984, after the approval of cyclosporine for use in transplantation in the U.S. in the autumn of 1983. Almost three-quarters of U.S. kidney transplant patients received cyclosporine as an immunosuppressant agent in 1984. Differential rates of transplantation between different groups resulted in an increasing proportion of Black patients receiving dialysis. Eggers noted that the cost of maintaining a patient with a functioning kidney graft was only about a third the cost of treating a patient with dialysis, that relatively few patients sixty-five years and older received kidney transplants, and that Black ESRD patients received transplants at about half the rate of White patients. He summarized the current situation as two ESRD populations: "those under 55 years old, who are increasingly likely to receive transplants, and those aged 55 and older, who are almost all on dialysis."

Advances in Matching in Kidney Transplantation: Were They Helping?

Several changes and trends in transplantation have occurred from the 1970s until now, most resulting in improved ESRD patient outcomes. In the 1980s, blood transfusions were recommended for patients receiving deceased donor transplants, as a result of studies published in the *NEJM* by Paul I. Terasaki and Gerhard Opelz in 1978.[21] The role of transfusions as well as the importance of HLA matching had become unclear and had to be reevaluated in the cyclosporine era, since use of the calcineurin inhibitor had resulted in dramatically improved outcomes for the recipients of kidneys from deceased donors. In addition, the importance of individual patient factors, preservation solutions, and time spent transporting organs, as well as the national allocation, matching, and distribution systems themselves, were uncertain in the absence of well-designed randomized controlled trials addressing clearly outlined questions, which obviously were not feasible given the clinical constraints. The complexity of the kidney transplant system created a kind of Heisenbergian uncertainty regarding its individual components, including tissue typing, especially in an era of new immunosuppressant drugs. Studies regarding the importance of HLA matching published between 1984 and 1990 yielded conflicting results, and the optimal clinical approaches to patient care and kidney allocation schemes were both controversial and unknown. Disturbing analyses also suggested that contemporary sharing practices using HLA matching systems discriminated against Black ESRD patients. The majority of patients transplanted did not have perfect HLA matches, but there was not good information regarding how the number of mismatches affected kidney transplant outcomes.

In 1992, Terasaki and colleagues, including those from the UNOS Transplant Registry, in a *NEJM* paper, stepped back from assertions made by his group more than twenty years earlier.[22] The authors noted that although short-term kidney transplant survival had increased over the previous two decades, the length of long-term kidney graft survival had barely changed, even in the cyclosporine era. The investigators noted that data linking HLA matching to outcomes was necessarily retrospective and dependent on administrative rather than clinical trial data. Their paper reported on outcomes of a large nationwide study of kidneys allocated by UNOS. The tissue typing was performed at more than one hundred centers across the country, using the standardized techniques pioneered by Terasaki and his group: 1,386 cadaveric kidneys were distributed among 1,004 first transplant recipients, with 362 patients receiving subsequent transplants, using an HLA matching system. A set of 26,138 transplant patients with information about HLA matches was used as a comparison group. The investigators found HLA-matched patients consistently fared better than those who were mismatched. The authors concluded that the "high success rates obtained when more than 1000 kidneys from matched cadaveric donors were shipped for transplantation, with a maximum of four years of follow-up, demonstrate that there can no longer be any doubt that HLA typing for the A, B, and DR loci is sufficiently standardized throughout the United States to serve as the sole basis for kidney allocation." The authors pointed out the low rate of kidneys obtained from Black donors. They emphasized that because racial groups shared HLA antigens, "minority recipients can receive matched transplants only when the number of minority donors increases." They urged a review of allocation systems to both ensure equity and enhance outcomes for kidney transplant recipients. (This was a tall order and still has not been adequately achieved.)

In 1994, Terasaki and colleagues illustrated how a change in the HLA system classification might be used to enhance local sharing of kidneys, in the *NEJM*, to increase equity.[23] The authors described the matching system presently in place.

> The current kidney-allocation system of the United Network for Organ Sharing incorporates elements of each philosophy, allotting points for waiting-time, presence of preformed anti-HLA antibodies, age, and levels of HLA compatibility. The patient with the most points rises to the top of the waiting list. The physician makes the final judgment whether or not that patient will receive an available kidney. When UNOS identifies a perfect match somewhere in the United States, the kidney is sent to that recipient. Otherwise, most kidneys are transplanted locally. Through the UNOS six-antigen matching program, in which the recipient is matched to the donor for two antigens each in the HLA-A, B, and DR loci, projected survival at 29 years is 50 percent for grafts functioning at 1 year.

The authors estimated only about 5% of patients received a perfect match, and that the "next best match does not yield a sufficiently high success rate to justify national sharing." The investigators quoted data suggesting that contemporary, as well as theoretically perfect HLA matching systems would result in decreased kidneys being available to Black recipients. Using a theoretical model, they proposed instituting new matching categories that might increase the number of patients who could be matched, including a higher proportion, and therefore number, of Black and Hispanic recipients.

In the succeeding paper in the same issue of the *Journal*, Philip J. Held, Ph.D., and a dream team of transplantation and biostatistical expert colleagues from a diverse group of institutions, including the University of Michigan, the University of Iowa, the University of Texas at Houston, the NIDDK, and the Urban Institute, among others, set out, using administrative registry databases, to evaluate the effect of HLA mismatches on outcomes in ESRD patients who received cadaveric transplants.[24] Held had a degree in physics, but had become a health economist and was respected for his wit and intellect. He had devoted much of his career to studying the ESRD program. Henry Krakauer of the Uniformed Services University of the Health Services was senior author. In addition, the investigators wished to quantify the potential ramifications of an allocation system in which HLA matching would be prioritized. To create a homogeneous group, the study sample included 30,564 recipients of cadaveric kidneys between 1984 and 1990, all of whom had previously been treated with dialysis, in whom the HLA tissue types of donors and recipients were known. As Terasaki had surmised, only a small number of patients had no mismatches. There were only 3.7% "perfect" matches between 1988 and 1990. The investigators found transplants with fewer HLA mismatches had longer survival and that transplantation without mismatches yielded better survival outcomes than those with one mismatch. It was difficult to define differences in outcome between transplantations with one to six mismatches. In alternative analyses, the investigators were able to show that graft survival correlated with the number of matches, incrementally, in a kind of dose-response curve. Five-year survival was estimated as 65% for those with no mismatches, 55% with four mismatches, and 52% with six mismatches.

The authors found that a system could be created in which almost one-fifth of the transplant recipient population had no mismatches. That would have resulted, theoretically, in the five-year survival of the grafts from deceased donors increasing from 58.5% to 62.9%. Such an allocation system would paradoxically also have increased the probability that the number and propor-tion of white kidney recipients would increase at the expense of candidates from other racial or ethnic groups. The authors noted, using a national per-spective, that longer organ preservation times, associated with better match-ing, but requiring more time spent in transit, might diminish the effects of better tissue typing. In many ways, although the findings contrasted with those from Terasaki's group decades before, Held and colleagues also showed that although HLA mismatches mattered, the differences better matching con-ferred in patients who received kidneys that were not perfectly matched, although statistically significant, were not large. The findings put the data from Terasaki and colleagues into perspective after twenty-five years but also had grave implications regarding the equity of our national transplant alloca-tion systems.

The distinguished transplant clinician scientist Dr. Fred Sanfilippo, then of Johns Hopkins University, tried to put these two papers into the context of contemporary clinical practice. He opined, in an editorial in the same *NEJM* issue,[25] commenting on the papers by Drs. Held, Kahan, and colleagues and Dr. Terasaki and colleagues, that HLA matching conveyed advantages to patients receiving both first and second cadaveric transplants. HLA matching had implications for both patients' clinical outcomes and the allocation of kidneys between patients of different racial and ethnic groups. It seemed the important remaining clinical questions could not be definitively settled in the absence of prospective carefully controlled randomized trials, which were clearly not fea-sible. Sanfilippo acknowledged that "in contrast, it is apparent that excellent outcomes can be obtained without good HLA matches for many recipients of a first graft, who may have weak immunologic response to alloantigens, espe-cially when conditioned by donor blood or bone marrow cells." Sanfilippo noted that in studies he, as well as others, had done, the outcomes of kidney transplantation were not as favorable in Black patients as they were in White patients. Although Sanfilippo endorsed changes in allocation systems, he noted, "The key to increasing the number of recipients with optimally matched kidneys and reducing waiting time is to increase the number of organs donated, especially from minority groups. As the debate on the role of HLA matching in cadaveric kidney transplantation continues, the most important measure of the appropriateness of the organ-allocation policy is a public perception of equity and utility, which in large part is manifested by the willingness to donate organs." UNOS has wrestled with the problem of creating an allocation system that will maximize good medical outcomes, be efficient, and sustain equity from that time until the present.

Over the ensuing years, determination of HLA types has moved from serologic methods to more precise molecular determinations, using nucleic acid rather than protein-based antibody interaction methods. The former molecular techniques have revealed an even greater complexity of the HLA system. The role of tissue typing has become less important for patients receiving kidneys from deceased donors, but the evaluation is still performed in patients receiving kidneys from deceased donors, across the nation, as perfect matches between donors and recipients are associated with better recipient outcomes. A different test, a positive cross match, often performed just before the surgery, suggests a high probability of rejection. Tissue typing is still acknowledged as critical for those receiving kidneys from a living donor, especially between family members.

The number of kidneys available each year (about 24,000—a little more than 75% from deceased donors and less than a quarter from living donors) is far lower than the approximately 75,000 patients joining the waiting list each year.[26] The number of living donors and the total number of kidney transplants, however, has increased over the years, as the population of the country with chronic kidney disease and the general population have increased. Transportation of kidneys for transplantation across the U.S. and intercontinentally was enhanced by preservative techniques promoted by Dr. Folkert Belzer, most notably after he joined the University of Wisconsin. Transfusions before transplantation are no longer suggested for recipients of kidneys from deceased donors.

Tacrolimus was approved for liver transplantation in the mid-1990s but shortly thereafter became the most common immunosuppressive medication for patients receiving kidney transplantation. Toxicities associated with tacrolimus are similar to those seen with cyclosporine (such as nephrotoxicity and development of diabetes), but the side effect profile of tacrolimus is more favorable. Three main eras have broadly characterized the kidney transplant program—those of azathioprine, cyclosporine, and tacrolimus. In general, better patient and graft survival has been seen across the eras and across time.

Kidney Transplantation: Where Are We Now?

USRDS statistics released in 2022 provide an overview of the long-term status of kidney transplantation over the last twenty years. Graft and patient survival for those receiving deceased donor kidneys has increased over the last decades. Women receiving deceased donor kidneys in most analyses have slightly better graft survival than men. Asian and White patients who receive kidneys from deceased donors have better graft survival than Black and Native American patients. Those who receive kidneys from living donors have better kidney graft survival. Comparable ESRD patients, when age, sex, and race are accounted for, have better survival with transplantation than those patients treated with dialysis. The present focus is on improving patient and graft survival for over ten years after transplantation, the new long-term goal.

A Patient from the 21st Century

As a scarce resource, kidneys for transplantation were always under scrutiny for potentially being allocated primarily to the privileged members of society. Such issues became more salient and urgent as transplantation has improved and increased numbers and proportions of patients with kidney failure waited for and sometimes received the "gift of life."

How kidney transplantation changed in the two decades after the introduction of cyclosporine (and subsequently other calcineurin inhibitors), as well as because of advances in tissue typing and surgery for living donors, is apparent considering the case of Dr. Sally Satel, who needed a kidney in 2005. Satel grew up in Queens, New York, and attended Cornell University. After graduate work at the University of Chicago, she enrolled in and graduated from the medical school at Brown University, in Providence, Rhode Island. She was a resident in psychiatry at Yale from 1985 to 1988 and was an assistant professor of psychiatry at Yale from 1988 to 1993. She then went to Washington, D.C., as a Robert Wood Johnson Fellow, assigned to the Senate Labor and Human Resources

Committee. Her areas of expertise include psychiatric issues associated with substance abuse and opioid therapy, as well as public policy. She contributes to journals of opinion, including the *New Republic*, the *Wall Street Journal*, and what was previously known as the Op-Ed page of the *New York Times*. She is currently a resident scholar at the American Enterprise Institute in Washington, D.C. Satel is a straight-talking person, with a razor-sharp intellect, a penchant for debate, and a lancinating but often self-deprecating sense of humor.

Satel told the story of her search for a kidney in the *New York Times Magazine* in December 2007 in a frank and poignant manner that perfectly but succinctly recapitulated the patient's view of ESKD while also outlining the societal implications of the illness. Satel had had a long history of kidney disease, first diagnosed by excellent nephrologists at Yale, perhaps associated with treatment of an unrelated medical disorder during her training as a physician. She had been cared for by several nephrologists in Washington, D.C., but over the years the illness had progressed, as was typically the case, and she was told that her kidney disease was nearing end-stage. She would need dialysis or transplantation to stay alive. Satel, as a physician, knowing the ins and outs, medical risks, and personal consequences of that modality of therapy, wanted to avoid treatment with dialysis at all costs. She had said, "No matter what happens, I'm never going to go on dialysis." And she was sophisticated enough to know what such a stance meant and what her options and chances were. Satel was referred to transplantation centers in Washington, D.C., and Maryland, and began the wait for a kidney from a deceased donor for a "preemptive" transplant, before starting dialysis. The trouble is the waiting period for such a kidney could be several years. Satel didn't have relatives to provide a kidney, so she set out to move things forward on her own. As a medical expert and public intellectual, she had a wide network of friends, acquaintances, and collaborators. Satel quietly and selectively put out word that she was in desperate need of a kidney. Several paths forward ended in roadblocks. A physician friend who previously said she would donate a kidney to Satel backed out after purportedly discussing the matter with a transplant surgeon. A person Satel corresponded with over the internet mysteriously went on radio silence as the time for donation approached. Yet another friend offered her a kidney and then demurred. Satel understandably grew frustrated and was exhausted by the emotional strain of the search and her race against time. Drs. Renée Fox and Judith Swazey had described just such scenarios in *The Courage to Fail* and *Spare Parts: Organ Replacement in American Society* when the transplant team provided medical excuses to give cover to people who really didn't want to be donors or who couldn't come to grips with donating a kidney. As Satel wrote, "I didn't want a gift, I wanted a kidney." She considered becoming a "transplant tourist," journeying to another country to buy a kidney from a donor. Wryly, considering her chances in the internet market, she quipped, "Were I a prospective donor, even I wouldn't have picked me."

She had accurately described the need, dependence, and anxiety of the patient seeking a donor for a kidney transplant and the reluctance of friends and families to provide an organ, summing up the major challenge faced by patients with advanced kidney disease and kidney transplant programs across the globe. In a stark illustration of the law of supply and demand, there is a significant disproportion between the number of people with kidney failure who need an organ and the number of deceased as well as living donors available to satisfy the need. This supply/demand inequity has generated many ethical quandaries over the years regarding transplantation and solutions varying in cost, feasibility, and moral integrity, such as donor kidney "auctions" and transplant tourism, where rich patients may impose financial pressures on poor people with two kidneys. (Current U.S. law prohibits the provision of kidneys for financial remuneration.) Anecdotes have been related about those who wished to donate even a single remaining kidney after a first nephrectomy (with or without understanding the predictable consequences). Altruism may provide a philosophical and ethical solution to such inequities, but the number of altruistic people is not unlimited.

Succor for Satel came in an email titled "Serious offer" from a friend in journalistic circles. Virginia Postrel was an author of several books, a contributor to the *New York Times*, and a columnist at *Forbes*. Postrel knew Satel, but she was not a close friend. Postrel heard about Satel's plight from a mutual friend during a casual conversation. Postrel told Satel, "If I'm compatible, I'll be a donor." In a true example of altruism, Satel received a kidney from Postrel when they both underwent surgery simultaneously in Washington, D.C. As Satel wrote, "On March 4, 2006, I became the proud owner of Virginia's right kidney." Postrel told Satel, "I felt intense empathy and imagined how desperate you must feel. I liked the idea of being able to help in a straightforward way to be able to cure a sick friend rather than just bring food or send a card." Postrel subsequently told her story in June 2006 in *Texas Monthly*. She outlined a supremely rational approach to an irrationally kind, radical, altruistic act—giving a kidney to a person she knew but to whom she was not related. In contrast to Brian Kampschroer's brother's experience, Postrel emphasized that her postoperative course, more than thirty years later, while not a walk in the park, was relatively benign. Her kidney was removed laparoscopically, through a small incision.

Satel wrote, "My story, it turns out, is a triumph of altruism . . . thousands of people have no donor at all nor relative who will do it out of love or obligation, no friend out of kindness, no stranger out of humane impulse. Alas, I have no kidney to give away. Instead I am urging . . . that society has a moral imperative to expand the idea of 'the gift.'"

Dr. Satel concluded her reminiscence by providing a prescription for the body politic.

Altruism is a beautiful virtue, but it has fallen painfully short of its goal. We must be bold and experiment with offering prospective donors other incentives for giving, not necessarily payment but material reward of some kind, perhaps something as simple as offering donors lifelong Medicare coverage. Or maybe Congress should grant waivers so that states can implement their own creative ways of giving something to donors: tax credits, tuition vouchers or a contribution to a donor's retirement account. In short, we should reward individuals who relinquish an organ to save a life because doing so would encourage others to do the same. Yes, splendid people like Virginia will always be moved to rescue in the face of suffering, and I did get my kidney. But unless we stop thinking of transplantable kidneys solely as gifts, we will never have enough of them.

After her successful transplantation, Satel had a party in Washington, D.C., to thank Postrel, her transplant surgeon and team, and her physicians, as well as the friends who supported her as she took charge of her care for ESRD during a harrowing year and a half. It was a grand occasion, where her numerous academic, intellectual, political, and journalistic colleagues gathered to toast her newfound well-being. After the surgery Postrel and Satel gave a joint interview on C-SPAN about the experience. In 2009, Satel edited *When Altruism Isn't Enough: The Case for Compensating Kidney Donors,*[27] a multiauthor text outlining the scarcity of kidneys for transplantation and considering various methods of potential donor compensation.

Satel's case contrasts with Brian Kampschroer's in that the donor's surgical operation was much less intrusive. Advances in retrieving a kidney using a laparoscope (a tube with a cutting edge that can be manipulated by a surgeon to safely remove a kidney through a small incision in the flank and repair the cuts made through the renal artery, renal vein, and ureter) allow the donor to have a much easier and shorter recovery. As Postrel noted, "I never had much pain and, once I left the hospital, took nothing stronger than aspirin, which my surgeon prescribed to prevent blood clots. But it took me about three weeks—longer than I expected—to get back to normal. The surgery left me easily exhausted.... Then suddenly I was myself again.... I caught up with my work and started traveling—short trips with light luggage. My all-purpose excuse, 'I just donated a kidney,' had expired."

Gender Inequality in Kidney Transplantation

A long-standing issue in transplantation programs has been sex and gender inequity in donation of kidneys (and other organs), being placed on the waitlist, and receiving a kidney transplant. The disparities have been noted since at least the late 1980s, including an article published in *Archives of Internal Medicine* in 1988 by Dr. Carl Kjellstrand. Kjellstrand was truly an international physician who had emerged as a powerful voice for the ESRD patient. He was born in 1936 and graduated from the University of Lund Medical School in Sweden in 1962. Kjellstrand did his residency at the University of Lund, where he trained under and did research with the legendary dialysis pioneer Professor Nils Alwall. Afterward, Kjellstrand pursued clinical training in the U.S. at

Bethesda Lutheran Hospital in St. Paul, Minnesota, where he directed the Artificial Kidney Unit from 1963 to 1964. Thereafter, he returned to the University of Lund, where he served in the Department of Nephrology until 1968. Kjellstrand returned to the U.S. to become the director of dialysis at the University of Minnesota in Minneapolis, a post he held from 1968 to 1981, as he became perhaps the world's preeminent expert on dialysis. Kjellstrand took over the post of director of the Division of Nephrology at UM in 1976 and served in this capacity until 1980. Thereafter, he did work at the Hennepin County Medical Center in Minneapolis before leaving to accept the position of chief of the Division of Nephrology at the Karolinska Hospital in Stockholm. While in Sweden, he earned a Ph.D. at the world-famous Karolinska Institute, in 1988. His thesis topic was "Ethical Problems of High Technology Medicine." He returned to Minneapolis to do clinical work but left shortly thereafter for an academic position at the University of Edmonton in Alberta, Canada. Kjellstrand worked in the University Hospital in the Departments of Nephrology and Bioethics from 1990 to 1997. Thereafter, he moved to industry, as the vice president for medical affairs at Aksys Ltd., based in Illinois.

At Minnesota, Kjellstrand became a leader in the ESRD program, locally, nationally, and internationally. While acknowledged as a superb physician, nephrologist, and physiologist at UM, he also made a name for himself across the country as a vocal champion of social issues related to ESRD patients. He started his article "Age, Race and Sex Inequality in Renal Transplantation" with the blunt assertion that "treatment of end-stage renal failure by dialysis is not distributed fairly."[28] Kjellstrand reviewed local organ-sharing practices and kidney transplant inclusion and exclusion criteria in the region in which the University of Minnesota was situated. More trenchantly, Kjellstrand reported on the characteristics of the medical staff in the region.

> In the Midwest, there are 11 transplant staff surgeons. One is a woman. There are no black or Native American transplant surgeons. There are approximately 60 practicing nephrologists who work with the transplant teams. Of these, three are women and one is black. There is no Native American transplant nephrologist.

In research largely preceding the establishment of national contracts for UNOS and the USRDS—and their ready ability to provide comprehensive, meaningful data to U.S. academic researchers—Kjellstrand went on to show, using U.S. nationwide data from HCFA from 1983 and regional data from his local ESRD network from 1979 to 1985, that of the 23,026 patients who started dialysis under the purview of the ESRD program, 6,112, or about 26.5%, received a kidney transplant. However, 31% of the men in the program received a transplant, compared to only 21% of the women. In the Midwest, approximately 39% of the men in the program received a transplant, compared to only about 30% of the women. Using Midwest data, Kjellstrand found non-White women between the ages of twenty-one and forty-five had about two-thirds the chance of receiving a kidney transplant compared to a White woman in that age group. Women between the ages of forty-six and sixty years had about half the chance of receiving a kidney compared to men of comparable age. Kjellstrand was unable to demonstrate definitively if these disparities were due to biological differences between the sexes, such as the presence of cytotoxic antibodies in women. In limited analyses, Kjellstrand was unable to show whether access for kidney transplantation for women had improved over time.

Kjellstrand's conclusions did not shy away from controversy. He commented, "There is inequality in renal transplantation, based on age, race and sex. Women receiving long-term dialysis in the United States and in the Midwest have three fourths the chance of men of receiving a kidney transplant." Kjellstrand wrote that such disparities were also present in Canadian and Swedish populations and appeared in access to treatment for women with heart disease. Taking an impartial, scientific stance, Kjellstrand opined the "causes of the observed imbalances are many. They may be morally neutral and based on biological, medical, sociological, economical, cultural, and geographic differences. However, they may also be caused by bias." Kjellstrand concluded that because of the scarcity of kidneys for transplantation that medical factors could not be the determining factor in the resultant differences in access. He cited that there were "distrust and communication difficulties between different racial groups." Kjellstrand summed up his findings, more than three decades ago, with a clarion call to social justice that would ring true today.

In transplantation, as in other medical and social services in society, there exists inequality caused by an unalterable hard fate. However, the imbalance that we have found among sex, age and race, independent of each other, and the similar differences that exist in the distribution of patients receiving long-term dialysis and cardiac catheterization is difficult to explain only by morally neutral biological, medical, geographical, or cultural differences. If there is actual bias, it is not possible to use our data to examine where the bias exists in patient, family, society in general, or in physicians and medical institutions. However, the most favored recipient of a transplant is similar to the physicians who make the final decision: a young, white man. Nephrologists and transplant surgeons should strive to correct the existing imbalances among renal transplants.

Kjellstrand's observations were amazingly prescient—including his observations regarding bias and trust between patients and health-care providers. One thinks back to the original days of Dr. Belding Scribner's Dialysis Program in Seattle. Many nephrologists and health policy experts had hoped that the enabling congressional ESRD legislation had solved those problems of scarcity and differential access to ESRD treatment over the succeeding decade and a half, but evidently the disparities still persisted on a national basis. Perhaps Kjellstand's status as a European helped him see the structures of the health system related to the U.S. ESRD program with a more disinterested, dispassionate view. Kjellstrand's research was supported by a grant from the Northwest Area Foundation to the University of Minnesota Bioethics Center and a grant from the Swedish Research Council.

Studies by many investigators between the 1990s and the first decade of the 21st century corroborated Kjellstrand's findings about sex biases in access to transplantation. In general, there is a greater proportion of female than male living donors, and these kidneys are more often given to men.[29] Female spouses are more likely to give their kidneys to their husbands with kidney disease than are wives with kidney disease likely to receive kidneys from their male spouses. Similarly, in general, women are proportionally more likely than men to donate kidneys to biologic relatives and unrelated recipients. While it is unclear whether medical factors contribute to such imbalances, it has been plausibly suggested that socioeconomic factors could be driving these differences. Studies show barriers to women achieving successful transplantation include differential placement on waitlists as well as the ultimate receipt of a functioning kidney.

These issues were reviewed by Drs. Phyllis August and Manikkam Suthanthiran of New York–Presbyterian Weill Cornell in 2017 in an editorial commenting on two papers on gender inequalities in kidney transplantation published in *JASN*, intriguingly entitled "Why Can't a Woman Be More Like a Man?"[30] The articles considered suggested that immunologic factors—in part related to sensitization during pregnancies, as well as other factors—may have precluded the ability of women to receive kidneys and to avoid graft failure after transplantation. August and Suthanthiran acknowledged that the factors underlying differences in outcomes between kidney transplant donors and recipients of different sexes were complex, including immunologic, anatomic, hormonal, and societal parameters. They noted that desensitization techniques and paired transplantation of incompatible live donors and recipients might somewhat ameliorate gender inequalities in kidney transplantation. Phyllis August, M.D., M.P.H., of Weill Cornell Medical Center received the 2022 Belding H. Scribner Memorial Award from the American Society of Nephrology.

The topic of gender inequality in kidney transplantation was also comprehensively reviewed in an article, "Equally Interchangeable? How Sex and Gender Affect Transplantation," in 2019 in *Transplantation*.[31] The paper was written by a multidisciplinary, international group of researchers, reporting on the findings of a conference held in Munich, Germany, in March 2018 on sex and gender influences on outcomes of transplantation. The authors considered differences in receiving living donations, being placed on a waitlist, time spent on the waitlist, and outcomes after kidney transplantation was performed. (For reference, the USRDS reported that in 2017, about 58.1% of ESRD patients were men. About 59.6% of prevalent patients with kidney transplants were men.)

The investigators reported that 60% of patients who received kidney transplants in the U.S. between 1988 and 2017 and 62% of patients with kidney transplants in Europe between 2008 and 2017 were men. At the time of publication, 61% of patients on the waitlist for a kidney in Europe and the U.S. were men. Although there were imbalances, the authors could not delineate whether they were disproportional or inequitable because of the larger fraction of men with kidney disease. The investigators cited studies suggesting imbalances between men and women throughout the process of qualifying for kidney transplantation and called for more fine-grained studies to evaluate access to deceased donor kidneys between the sexes.

While the authors cited variability in studies and across geographic regions, they opined that in general, outcomes were worse for women after receiving a kidney transplant than for men. Because of differences in donor characteristics, including sex, and in characteristics of recipients, the authors suggested that in studies from different populations, it was difficult to come to clear conclusions regarding differential outcomes between patients of different sexes with kidney failure. The authors reviewed the many biological differences between men and women that might affect the outcomes of kidney transplantation, including those related to sex hormones and the genetics related to the X chromosome, which are typically unavailable for analyses in large, administrative databases. The investigators noted the key roles of social determinants of health, including insurance coverage and marital and socioeconomic status, that might affect representation of groups at every step of the process involved in successful transplantation and maintenance of kidney function afterward. The authors suggested in their conclusions that although prevalent research often showed that access to transplantation differed by sex, further detailed research on sex differences in transplantation access and outcomes might be enhanced by attention to age differences in populations and studies on the biologic, as well as social, mechanisms, underlying disparate outcomes between the sexes. Nevertheless, in kidney transplantation, women are the givers and men are the takers.

Race Inequities in the Transplantation Program

Kjellstrand had reported on disparities in access to kidney transplantation by race in his paper in 1988, and Krakauer and colleagues noted differences in outcomes in Black and White patients receiving kidney transplants in 1983. Eggers followed his earlier observations on kidney allocation for transplantation in 1995 in an article entitled "Racial Differences in Access to Kidney

Transplantation" published in *HCFR*.[32] After acknowledging that previous work had pointed out disparities in access to transplantation between Black and White ESRD patients, Eggers concluded, "No matter what measure of transplant access is used, Black . . . ESRD beneficiaries fare worse than white, Asian-American, or Native American ESRD beneficiaries. Second, because the rate of renal failure exceeds the number of cadaver organs, access to kidney transplantation will deteriorate in future years for all races."

Dr. Friedrich K. Port, along with colleagues, reported in 1987 differential survival when Michigan kidney transplant donors and recipients, between 1972 and 1981, were of the same or different races.[33] The investigators found graft and patient survival were higher when the race of donor and recipient were concordant. Patient survival was poorer when a kidney from a Black donor was given to a White recipient. Although other studies from single centers disputed these results, the finding of Port's group was corroborated in several more contemporary populations. Dr. Kevin Abbott and colleagues showed in 2002 in a paper in *AJT* that kidney transplant survival was shorter in patients who received kidneys from donors of African ancestry, compared to those who received kidneys from donors of other race groups.[34]

Dr. Bertram Kasiske was the lead author of a report from the Patient Care and Education Committee of the American Society of Transplant Physicians, on racial inequality in transplantation. "The Effect of Race on Access and Outcome in Transplantation" in the *NEJM* in 1991 summarized the group's conclusions as well as the recommendations of the committee.[35] The authors reviewed that the risk of ESRD was about four times as great in Black compared with White patients, and that Native Americans had a threefold greater risk of developing ESRD than White patients. The committee noted that comorbid illnesses might explain the disparities for Native Americans, but coexisting illnesses did not account for all the differences between Black and White patients. The group confirmed that tissue typing results yielded more matches for White than Black patients. The committee found

> a major proportion of the racial differences in the overall rate of transplantation reflected differences in the rate of transplantation from living related donors.

Why proportionally fewer blacks have received kidney transplants is unknown. However, differences in the frequencies of ABO blood groups and the major-histocompatibility-complex (MHC) antigens, inadequate financial coverage, knowledge that the outcome after transplantation is worse in blacks than in whites, cultural barriers and other socioeconomic factors could all affect the rate of transplantation.

The authors, although they acknowledged that many social factors might underlie inequities in access to kidney transplantation, did not explicitly consider (or, if they did, did not write) that systematic or institutional racial biases could have played a role in creating or exacerbating differences between patients of different races. They noted that matching for the ABO blood type system and HLA (MHC) loci made it more likely that patients would receive kidneys from donors of the same race. They admitted that there had been "no systematic studies to determine how the subject of transplantation has been presented to and perceived by minority patients on dialysis." The committee recommended analyses of the interactions of ABO and MHC matches and patient characteristics, evaluations of availability of insurance coverage, education and compliance programs, and scrutiny of practices regarding wait-listing, as well as performing in-depth interviews of health providers and dialysis patients eligible for transplantation. The committee concluded,

Fewer blacks than whites in the United States undergo kidney transplantation. It is likely that both biologic and socioeconomic differences between blacks and whites contribute to this inequality....

... Although it is important to collect the information needed to answer critical questions regarding race and transplantation, the present lack of data should not delay potentially beneficial action. Efforts to increase the number of organ donations . . . from members of racial minorities . . . should yield immediate dividends. This approach should increase the number of suitable organs available for minority candidates without sacrificing the benefits of matching. Finally, health care providers should increase their advocacy role to assist patients in obtaining the most suitable form of treatment. This duty is greater for advocates of patients ill equipped to understand, accept or comply with the complicated issues of transplantation and its follow-up. Any and all barriers imposed by ignorance or misunderstanding on the part of health care givers and patients alike must be identified and eliminated by an intensive educational process.

Drs. G. Caleb Alexander and Ashwini R. Sehgal of Case Western Reserve University in Cleveland, Ohio, showed, subsequently, in *JAMA* in 1998, that Black patients were less likely to surmount the barriers posed at every step in the transplantation process.[36] They studied more than 7,000 ESRD patients beginning treatment with dialysis in Kentucky, Ohio, and Indiana between 1993 and 1996. The transplantation rate for Black patients was about 44% that of White patients. Systematic obstructions were present throughout the process—from being definitely interested in transplantation, through completing the evaluations necessary to qualify for kidney transplantation, up to getting a place on the waiting list, and finally receiving a kidney for transplantation— for Black compared to White dialysis patients. The investigators documented that women and poorer patients were also less likely to complete the steps necessary to achieve kidney transplantation. Their research was supported by NIDDK.

The extent of racial inequity in the U.S. ESRD program, however, became headline news for American physicians in the late autumn of 1999. On Thanksgiving Day, the issue of racial injustice in access to kidney transplantation was made apparent to all U.S. physicians in two adjoining articles covering seventeen pages in volume 341 of the *NEJM*, accompanied by a scathing editorial written by one of the deans of American nephrology at the time, Dr. Norman Levinsky (1929–2004), of Boston University. Levinsky had previously chaired a blue-ribbon committee of the prestigious Institute of Medicine charged with evaluating the U.S. ESRD program as it blossomed into maturity.

At the time, almost three decades after Medicare coverage was provided for U.S. ESRD patients as an entitlement, more than 200,000 people were treated for ESRD in the United States. A recurring concern for policymakers, physicians, and patients was that proprietary dialysis units, run for profit, might cut corners on patient care to protect corporate finances. For-profit units constituted more than two-thirds of dialysis providers at the time nationally. The first article, by Dr. Neil Powe (who held both an M.P.H. and an M.B.A.) and colleagues at Harvard and Johns Hopkins, bluntly speculated that for-profit dialysis facilities might not refer their patients for transplantation since that would cut into their corporate bottom line.[37] After all, a successfully transplanted patient was one lost to dialysis care and dialysis corporation billing. Payments for dialysis treatment had not increased since 1973. The investigators quoted the report from the Institute of Medicine by Drs. Norman Levinsky and Richard Rettig, the IOM study director, and colleagues, *Kidney Failure and the Federal Government*,[38] suggesting the "declining inflation-adjusted value of this reimbursement has aroused concern that attempts by dialysis providers to maintain income by cost containment may compromise the quality of care and lead to increased mortality among patients." The investigators, using publicly available information from the USRDS, funded by NIDDK, analyzed the association of for-profit dialysis unit management with dialysis patient referral for kidney transplantation and survival, while carefully controlling for the effects of patient age, race, sex, and zip code median household income, educational, employment, and marital status, as well as clinical considerations, such as type of kidney disease and comorbid illnesses and the characteristics of the individual dialysis units in the study. The authors showed, in a population of 3,681 patients across the U.S., for-profit dialysis units had a mortality rate of 21.2 deaths per 100 person-years of ESRD, compared with a rate of 17.1 deaths per 100 person-years of ESRD in not-for-profit centers, about a 20% difference. In analyses using all the adjusted variables, patients treated in for-profit facilities similarly had 20% higher mortality. Patients treated in for-profit units were 26% less likely to be placed on the waiting list for kidney transplantation than their counterparts treated in not-for-profit dialysis units. The authors wondered if cost-cutting measures, such as reductions in staff and time allotted for dialysis treatments and reused dialyzer practices, might underlie the mortality differences. They opined that decreased staffing might affect patient education regarding transplant options and that financial considerations may have led to fewer referrals of dialysis patients for transplantation from for-profit units. The investigators proposed that the financial incentives inherent in the government payment system did not necessarily work to enhance patient outcomes. The research was supported by the Robert Wood Johnson Clinical Scholars program and by a grant from NIDDK to Dr. Powe. Although the investigators had used the public USRDS for their research, they hastened to note that "the interpretation and reporting of these data are the responsibility of the authors and should in no way be seen as an official policy of or interpretation by the U.S. government." (Neil Powe received the Belding Scribner Memorial Award from the American Society of Nephrology in 2011.)

In the accompanying article in the *Journal*, "The Effect of Patients' Preferences on Racial Differences in Access to Renal Transplantation," Drs. John Ayanian, Paul Cleary, Joel Weisman, and Arnold Epstein,[39] a multidisciplinary team of investigators from Boston, assessed ESRD patients' access to transplantation after starting dialysis. The investigators addressed the very issue the Patient Care and Education Committee of the American Society of Transplant Physicians had raised in their *NEJM* article eight years previously. The authors began their article by citing a long history of differences in access to many kinds of salutary health care in the U.S. according to race. They noted that in 1996, more than 70,000 people started ESRD therapy, and almost 12,000 (or about 17%) received a kidney transplant. The investigators quoted the Eggers and the Alexander and Sehgal papers on disparities in access to kidney transplantation by race.

They interviewed almost 1,400 Black and White men and women from a random sample of those treated with dialysis, across several regions of the country, about their preferences regarding kidney transplantation. Their analyses were adjusted for differences in patients' preferences about transplantation, age, and socioeconomic status (such as marital status, education, income, health insurance coverage, and employment), as well as their perceptions of their quality of life and quality of health care, the type of dialysis facility in which they were treated, the region of the country in which the unit was located, the cause of the patients' kidney disease, and the coexisting illnesses of the patients between the groups.

Surprisingly, the authors found Black patients were less likely to want a kidney transplant than White patients. Not surprisingly, the findings suggested that was because Black patients were less informed about the potential benefits of transplantation than were White patients. Black patients were less likely to trust their physician than White patients. Large differences in the rates of referral for transplant evaluation and placement on a waiting list or actual kidney transplantation between Black and White patients were documented. "Black patients were much less likely than white patients to have been referred to a transplantation center for evaluation; they were also much less likely to have been placed on a waiting list or to have received a transplant within 18 months after the initiation of dialysis." The substantial differences between Black and White patients regarding outcomes related to kidney transplantation were significant after controlling for differences in socioeconomic and demographic characteristics, type of dialysis facility, patients' preferences, health, cause of kidney failure and comorbid illnesses, as well as perceptions of care between patients in the four groups.

The investigators concluded:

> Racial differences in access to renal transplantation are pervasive, but they are not immutable. Approaches to improving black patients' access include providing more systematic education about transplantation, offering greater encouragement to undergo evaluation for transplantation and to consider potential living donors, and monitoring and informing physicians and medical groups about racial differences in referral rates among their own patients. By making renal transplantation available to all clinically appropriate candidates who desire it, such efforts would foster greater effectiveness and equity in the use of this valuable procedure.

The authors did not mention that financial disincentives regarding transplant referrals may have mediated the results their research uncovered. Their research was supported by the Robert Wood Johnson Foundation.

Levinsky, in an accompanying editorial in the same *NEJM* issue, commented on the Powe and Ayanian papers.[40] He began with observations regarding the growth in the number of patients and outlay of funds over the approximately twenty-five-year history of the ESRD program. Levinsky noted reimbursements for dialysis treatments had fallen about two-thirds in real dollars over that time, and those exigencies forced dialysis providers to make tough economic choices to stay in business and provide necessary care. Levin-sky questioned whether despite economies of scale and technologic advances, decreased reimbursements may have compromised the quality of care and adversely affected patient outcomes. He pointed out that as the ESRD program developed over time, more minority patients and poorer individuals were treated, rendering the program much more representative of the U.S. popula-tion. Levinsky reviewed the two published papers and summarized them as showing that access to transplantation in the ESRD program was not equitable for Black patients. Levinsky clearly stated,

> Such differences, whether they are due to bias, to difficulties in commu-nication between black patients and their physicians, or to other unknown factors, are especially unconscionable in a program paid for largely by the U.S. government. . . . The federal government should expect dialysis programs to meet reasonable standards for equitable access to transplantation, for all patients, regardless of race, sex or social status. The government should also encourage and facilitate research on methods to overcome the persistent inequity in the ESRD program.

I vividly remember reading these papers in a bar on the Wednesday before Thanksgiving while waiting for the beginning of a movie next door. Tears came to my eyes as I realized the stark implications of the articles. Collectively, these three papers formed a condemnation of inequity in the U.S. ESRD pro-gram. Although Black patients had ESRD far out of proportion to their repre-sentation in the general population, access to the treatment that was cost effective and provided improved quality of life and length of survival was less available to them. Now all American physicians should have been aware of the facts. And all Americans, and the government, should have made efforts to rectify inequities.

One week later, in the December 2 issue of the *Journal*, Robert A. Wolfe, Philip J. Held, and Friedrich K. Port, with help from colleagues in academia and at the USRDS, settled a decade-old question.[41] Their paper showed definitively, using elegant statistical and comparative techniques, albeit with observa-tional data, that kidney transplantation clearly extended the lives of ESRD patients as compared with similar patients treated with dialysis. The investigators were able to deal with some issues of comparability by evaluating ESRD patients treated with dialysis on the transplant waiting list who did and did not get a kidney transplant, short-circuiting some of the analytic problems related to selection bias. The analysis confirmed that women and Black patients were underrepresented in the group that went from the waitlist to receiving a kidney transplant. These findings made the lack of access to kidney transplantation for Black patients even more galling—those patients were being deprived of life. On a bright note, the study revealed that Black patients who received a kidney transplant had comparable or slightly better survival than people of other comparison groups. (Wolfe, Held and Port received the Belding Scribner Memorial Award from the American Society of Nephrology in 2004.)

These *NEJM* articles from the end of the 20th century suggested kidney transplantation meaningfully extended the lives of patients over dialysis treatment, and that Black patients around the country had been systematically denied access to transplantation, a lifesaving therapy, to which they were entitled as U.S. citizens. Taken together, the four articles implied that the search for profits and institutional biases underlay the disparities in access to better therapies for patients in different groups with similar chronic illnesses and insurance coverage. Lamentably, an article published in 2021 in *JASN*, by Drs. Jesse Schold, John Sedor, Emilio Poggio, and colleagues,[42] frankly pointed out that little progress has been made in achieving equitable solutions to the issue of differential access to kidney transplantation between the poor and the rich and between White and Black patients in the U.S. in the more than twenty years since those seminal articles highlighting the problem were published in the *NEJM*.

Children as Kidney Transplant Patients

Kidney transplantation in children poses challenges not present in adults. William Harmon (1943–2016) received an M.D. from Case Western Reserve University and trained in pediatric kidney disease and transplantation in the Harvard system before joining its faculty. He pointed out, with coauthors Drs. Vikas Dharnidharka and Paolo Fiorina, in a review article in the *NEJM* in

2014,[43] that the early results of kidney transplantation in children were subop-timal, but outcomes for patients had improved dramatically in the first decade and a half of the 21st century. Kidney allocation systems in the U.S. were revised to favor children, whose growth and neurocognitive development are dependent on kidney function. Younger children with ESRD most often have congenital abnormalities of the kidney, while adolescents typically have a vari-ety of glomerular diseases (primarily affecting the filtering apparatus of kid-neys). Pediatric kidney transplant candidates usually do not have the multisystem diseases of the aging, primarily hypertension and diabetes, that account for so much kidney disease, as well as morbidity, in the adult population.

Harmon and colleagues noted kidney graft survival in children increased when results from 1987 to 1995 were compared to those of children who received kidney transplants between 1996 and 2010. These beneficial changes were thought to be the result of the interplay of several factors. In pediatric ESRD patients, surgical techniques, identification and matching of donors for specific recipients, and the development and understanding of optimal immu-nosuppressive drugs and regimens had all improved. The management of transplant rejection in children had changed for the better over time, resulting in decreased rejection rates, culminating in better graft survival. Since, in large patient populations, the most important factor determining mortality is a patient's age, all things being equal, pediatric ESRD patients, especially if transplanted, had excellent survival.

A comprehensive study using observational data by Maria E. Diaz-Gonzalez de Ferris, M.D., M.P.H., Ph.D., and collaborators in 2006, encompass-ing the outcomes of children who started ESRD therapy over the years between 1978 to 2002, showed nearly 80% of children between the ages of twelve and nineteen in the U.S. who received renal replacement therapy over the almost twenty-five years covered by the investigation survived.[44] Unfortunately, even though the survival of this cohort was so good, adolescents with ESRD were thirty times more likely to die than their counterparts without kidney disease. Three-fourths of adolescents with ESRD in the U.S. received a kidney trans-plant between 1978 and 2002. A bit fewer than two-thirds of the children at any point of time had functioning transplants (while more than one-third were treated with various dialysis modalities). As in the adult population, Black, Native American, and Asian patients were less likely to receive a kidney transplant compared with White patients, and boys were more likely to be transplanted than girls. Estimates suggested adolescents who received kidney transplants would enjoy an additional forty years of life, on average.

Ferris, a professor of pediatrics at the University of North Carolina and the mother of a child with ESRD, has emerged as a champion of children transitioning to adult care in the ESRD program. She is the director of the UNC Transition Program in the Department of Pediatrics. Ferris always knew she wanted to be a pediatrician but was first attracted to the care of critically ill infants. She was intrigued by nephrology when she first learned its principles in her second year of medical school. Shortly thereafter, she learned that her eldest child, who had had infections and was not growing as fast as his peers, had kidney disease. Because of the time constraints the care of a sick child imposed on a busy student about to become a physician, Ferris decided to abandon intensive care and focus on nephrology as a career, which would let her spend more time with her family. Ferris received a master's degree in public health, undertook fellowship training in nephrology at the University of North Carolina, and eventually started studies for her Ph.D. in 2006.

Her son Ted's illness progressed to ESKD when he was fifteen years old. Ferris donated a kidney to him when he was fifteen, but unfortunately, the transplant didn't function. Ted had to be treated with hemodialysis. His father donated a kidney to him in April 1997. Shortly thereafter, Ted was diagnosed with a complication of immunosuppression, post-transplant lymphoproliferative disorder, or PTLD. Ferris sought experimental therapy for her son in the form of an antibody directed against the CD20 molecule, primarily found on the surface of B-cells, which was in trials to determine whether it could safely alter the immune response. The treatment successfully addressed the complication and saved both the kidney and the patient. The experimental drug, subsequently released as rituximab, is now often used in clinical practice for patients with a variety of immunologically related disorders. Fifteen years later, a viral infection was associated with the loss of Ted's second transplant. He received a kidney from a cousin in 2017 and is now healthy. Ted is the father of two children, and Maria, an expert in the medical field that so deeply affected her family, is a proud grandmother. Ted Ferris is a consultant and a manager of hospice services.

Ted Ferris, born in 1981, attributes his success to his family. "I got to become an adult with a family and a professional career because I'm upper middle class. Because of my socioeconomic status, and the attributes of my family members, I had opportunities that others didn't have. My parents were encouraging, strong, loving and supportive every day. I hit the jackpot!"

Interestingly enough, Ted did not feel that he was different as a child growing up with kidney disease who underwent many procedures and operations:

My parents made me feel like I was normal—there was nothing wrong with me. Although I had had 30 surgeries by the time I was 20, I was told "Be optimistic. It will all work out." I was a "normal" kid. When I was 9 years old, I had surgery on my bladder. I was in Little League. (My Dad was the Little League coach.) I went out and played third base that afternoon. Nothing was going to stop me from living a normal life. Being optimistic—positive—carried me through some difficult times.

Ted started hemodialysis at a pediatric unit at the age of fifteen, after his first transplant, a gift from his mother, failed. Ted wanted to be an "easy" patient, and the experience further helped him "come out of my shell. I was their favorite patient." Dialysis imposed the challenge of a significant time burden, and his grades suffered a little. Ted felt he was never going to be a doctor, but his life had taught him he wanted to help others. "I care about others, like my mother." He received a second kidney transplant, a gift from his father, about a year after the failure of his first transplant. Within the next year, he developed PTLD and faced this new medical problem without fear. In retrospect, Ted realized what a grave complication PTLD is. However, with family support, particularly from an indomitable mother, he weathered the challenge.

Ted graduated from college and started a career as a manager in the film industry in Los Angeles. He experienced an episode of rejection at the age of twenty-five and successfully got through it. While back home for treatment, he started work at the University of North Carolina as a "transition coordinator" for patients with kidney disease. Ted found more meaning in this manner of "helping others, working with patients." Ted started to work with his father as a consultant in all aspects of the management of hospice care. Over the next several years, Ted got married and worked in several capacities in hospice care. He found this work very fulfilling and felt his experience as a patient helped him empathize with and help others.

In his early thirties, his second kidney began to fail. Eventually, the kidney lacked enough function to sustain him, and Ted resumed treatment with peritoneal dialysis. He defaulted to his childhood attitudes, thinking "this is just like before. Just another hurdle." Unfortunately, as he was preparing to receive a third transplant, his marriage failed. At the age of thirty-three, Ted received a kidney from his cousin, a dancer, who was ten years younger. The two cousins had been "very close." Ted recalled, "My cousin took the risk of major surgery. It was a big step to take, as it might have affected her career as a dancer. She did it out of love." Both Ted and his cousin resumed work shortly after the successful transplantation.

Ted Ferris was reunited with his high school sweetheart, and they are the proud parents of two girls. At the age of forty-one, Ted attributed his success to his parents and acknowledged the roles of socioeconomic status and support from others in his ability to become an adult, although he had a grievous childhood chronic illness.

Michael Mittelman also knew from an early age that he had kidney disease, but like Ferris, he felt "normal" as a child. He attributed this feeling to his parents' desire to have everyone treat him as a person and not as a patient. His kidney disease was diagnosed at the age of three. Mittelman remembers "getting puffy, and having things on my legs." He recalls being told by his mother that when he was taken to his pediatrician, "the doctor's jaw dropped." The physician, an old-timer, had been Michael's mother's pediatrician as well. "He instantly knew I had kidney disease, by looking at me." Mittelman remembers that he wasn't allowed to eat certain foods. His family changed to a low salt diet, and his friends' families accommodated his needs related to meals and snacks. He was often tired.

Laboratory tests were an "ordeal. They got blood all over my new sweat suit." At the age of five, Michael started peritoneal dialysis. Dialysis was performed at night, using a cycler machine (which Michael called "Alf"), administered with such care by his mother that he never came down with peritonitis. Because of urinary protein losses and severe hypertension, shortly after starting PD, both his kidneys were surgically removed. Michael remembers enduring severe headaches before the nephrectomies, characterized as "like elephants trampling on my head."

Nevertheless, Michael felt like other kids. "I was a normal kid during the day. At night, I did dialysis. I did sleepovers on weekends. I played baseball in Little League." Although family members wished to be donors, no one was suitable. "My mother was devastated that she couldn't be a donor, because our blood types were incompatible." Before the introduction of erythropoietin into clinical practice, Mittelman was anemic and needed frequent red blood cell transfusions. His family was concerned because at the beginning of the AIDS epidemic, the safety of the U.S. blood supply was a serious issue for patients, families, and physicians. Michael remained on dialysis for a year while receiving several "false calls" for a transplant kidney. "There were multiple disappointments that first year." About a year after starting dialysis, Michael "got the call." The donor was a teenage African American girl, from the Philadelphia area, "who died as a result of a tragic shooting on New Year's Eve." The Mittelman family tried to make contact to thank the donor family but were unsuccessful. Michael remembers his nephrologist, Dr. Jorge Baluarte, fondly for his care and uplifting bedside manner.

Michael initially did well, but he gained weight on steroids. He was not allowed back in school at first and remembers having to wear a mask in public. One of his elementary public school teachers helped by providing home tutoring services for him for three or four months after the transplant. Mittelman remembers, "It was wonderful to pee again. I had to learn how to use my bladder." With the help of his parents, Mittelman focused on school and sports. He played baseball, basketball, and soccer. His father was his coach. In 1990, at the age of nine, Mittelman was the youngest participant in the Transplant Games when he was in the fourth grade and won several medals. About that time, however, his transplant began to fail. He received a call to report to St. Christopher's Hospital in Philadelphia to receive a transplant in December 1990. The donor was a young man who had been hit by a train in a traffic accident. Once again, the Mittelman family was unable to contact the donor family to thank them. The transplant did well, but Mittelman remembers being teased by fellow students about his appearance. Because of his height, he started to receive injections of growth hormone. As he navigated middle and high school, he enjoyed academics, got excellent grades, and continued with sports, concentrating on golf. Michael was on the varsity golf team throughout his four years of high school and was also elected the president of the student body. He got a driver's license. But during his senior year of high school, as he was applying to colleges, Mittelman was told he "would need to start dialysis soon." His kidney was failing. To treat anemia, he was started on erythropoietin. A graft was inserted to prepare him for hemodialysis. Mittelman was about to matriculate at the University of Pennsylvania after graduation and started work during the summer as a golf pro at a local country club.

Mittelman started dialysis at Childrens' Hospital in Philadelphia as he was beginning college, working in his treatments between classes. During his freshman and sophomore years, he "was in and out of the hospital frequently for access procedures." Mittelman credits his father for ensuring he could be a full-time student and receive care on campus. He remembers that the professors made accommodations for his illness and his need for time on dialysis as well as his hospital stays. During that time, in 2001, Mittelman's mother read about experimental studies occurring at Johns Hopkins that were evaluating treatments to allow donation between ABO incompatible donors and recipients. The studies were being conducted by Drs. Lloyd Ratner and Robert Montgomery. Mike's mother was blood type A, and he was O+. Intrigued, Mrs. Mittelman consulted several physicians regarding the safety and feasibility of such procedures and heard contradictory optimistic and pessimistic viewpoints about its advisability. Mother and son decided to make an appointment at Johns Hopkins with Dr. Ratner.

Mrs. Mittelman was determined to be a good HLA match for her son. Dr. Ratner explained to them that this was to be an experimental procedure, based on early studies from Japanese transplant physicians. Mrs. Mittelman underwent rigorous testing to ensure that she was healthy and could donate a kidney. They were told that Mrs. Mittelman had had cytomegalovirus infection, a common viral illness, but that Michael had not. Subsequently, Michael was one of the first patients at Hopkins to undergo kidney transplantation from an incompatible living donor. He underwent three plasmaphereses, a treatment to remove plasma and replace it with pooled donor plasma, often used in the treatment of immune disorders, and received a kidney transplant from his mother. His mother had had the kidney removed by the relatively newfangled laparoscopic surgery, conducted by Dr. Robert Montgomery. Mittelman had one or two plasmapheresis treatments after surgery and received intravenous treatment with immunoglobulins to modify his immune responses to his mother's incompatible kidney. The kidney functioned perfectly after surgery, and began to produce urine during the operation. Mittelman noted that he hadn't urinated in two years. It was not until years later that Mittelman learned about the expenses entailed by the living donor. (These include the costs of medical supplies, income lost from days off work, and temporary loss of ability to provide for others. Some of these issues are considered in the epilogue as well.)

He returned to Penn to start his junior year. Mittelman had a new life, with more emphasis on social relationships and interactions. However, shortly after beginning school, he became ill with an acute, life-threatening cytomegalovirus infection, a disease transmitted through his mother's kidney. After intensive treatment, he once again became well and tackled his studies. Mittelman decided to achieve his goal of becoming a transplant surgeon.

Toward the end of his junior year, Mrs. Mittelman developed symptoms suggesting a gastrointestinal illness. After an extensive evaluation that was largely negative, ovarian cancer was diagnosed. Mittelman still remembers the intense emotions he and his family experienced at that time. His mother had been his savior and had undergone an extensive medical evaluation just a year earlier to prove she was in perfect health, fit enough to be a kidney donor for her son in an experimental procedure. If the cancer had been detected at that time, she would have been unable to give her son a kidney. If the family had waited, the donation would have been impossible. Their health conditions were inextricably ironic. So much in Mittelman's life had depended on timing and fate.

Mrs. Mittelman's treatment for cancer started, and Michael helped in her care over the next several years. Although Michael had some medical complications, he finished his schoolwork, graduating with a bachelor's degree in the biological basis of behavior. After graduation, Michael planned his course to achieve his dream of becoming a transplant surgeon. He embarked on completing the science courses necessary for medical school admission and started work as a research associate in the Division of Pulmonary Medicine, Allergy, and Critical Care at the University of Pennsylvania. Mittelman did basic research on human airway cells subjected to different pathologic environments, preparing to apply to medical schools.

The summer after graduation, Mittelman applied for and started an externship with Dr. Ratner, designed to show him what his planned career would entail. He would shadow Dr. Ratner and "live the life of a transplant surgeon." He spent long days with Ratner in the clinic, in the operating room, on rounds, and in organ recovery. Although the work was exciting and exhilarating, in a stunning but disappointing revelation, the athletic young transplant patient realized that the many hours spent standing up, without meals or water, and frequent night calls would be too physically taxing for him. He sadly made a snap decision to abandon plans for a career in medicine. Another blow came when Mrs. Mittelman died, two years after Michael graduated from the University of Pennsylvania. Mittelman needed a new path forward. He decided to apply for graduate training in healthcare management sciences. He notes his sister and father helped him find a path forward.

Mittelman liked the subject matter, and enjoyed learning new perspectives about the health-care system and its finances. He became interested in entrepreneurship. He won a business competition, and he and colleagues started a digital health company after his graduation, tracking home health-care utilization. He gained experience as the patient editor at the *British Medical Journal*, worked for a health insurance company, and did independent consulting work. He used his business and personal experience to start the American Living Organ Donor Fund. The foundation, inspired by his mother's gift, is devoted to protecting and supporting living donors by addressing their financial, mental health, and other needs. Mittelman serves as the founder, director, and president of the board of the organization. He currently works as a cybersecurity researcher for a health-care system. Mittelman describes himself as a patient advocate and advisor and a health-care consultant. He is a sought-after speaker at medical and health-care conferences.

Mittelman attributes his success to a supportive family and perseverance in the face of numerous obstacles. He remains fascinated by medicine because of his own medical illness and experiences as a patient. He considers his work at the fund meaningful, as "it helps at least one person every day." Mittelman, at the age of forty-one, recently celebrated the twenty-first anniversary of his third kidney transplant.

Austin Lee mentors children who have received kidney transplants at the Children's National Hospital in Washington, D.C. An air force "brat," he was born, the youngest of five children, in Germany in 1989, with abnormal urethral valves, revealed on a prenatal ultrasound that showed an abdominal mass. His mother was advised to have an abortion because of the baby's poor prognosis. Lee recalls his mother "fought back" because she wanted the baby despite the obstacles. The family returned to the U.S. in 1990. He started peritoneal dialysis when he was one and a half years old and had a ureterostomy tube to drain the kidney. Lee started walking late because of kidney metabolic bone disease. His mother was advised she would not be able to donate a kidney to Lee until she lost a great deal of weight. She lost almost fifty pounds, and Lee underwent a successful living donor transplant in 1993, at the age of four. The kidney functioned for fourteen years. Lee remembered that he felt different as a child because he couldn't compete in sports, but by seventh grade he felt "normal." Lee and his family fought for Social Security disability support.

When Lee was seventeen, his kidney failed, and his family "took it very hard." Lee missed his last two months of high school and was "embarrassed." He had "wanted to go to college, to work in the medical field, but now everything was on hold." Lee graduated from medical technical school while he was still treated with peritoneal dialysis and had started working at CVS, but he couldn't keep up with the workload. He was highly sensitized and underwent intravenous immunoglobulin treatments at Children's National Hospital to prepare for another transplant. His kidney was given to him by Ms. Stella, an altruistic donor who originally wanted to give a kidney to a member of her church in Prince George's County. The presumed donor was incompatible, so Ms. Stella and Lee participated in a paired exchange that involved fourteen recipients. Lee received Ms. Stella's kidney. Lee did not know Ms. Stella, but her church was located close to his. Although Lee longed to meet his donor, Ms. Stella was initially reluctant. They finally met on an Easter Sunday at Lee's church. Lee recalled, "It was one of the best days of my life."

Lee began mentoring children at Children's National Hospital about a year after his transplant. "My way of thanking Ms. Stella is my work. My work on social media has encouraged living donors." Lee pursued a career in childcare and has become a preschool teacher in the public school system. He works as an adviser with the NKF, the American Kidney Fund, and corporations involved in the care of people with kidney disease.

As a person of color, he wonders whether the travails his mother had to put up with during his birth and on receiving transplantation may have involved discrimination. He acknowledged his luck in having been a member of a close-knit, loving family. Lee attributed his success "to faith. . . . For me, transplantation meant no excuses anymore. There were no excuses why I shouldn't be successful and give back to others. I attribute my success to my donors." Lee noted, "Everyone outside my family views me as a normal person, but my family treats me as a transplant recipient, and they were always there to help me."

The stories of Ted Ferris, Michael Mittelman, and Austin Lee show children with ESRD are resilient and have long life expectancies, but their road is not easy. Children with kidney failure often have several transplants and many surgeries over the course of their lives. The close bond between parents and children with ESRD is critical, especially when the parent is a donor. Pediatric ESRD and transitions to adulthood are truly a family affair. Patients have to work hard throughout their lifetimes to make things work.

Susan Mendley graduated from the Boston University School of Medicine and did residency work at the University of Chicago before undertaking fellowship training in adult and pediatric nephrology at Chicago Hospitals. She spent the bulk of her career at the University of Maryland in Baltimore, before joining NIDDK as a senior adviser. She had been interested in the cognitive function of children with CKD, participating in a longitudinal evaluation of such patients, called the Chronic Kidney Disease in Children (CKiD) study. After starting at NIDDK, she became interested in the long-term outcomes of U.S. pediatric ESRD patients. Her recent work in *JASN* showed the survival of Black pediatric ESRD patients was shorter than that of White patients.[45]

Survival depended on the time the pediatric ESRD patient had a functioning kidney transplant. Black children had less access to transplantation and had fewer kidney transplants, which functioned for shorter periods of time. Mendley and colleagues noted that such glaring disparities in care and outcomes between these groups of children needed to be addressed.

More than 10,000 children with ESRD are living with a functioning kidney transplant as of 2019, according to the Scientific Registry of Transplant Recipients (SRTR).[46] Challenges remain for children and adolescents with ESRD treated with transplantation. Growth, while improved, is not as optimal as in children without renal disease. Bone and joint disease may occur despite excellent maintenance of kidney transplant function. Pediatric kidney transplant patients must follow a complex, lifelong daily drug regimen, which may become problematic for teenagers. Immunosuppressive drugs may change a child's appearance. Coping with such changes can be difficult in patients transitioning to adulthood, beginning sexual relationships, and experiencing peer pressure, resulting in difficulties with adherence to a challenging medication schedule. Indeed, adherence to immunosuppressive regimens remains a great obstacle to continued successful transplantation in young people and adults. Becoming an adult, even with a functioning kidney transplant, may be problematic for those whose childhood was centered on receiving medical care and who may have been more dependent on their parents and members of the health and social care systems than their peers. This may be a particular problem for former pediatric kidney transplant patients trying to establish themselves in the workforce. Long-term exposure to immunosuppressive medications may result in the development of infections or malignancies in patients with well-functioning kidney transplants. Successful pregnancies are a benefit of transplantation, compared with the relative infertility of ESRD patients treated with dialysis, but parenthood may present difficulties for those who start life as pediatric transplant patients. On an optimistic note, in 2003 Sharon M. Bartosh and colleagues, pointed out that of the mostly White childhood transplant patients who reached adulthood who they evaluated, about half were married, and the overwhelming majority were employed and reported fair to good health.[47] About seven to eight hundred children receive kidney transplants in the U.S. each year.

Liquid Biopsies

One of the key objectives in the care of kidney transplant patients since the beginnings of the procedure is the rapid diagnosis of rejection, so that therapy can be initiated as efficiently and as soon as possible. Over the first couple of decades of transplantation, the clinical diagnosis of rejection was established using clinical signs and symptoms, validated by the results of kidney biopsy. The rather obvious signs of rejection were altered, becoming more subtle as immunosuppression moved from azathioprine to cyclosporine and other calcineurin therapies. Some kidney transplant programs used protocol kidney biopsies, to provide periodic systematic assessment of signs of rejection using the gold standard of examination of kidney tissue under the microscope by pathologists. The Banff criteria, developed by a group of transplant clinicians and pathologists, were subsequently accepted to provide uniform guidelines for changes in transplant status according to histologic characteristics noted on renal transplant biopsies.

Dr. Phillip F. Halloran, a nephrologist at the University of Alberta, in Edmonton, Canada, has worked over the past several decades to use material from kidney biopsies for molecular analyses to predict outcomes in patients, as well as establishing clinical correlations from biopsy findings.[48] He spearheaded the Alberta Transplant Applied Genomics Centre to pursue such studies. Halloran was the first recipient of the Paul Terasaki Award from the American Society for Histocompatibility and Immunogenetics.

On the other hand, clinician scientists have long sought markers that might be available noninvasively, perhaps from the blood or urine, that could provide diagnostic clues to the presence of rejection of the kidney transplant or signaling irreversible graft loss in the form of a "liquid biopsy." For almost three decades, Manikkam Suthanthiran, M.D., of Cornell University has studied the molecular profile of cells in the urine, to provide noninvasive measures to predict outcomes of patients who have received kidney transplants. Suthanthiran was born in Madras, India, and graduated from the University of Madras. After residency in internal medicine at Wayne State University in Detroit, Michigan, he joined the fellowship program in nephrology at the Peter Bent Brigham Hospital. In 1998, Suthanthiran wrote a review article on "Renal

Transplantation" in the *NEJM* with the renowned transplant physician scientist Dr. Terry B. Strom.[49] In landmark *NEJM* articles published in 2001, 2005, and 2013, Suthanthiran and colleagues described the correlation of molecular findings in the urine of kidney transplant patients with outcomes of their grafts. The 2001 paper[50] linked the finding of molecular signatures of the active biochemical products of T-cells in the urine to the clinical outcome of rejection in kidney transplant patients. In 2005, Suthanthiran's group showed the measurement of FOXP3 (a protein produced by regulatory T-cells) mRNA in the urine of kidney transplant patients could differentiate those with acute kidney transplant rejection, chronic allograft nephropathy, and a benign clinical course.[51] In 2013, Suthanthiran, as the first and corresponding author, reported for a multicenter observational study that specific RNA levels in urinary cells from kidney transplant patients differentiated patients who had acute cellular rejection from those who did not.[52] These research endeavors were supported by the NIH as well as various other funding agencies.

Dr. Suthanthiran is currently the Stanton Griffis Distinguished Professor of Medicine and professor of biochemistry and surgery in medicine at Cornell University Medical College in New York City, and the founding chairman of transplantation medicine and chief of nephrology at the New York Presbyterian/Weill Cornell Medical Center.

Dr. Barbara T. Murphy started training at the Brigham and Women's Hospital after graduating from the Royal College of Surgeons in 1989 and subsequently doing medical postgraduate work in Ireland. Her research at the Brigham focused on clinical and immunologic aspects of kidney transplantation. She joined the Mount Sinai School of Medicine faculty in New York City in 1997 as a transplant nephrologist. At Mount Sinai, Murphy had a meteoric career trajectory. She was part of the Stock multicenter grant studying transplantation in patients with HIV (see below). She became the head of the Division of Nephrology at Mount Sinai in 2003. In 2012, Murphy became the head of the Department of Medicine at the Icahn School of Medicine at Mount Sinai. Murphy participated in the NIH-supported APOLLO Consortium, studying the outcomes of those who had received a kidney transplant with *APOL1* gene variants. Her later research involved using patients' genetic makeup and gene expression algorithms to predict transplant patient outcomes, and she collaborated with commercial entities to make such findings available clinically. Dr. Murphy died an untimely death at the age of fifty-six in 2021. She was on track to become the president of the American Society of Nephrology.

The work of Halloran, Suthanthiran, and Murphy represents only some of the efforts of the research community to develop noninvasive ways to evaluate the status of kidney transplants in patients.

Continuing Inequities—Addressing the Kidney Donor Shortage

Over the past decades, advances have been made in facing perhaps the greatest challenge to kidney transplantation: the critical shortage of kidneys available to the many ESRD patients who need them. In 2018 in the U.S., 5,645 kidneys—or about 28% of the total available—were provided by living donors, while almost three times as many, 14,516 kidneys, or 72%, came from deceased donors. Up to one-fifth of kidneys procured from 2007 to 2019, however, were discarded, because of varying concerns of the doctors and patients involved regarding the lifestyle of or infections in the donor or the substandard quality of the organ. While problems in xenotransplantation (the use of organs from other species, such as swine, for transplantation into humans) had been addressed experimentally for more than fifty years, in many laboratories, the science was not at a stage that would allow clinical trials in patients with kidney disease. Although recent advances using CRISPR-Cas9 gene editing technology may result in the elimination of porcine viruses transmitted to humans, the possibility of hyperacute rejection of cross-species tissue by humans remains a paramount problem that has stymied progress in this area of research. The landscape of xenotransplantation, however, would soon change.

Concurrently, interest has surged in the manufacture of organoids, or "kidneys in a dish." Techniques for growing human kidney cells into tissues, such as glomeruli and tubules and the blood vessels that feed them, have been tested and evaluated in research ongoing in laboratories around the world.[53] This stunning achievement in basic science, however, is still in its infancy. Decades of research will be necessary before the individual parts of tissues grown in laboratories as organoids can be assembled into an organ that can be placed into a human as a functioning kidney with blood supply and nerve inputs sufficient to sustain the life of a person with uremia.

Another way to address the organ shortage is to use kidneys that were not previously considered suitable for transplantation. Approximately one-fifth of kidneys available for donation are discarded because transplant physicians or ESRD patients on the waitlist will not accept them based on information provided by Organ Procurement Organizations (OPOs). Such actions contribute to longer waiting times for patients in need. Reasons for discarding kidneys include perceptions of risk regarding coexisting conditions that may be present in the donor (because of behaviors such as substance use) or because of reliance on algorithms such as the Kidney Donor Profile Index (KDPI). These may include kidneys from older donors, or from patients with hepatitis, HIV, or other viral infections. Consultants have claimed that current allocation systems and metrics employed by CMS wrongly encourage the use of only the best kidneys, resulting in the unnecessary rejection of organs that might be suitable because they may not pass restrictive clinical quality measures imposed by the government, such as achievement of criterion one-year survival rates. But such approaches engender controversy. Organ Procurement Organizations and transplant physicians, possibly with the support of conservative patients, were encouraged to play it safe rather than maximize the number of kidney transplants, perhaps as an unintended consequence of government regulations designed to ensure medical excellence. Protocols have been developed and tested so that donors with chronic infections, such as those with human immunodeficiency virus (HIV) or hepatitis C virus (HCV), which previously precluded the use of their organs for transplantation, can be accepted to sustain the lives of recipients with kidney failure.

Hepatitis C Viral Infection

Transplant teams were traditionally reluctant to use kidneys from patients infected with hepatitis B or C virus. Dr. Peter Reese and colleagues at the University of Pennsylvania had been interested for many years in the possibility of transplanting kidneys from people with HCV infection into uninfected recipients with ESRD languishing or dying on the waitlist. The development of antiviral drugs that could eradicate HCV infection, safely and effectively, allowed the investigators to conceive of a study in which kidneys from HCV-infected donors could be transplanted into uninfected recipients who would subsequently be treated. Reese and colleagues wrote a Perspective article in 2015 in the *NEJM*, proposing just such a study, emphasizing the size of the waiting list for kidneys and the waits of five or more years for patients to be transplanted.[54] They noted that 63% of otherwise acceptable kidneys from HCV-infected donors had been discarded. Reese and coauthors highlighted that ethical and safety concerns were of paramount importance and that informed consent approaches to patients had to be transparent, clear, and comprehensive. In 2017, Goldberg, Reese, and a great many colleagues reported, in a letter to the *Journal*, on a small pilot trial of HCV-negative ESRD patients who had consented to receive kidneys from HCV-infected donors and be treated with the new potent antiviral drugs thereafter.[55] The kidneys were from HCV genotype 1–infected donors, and the ten recipients were treated with the antiviral combination drug elbasvir-grazoprevir (Zepatier). The results were gratifying. The infections were eradicated without side effects, and kidney function was excellent in the recipients. The investigators are currently performing a larger study of kidneys from HCV+ donors with the support of the NIDDK.

Advances in research and policy initiatives have allowed an increasing number of HCV-positive donors to participate in kidney transplantation, but their cumulative number is relatively small compared to the need. There are fewer than 2,000 HCV-positive deceased kidney donors a year, making up only a small minority of successful deceased kidney donors. The proportion of adult kidney transplant candidates willing to consider a kidney from a HCV-positive donor has increased over the last decade (from 2008 to 2019) from near zero to about one-third. Peter Reese received the Midcareer Distinguished Research Award of the American Society of Nephrology in 2022.

HIV Infection

Since 1986, reports in the medical literature acknowledged the problem of HIV infection in kidney transplant recipients. In several early cases, transplantation of patients with infected kidneys occurred before the disease could be diagnosed, with catastrophic results. Concern also existed that the immuno-suppression necessary to prevent rejection of a transplanted kidney might cause the viral infection to progress in a previously uninfected recipient in an accelerated, uncontrolled fashion. Another fear was aggressive opportunistic infections would supervene in patients who would need immunosuppression to maintain a transplanted kidney. Kumar and colleagues reported the case of an uninfected patient in whom HIV infection was transmitted by transplant-ing a kidney from an infected donor in 1987.[56] The recipient developed AIDS. Similar reports and case series followed in other journals. Some investigators reported that HIV infection as well as kidney function could be controlled in patients, but the general consensus was that patients with HIV and kidney dis-ease should not be treated by transplantation, especially since effective thera-pies did not exist for the treatment of HIV infection at the time. The recipients' life span might be short, and kidney transplantation outcomes were not excellent.

The advent of HIV protease inhibitors as effective drugs for people living with HIV in the mid-1990s may have started to change clinical perceptions. In 1998, however, Dr. Aaron Spital, a nephrologist, at that time at the University of Rochester, published a national survey on the possibility of transplantation in patients with HIV in *Transplantation*.[57] The overwhelming majority of U.S. transplant centers would not transplant a person with HIV. The contribution of stigma, racism, or other medical and nonmedical biases to this clinical deci-sion-making process cannot be determined from the findings. More hard clin-ical data regarding population life spans and other outcomes would be necessary to move the field forward.

Two surgeons, Dr. Paul C. Kuo of Georgetown University and Dr. Peter G. Stock of the University of California, San Francisco (UCSF), were among the first to challenge the conventional wisdom regarding transplantation of patients with HIV with kidney disease. They published their results in the *AJT* in 2001.[58] They reviewed the outcome of kidney transplantation in patients with HIV before the use of protease inhibitors and combination antiretroviral therapy, which they termed "sub-optimal." Kuo and Stock outlined what they perceived as the ethical issues associated with transplantation in this patient population, and described some of the studies of drug-drug interactions that were necessary to provide useful medical information in the absence of clinical experience. They presented a clinical plan for starting transplantation in patients with HIV with end-stage kidney or liver disease. They concluded that although "many questions about HIV and transplantation remain unanswered, enough data exist to warrant reconsideration of HIV disease in transplantation." Paul J. Gow, Deenan Pillay, and David Mutimer published a short article on transplantation of solid organs in patients with HIV infection shortly thereafter, in 2001, in *Transplantation*.[59] A shift in the paradigm had begun.

In 2003, Stock and UCSF colleagues published a pilot study in *Transplantation* including ten ESRD patients with HIV who received kidney transplants.[60] Average follow-up was more than a year, and all the patients were alive and had transplanted kidneys that functioned at that time. Rejection occurred and was treated in half the patients with kidney transplants. HIV infection was successfully treated with antiretroviral drugs in the patients in the presence of immunosuppressive medications. In 2008, Stock and colleagues published in *AJT* one- and three-year outcomes of eighteen patients with HIV who received kidney transplants.[61] Patients were followed for a median of four years. Three-year kidney survival was about 83%, which the authors deemed comparable to the findings in the uninfected population. Kidney transplant rejection was a common event and sometimes resulted in graft loss, but patient survival at three years was excellent at 94.4%. Although HIV infection seemed well-controlled, it was difficult to evaluate outcomes in the absence of a prospective, randomized controlled study design.

In 2010, Stock and colleagues published another study of transplantation of patients with HIV who required kidney transplants in the *NEJM*.[62] This time the study involved nineteen medical centers around the U.S. The investigators recruited 150 patients with HIV and ESRD who received kidney transplants. Patients had to have adequate circulating T-cell counts and undetectable virus while they were treated with antiretroviral drugs, suggesting HIV infection was under good control, in order to enter the study. The patients received immunosuppression with steroids, tacrolimus or cyclosporine, and mycophenolate mofetil as determined by the center and continued antiretroviral therapy after transplantation. The kidneys came from both deceased and living donors. Transplanted patients were closely monitored for the incidence of opportunistic infections and rejection. One- and three-year patient and graft survival were excellent, at 94.6% ± 2.0% and 88.2% ± 3.8%, and 90.4% and 73.7%, respectively. The authors claimed these rates were comparable to those in older patients in the general population who received kidney transplants. Rejection appeared to be more common in the patients than in those in a reference group without HIV infection, and remained a challenge in the treatment of HIV-positive patients undergoing kidney transplantation. Few unexpected adverse events related to the underlying viral infection and immunocompromised state of the patients were noted. The chance of maintaining graft survival was markedly improved if the transplanted kidney came from a living donor. The main limitation of the study was that although it was prospective, it was neither randomized nor controlled. It was difficult to put the rates of rejection, and the rates of complications associated with HIV infection, such as opportunistic infections and death, into proper perspective. The study, deemed a success and funded by NIAID, showed transplantation of patients with HIV with ESRD was feasible. The results led to greater access to transplantation for ESRD patients with HIV. The authors noted that careful selection of candidates was imperative and that precise drug regimen choice, close monitoring of clinical events after transplantation, and the presence of an experienced interdisciplinary care team were essential in the care of such complicated patients. The study did not consider the donor pool, which would now be diminished for patients without HIV infection.

To address this issue, in 2010 Elmi Muller, Delawir Kahn, and Marc Mendelson from Groote Schuur Hospital in Cape Town, South Africa, building on the work of Stock and colleagues, reported the preliminary results of transplantation in 2008 of kidneys from two donors with HIV into four recipients with ESKD and HIV in a letter to the *NEJM*.[63] South Africa was a particularly good place to do such research since their facilities for providing treatment to patients by dialysis were limited. In three patients, the kidney disease was clearly linked to the HIV infection. All four patients were treated with antiretroviral drugs for HIV infection before as well as after receiving a kidney transplant. The patients had excellent control of HIV infection after transplantation while initially receiving standard immunosuppressant drugs (steroids, tacrolimus, and mycophenolate mofetil). All four had relatively good renal function, assessed one year after transplantation. In three patients renal biopsy results after transplantation were described as normal. In one patient, kidney biopsy findings were abnormal, described as "early collapsing glomerulonephritis." The authors speculated that the use of kidneys from donors with HIV might add to the donor pool since they otherwise would be discarded. They noted the potential problem of infecting the recipient with another strain of HIV, which might not be as amenable to treatment.

In a landmark *NEJM* paper in 2015, Muller, Zunaid Barday, Mendelson, and Kahn, advancing on their earlier studies, reported optimistic results of transplantation of kidneys from deceased donors with HIV into twenty-seven recipients with HIV and ESKD.[64] In 2009, the Groote Schuur Hospital had removed its restriction on HIV-positive patients donating kidneys to ESRD patient recipients with HIV. The design of the study was similar to the work of Stock and colleagues. One-, three-, and five-year patient survival rates were excellent, at 84%, 84%, and 74%, respectively, comparable to but perhaps somewhat lower than the results reported by Stock and colleagues. One-, three-, and five-year graft survival rates were also excellent, at 93%, 84%, and 84%, perhaps better than the results of the studies by Stock and colleagues. Rejection rates were lower than those reported by Stock and colleagues. The authors concluded, "Our study showed that kidneys from HIV+ deceased donors can be transplanted into carefully selected HIV+ recipients, with the expectation that the outcome would be similar to that observed in kidney transplantation programs involving high-risk patients without HIV infection." The study was supported by grants from Sanofi South Africa and the Roche Organ Transplantation Research Foundation. Muller and colleagues subsequently sent a letter to the *NEJM* in 2019, supporting and extending previous findings.[65]

Meanwhile the implications of the study were not lost on American transplant professionals as well as the U.S. government. Use of kidneys from HIV-positive donors could expand the donor pool but was impossible at the time under U.S. law. Dr. Dorry L. Segev, then of Johns Hopkins Hospital, led a campaign to study and realize transplantation in the U.S. using organs from HIV-positive donors. Segev was born in Israel, completed undergraduate studies at Rice University, and received his M.D. degree from Johns Hopkins School of Medicine in 1996. Thereafter, he completed a residency in surgery and further training at the Johns Hopkins Hospital and subsequently joined the medical school faculty. Segev also had engaged in policy work in the federal government. He completed postgraduate work in epidemiology at the Bloomberg School of Public Health of Johns Hopkins University. Segev started his research career working with Dr. Robert Montgomery. Segev published an opinion paper in 2009 in the *Archives of Surgery*, with coauthors including Drs. Jayme Locke and Robert A. Montgomery, on the feasibility of transplanting HIV-positive ESRD patients.[66] In 2011, with Drs. Brian J. Boyarsky and Montgomery, as well as other collaborators, Segev published a paper in *AJT* highlighting the feasibility of transplanting HIV-positive patients.[67] In the paper, which cited a diverse set of other papers, including his own and the Stock and Muller papers recently published in the *NEJM*, Segev set out to estimate the number of deceased donors with HIV who would be theoretically available for kidney transplants. The authors posited such an approach would "attenuate the organ shortage and waitlist mortality." The authors also pointed out that the National Organ Transplant Act of 1984 stated:

> "The Organ Procurement and Transplantation Network shall ... adopt and use standards of quality for the acquisition and transportation of donated organs, including standards for preventing the acquisition of organs that are infected with the etiologic agent for acquired immune deficiency syndrome." As such, based on the OPTN Final Rule, HIV infection is an absolute contraindication to deceased organ donation in the United States.

The paper included a great deal of well-grounded assumptions regarding the status of the proposed population, but the study was designed as an estimate, not a census. In an unusually political stance for an article published in a medical journal, the authors opined that deceased HIV-positive patients could "represent approximately 500–600 donors per year for HIV-infected transplant candidates. In the current era of HIV management, a legal ban on the use of these organs seems unwarranted and likely harmful."

The Hopkins team conducted focus groups among patients regarding the possibility of transplanting people with kidneys obtained from patients with

HIV while they pursued complementary studies of outcomes of transplantation in HIV-positive patients with kidney disease. In 2015 in *AJT*, Boyarsky and Segev published another article proposing transplantation of organs from patients with HIV into HIV-positive recipients.[68] They noted that Congress had passed the HIV Organ Policy Equity (HOPE) Act in 2013, allowing such procedures under the auspices of research protocols supervised by the NIH. The authors wrote, "The growing need for transplantation in HIV+ individuals led our group to propose the HOPE Act." They outlined:

> The HOPE Act mandates that the Secretary of DHHS develop and publish criteria for the conduct of clinical research involving HIVDD [deceased donor] organs. This process . . . involves input from the Centers for Disease Control (CDC), National Institutes of Health, Health Resources and Services Administration (HRSA), Centers for Medicare and Medicaid Services (CMS), Food and Drug Administration (FDA), OPTN [Organ Procurement and Transplantation Network], the professional transplantation societies and the opportunity for public comment. . . . Only after the research criteria are established will HIVDD transplants occur in the United States, and initially they will only be permitted in the context of clinical research studies. Two years after the criteria are published, the Secretary of DHHS will review the results of the clinical research to determine whether the practice of using HIVDD can occur in the United States outside of the context of clinical research.

In 2016, in an *Annals of Surgery* article entitled "How a Transplant Nuance Became 1 of Only 57 Laws Passed in 2013," Boyarsky and Segev further detailed for the medical profession the strategies that allowed the HOPE Act to be signed into law.[69] Getting HOPE enacted involved performing medical research, engaging advocacy groups, and communicating with legislative aides and politicians, as well as working with the mainstream press. Their article included bold timelines for medical advances in the field, as well as for legislative activities. Segev and colleagues then published a paper in the prestigious *AIM* so general internists and medical subspecialists would be aware of their work and the ethical and clinical changes they had engendered in the care of patients with infectious and kidney diseases.[70] They emphasized that clinical efforts would first be conducted under strict research protocols supervised by NIH and that ethical issues existed for both donors and recipients in the program.

In 2018, Segev and colleagues reviewed progress made in studies conducted under the auspices of the HOPE Act, in *Current Opinion in Organ Transplantation*.[71] The first HIV-to-HIV kidney transplant was performed at Johns Hopkins in March 2016. Researchers around the U.S. joined to perform studies under the constraints of the HOPE Act, supported by NIH, with the cooperation of UNOS and Organ Procurement Organizations. Other investigators supported the efforts.[72] In a 2019 paper in *Current Opinion in Organ Transplantation*, Boyarsky, Segev, and colleagues announced that through March 2019, fifty-seven donors participated in studies conducted within the guidelines of the HOPE Act, providing organs to more than 120 transplant recipients.[73] In 2021, a large number of authors, including Drs. Segev, Peter Stock, Elmi Muller, and Jonah Odim (of the NIAID of NIH), representing fourteen centers, reported in *AJT* that twenty-five HIV-positive donors had provided kidneys in a prospective pilot study.[74] There were no deaths in the study at the time of the report (with median patient follow-up of 1.7 years). Patients who received kidneys from HIV-positive donors had similar graft survival at one year (91%) as those who received a kidney from an uninfected donor. Kidney function was similar in recipients who had received kidneys from infected and uninfected donors. Rejection rates at one year were numerically higher in patients who received kidneys from infected (50%) compared with uninfected donors (29%) but not statistically significantly different, perhaps because of the relatively small number of participants. Infectious disease complications appeared to be similar in both groups. The authors noted the studies were ongoing and that attention had to be paid to potential differences in rejection rates between the two groups.

Segev joined Dr. Robert Montgomery in March 2022 as the vice chair of research in the Department of Surgery at NYU Grossman School of Medicine.

Another way to increase the number of donors could involve reducing the number of incompatible living donors and making the use of transplant centers' facilities for such donations more efficient. Over many years, Dr. Robert Montgomery achieved those goals. Montgomery knew more about transplantation than any other transplant physician. He knew what it was like to be a transplant patient, giving him a unique perspective for a physician. Montgomery went to the University of Rochester School of Medicine, graduating in 1987, and thereafter received a doctor of philosophy degree in molecular immunology from Balliol College, Oxford. He trained in general surgery and transplant surgery, as well as in human molecular genetics, at Johns Hopkins, eventually becoming the chief of transplant surgery and the director of the Comprehensive Transplant Center at Hopkins.

Montgomery and colleagues published an article in March 2009 in the *NEJM*, describing a program involving changes in procedures whereby multiple kidney donors, incompatible with their intended paired recipients, participated in a series of orchestrated transplants of ESRD patients across the country.[75] The key was that altruistic donors would forego giving a kidney to their designated patient and agree to donate to any patient, allowing another incompatible donor to present a kidney to the original patient needing a transplant. In the instance cited in the paper, the gift of one altruistic incompatible donor resulted in ten successful, coordinated kidney transplants, described as a "daisy chain." The authors called the procedure a nonsimultaneous, extended, altruistic donor (NEAD) chain. Presumably, a donor who would have been unable to make a gift was now not only able to give a kidney successfully but in turn potentially enabled many other such incompatible pairs to have comparably beneficial outcomes. The ten transplants described in the paper took almost two years to be realized. The authors pointed out that not requiring all the procedures to be done at one time increased the flexibility of the chain. Austin Lee benefited from such a scheme.

Montgomery credits a patient-centered approach and the work of individual patients for having provided much of the impetus for his research. He recalls that

> the inspiration for the daisy chain stemmed from the deeds of two altruistic donors. Joyce Rauch, a transplant coordinator, motivated by a lecture given by Dr. Lloyd Ratner, on laparoscopic retrieval of donor kidneys, decided to give a kidney to an undesignated recipient. Another donor, the mother of a child, tragically killed in an auto accident,

determined to give one of her kidneys to a patient in need. She also did not have a recipient in mind. She ultimately gave her kidney to a recipient who had an incompatible donor. At that time I conceived of the daisy chain. If she gave a kidney to another donor's incompatible recipient, she could set up a chain, a daisy chain, carried on through many pairs. I realized that with the right information and planning, a large number of patients who had previously been incompatible could be matched with the right donor, extending transplantation to many who had previously been confined to long waiting lists. We kept a magnetic board on the wall at an office at Hopkins to track incompatible pairs, for many years, until the registry took over this function nationally.

Montgomery did key research on the desensitization of incompatible kidney transplant donor recipient pairs. These early efforts involved carefully choosing red blood cell ABO incompatible donors with recipients who would not mount a vigorous or catastrophic immune response.[76] Montgomery acknowledged the help of Japanese colleagues who taught him much about ABO system incompatibilities. In addition, in selected patients, Montgomery removed antibodies with a blood cleansing technique called plasmapheresis and used drugs that neutralized antibody effectiveness, which increased the likelihood of successful transplantations in incompatible recipients.[77] Michael Mittelman was one of the first patients to participate in these studies. (Montgomery removed Mittelman's mother's kidney using laparoscopic techniques.) Such procedures, because of the distribution of ABO blood types in the population, also increase accessibility to kidney transplantation for African American and Asian ESRD patients and, therefore, enhance patient equity. (Austin Lee also underwent this type of treatment.) Montgomery estimated that such advances might increase the number of transplant recipients in the U.S. by six or seven hundred people a year. Montgomery envisions new immunoactive treatments, such as those using CAR (chimeric antigen receptor) T-cell technologies, presently studied in patients with several types of cancer, to disarm specific cells in order to modify the immune response. These could be deployed to increase the number of successful transplants in previously incompatible kidney donor/recipient pairs.

A vigorous proponent of increasing equity in the U.S. transplant patient population, Montgomery hopes well thought-out changes in the UNOS allocation system will in the future decrease waiting times and enhance equity. Noting the changes in HLA matching from protein-based to nucleic acid–centered analyses, Montgomery feels matching according to immunogenetics will be greatly improved as molecular techniques define the smaller regions of genes, or "eplets," that may most directly determine immune reactions between donor tissues and recipient responses. He is a champion of preemptive transplantation.

Montgomery's pathway in medicine has been influenced by family history and genetics. His father had heart disease, which was largely genetically determined. He, in turn, from an early age, has had life-threatening disturbances of heart rhythm, or arrythmias. In 1989, at the age of twenty-nine, he had one of the earliest implantable devices surgically placed in his abdomen to ablate a potentially fatal arrythmia. He was told his heart disease might jeopardize his ability to participate in a demanding medical career, such as specializing in surgery. In 2018, Montgomery underwent heart transplantation. His new heart was donated by a HCV-positive patient, and Montgomery successfully completed treatment for the infection with newly developed antiviral drugs. He subsequently returned to work as the director of the NYU Langone Transplant Institute. Montgomery noted that his experiences as a patient changed his perspective and the way he talked to and listened to patients. He developed better sensitivities for appreciating the patient voice. Montgomery feels that "long-term patient outcomes, rather than one year metrics, are more important. Long-term outcomes over decades are hard to determine, because of the current incentives in the payment system. The key goal for patients is long-term survival, with a concomitant good quality of life." Among his many accolades, Montgomery received the 2022 Medal of Excellence Award from the American Association of Kidney Patients.

In addition, the genetics involved in successful kidney donation and excellent long-term outcomes are being explored. After the discovery that variants in the *APOL1* gene, present only in people of recent African descent, were associated with increased risk of the development and progression of kidney disease, in light of efforts to increase living and deceased donors of kidneys in the

African American community, it became imperative that research to elucidate whether receipt of a kidney from a donor with two risk variants would result in poorer transplantation outcomes was needed. The notion that *APOL1* variants conferred risk in donated kidneys was consistent with the findings of Port and colleagues in 1987 and with those of Abbott and colleagues in 2002. In 2011 in *AJT*, Dr. Amber Reeves-Daniel, with Dr. Barry Freedman of Wake Forest School of Medicine, and colleagues from other institutions presented retrospective evidence showing that recipients of kidneys donated from donors who had two *APOL1* variants had worse outcomes than those who received kidneys from people with no or only one variant.[78]

In 2016, the NIH released a Request for Applications to form a consortium to study the outcomes of transplantation for recipients of kidneys donated by African Americans. The APOLLO (*APOL1* Long-Term Outcomes) Consortium first met in 2017 to start to collect information on the clinical course of recipients of kidneys donated by African Americans. The study involves thirteen sites, representing the majority of U.S. transplant programs. Patients and families participating in this key effort will help improve outcomes for kidney transplant recipients across the country. Organ Procurement Organizations across the country are providing invaluable assistance to the researchers. The findings of the APOLLO study will make the allocation of kidneys across the U.S. more efficient and, perhaps more importantly, potentially more precise by replacing the race factor in national UNOS sharing algorithms with more pertinent and meaningful information about the genetic makeup of the donors.[79] The APOLLO Consortium is expected to report its results in 2026.

Current Status and Future Prospects

Belatacept, a novel noncalcineurin inhibitor immunosuppressive drug, had been studied in clinical trials for several years and was approved for use in kidney transplant patients in the U.S. by the FDA and in Europe in 2011. Belatacept is in a different class of immunosuppressant drugs than the calcineurin inhibitors (such as cyclosporine and tacrolimus). Belatacept is a designer molecule that blocks the interaction of T-cells with costimulators, inhibiting their immune reactive responses. This blockade limits the ability of kidney transplant recipients to mount a powerful rejection response directed against transplanted tissues. Investigators and pharmaceutical companies were interested in regimens other than those based on calcineurin inhibitors and antiproliferative drugs, such as mycophenolate mofetil, in the presence or absence of steroids. Because calcineurin inhibitors, to greater or lesser extents over time, cause kidney damage, clinical trials that could meet the costs were also needed to evaluate long-term outcomes in patients who received kidney transplants.

In 2016 in the *NEJM*, an international group of scientists published the results of a trial of belatacept in ESRD patients receiving kidney transplants over a relatively long period of time.[80] Dr. Flavio Vicenti, a senior transplant nephrologist at the University of California, San Francisco, served as the first (and corresponding author). In addition to U.S. centers, physicians and patients in France, Spain, Mexico, Argentina, and India participated. More than 660 patients were randomized to receive either more or less intensive treatment with belatacept, compared with a control group of patients treated with cyclosporine. Patients were followed for seven years. At the seven-year time point, 447 of the patients in the study were able to be evaluated. Patients treated with belatacept had a 43% lower risk of death or graft loss during the study period than those treated with cyclosporine. In the belatacept groups, the composite end point of graft loss or death at seven years was a little less than 13%, while 21.7% of patients treated with cyclosporine died or lost their graft over the same observation period. Average renal function, measured using S[Cr] (by evaluating eGFR, or estimated glomerular filtration rate) increased in patients treated with belatacept but worsened in those treated with cyclosporine over the course of the study. Average eGFRs at seven years in the more intensive and less intensive belatacept groups were 70.4 and 72.3 ml/min/1.73m^2, while the comparable value in the cyclosporine group was 44.9 ml/min/1.73m^2. The rates of serious adverse events in the groups were the same. Patients treated with belatacept had lower rates of producing antibodies that might interfere with graft survival. Consistent with current viewpoints, the authors pointed out that this study provided important information about relatively long-term outcomes after kidney transplantation. The investigators confirmed that the results in the study were better than those in another study with belatacept in which sicker and older recipients had received "expanded criteria" kidneys from donors who were older and had more coexisting medical conditions.

They admitted that the design of the study precluded them from making comparisons with kidney transplant patients treated with tacrolimus, which had become the contemporary standard of care. The authors also acknowledged that belatacept required intravenous, rather than oral, administration, although it was given only at four-week intervals by the latter part of the study. The study was supported by the maker of the drug, Bristol-Myers Squibb.

So a new wonder drug, with potential advantages for patients, had come on the scene. Belatacept, however, is used in only a small minority of patients receiving kidney transplants. Aside from belatacept needing to be administered in an infusion center, its cost is undoubtedly a key issue in the lack of uptake for this drug. Paul Eggers found that in 2015, only seventy-two Medicare beneficiaries received the drug at an average cost of about $12,000 a patient. At that time, belatacept was not covered by most Medicare Part D (or pharmacy benefit) plans. In some databases, belatacept appears as an "injectable," not an immunosuppressive drug. That designation enhances potential revenues for physicians and treatment centers. As is the case quite often recently, molecular pharmaceutical advances come at a cost that cannot benefit patients.

According to the USRDS 2022 Annual Data Report, as of 2020, approximately 808,000 patients in the United States had ESRD.[81] About 480,000 people were treated with in-center hemodialysis, 65,000 patients with peritoneal dialysis, and about 12,000 people with home hemodialysis, accounting for about 69% of the ESRD patient population. Although there were only 23,853 patients who received a kidney transplant in 2020, because of better survival, about 31% of the total ESRD population (or about 246,000 people) have transplants. This percentage, as expected, has been increasing over the years. Tragically, 25,129 newly qualified patients who could not obtain a kidney remained on the waiting list in 2020. The total number of active patients on the waiting list in the U.S. is typically about 100,000 patients each year. (This represents about 18%, or almost 1 in 5, dialysis patients.) The median wait time for patients to receive a kidney transplant is about four years. White patients have a wait of about three and a half years, while Black patients face a longer wait time, about five years. For patients waiting to receive a kidney from a deceased donor, recent statistics show about 1 in 4 to 5 people get their transplant after one year. A little more than a third get a transplant after three years and about half after five years. (The COVID pandemic has rendered recent statistics not entirely comparable to preceding years.) Over the last approximately twenty years, the proportion of White patients who received transplants decreased slightly, and the percentage of Asian and Black patients who received kidney transplants increased somewhat. Strikingly, as the age of the general population and ESRD patients has increased, and perhaps as health outcomes have improved, the proportion of elderly ESRD patients (those sixty-five or older) who received kidney transplants doubled, to about one-fifth of the recipients. In the group of people getting a kidney transplant between 2014 and 2017, the cost of drugs during the first year of transplantation was about $25,000 per patient.

In 2017, of the 5,870 living donations, 12% were paired exchanges, 4% were nondirected, and 26% were unrelated directed, highlighting the influence of Montgomery's work. Of the prevalent functioning kidney graft population followed by the USRDS in 2017, the current (unadjusted) life expectancy is 17.9 years, far longer than that of dialysis patients. Of the 222,848 people living with a functioning kidney transplant, 18,280 (8.2%) had that transplant for over 20 years; 4,111 patients (1.84%) have had the same transplant for more than 30 years.

The vast majority of organs transplanted have been kidneys. UNOS recently celebrated its estimates of 1 million transplants having been performed in the U.S.

———— ✦ ————

In 2014, Sally Satel became aware that decreased function of her transplant kidney would necessitate her becoming an ESRD patient again in the future. She underwent a second transplant in June 2016. Her donor was a coworker who agreed to give Satel a kidney, but they had incompatible ABO blood groups. This not uncommon scenario, the requirement for retransplant, is particularly instructive in that Satel was able to receive a second kidney from a living donor, a testament to altruism and the personal characteristics of the patient who inspired people to make exceptional gifts to her. In addition, the case illustrates progress made in addressing incompatibilities that previously were viewed as insurmountable, pioneered by researchers in Japan and by Dr. Montgomery in the U.S. Satel continues in good health in Washington and contributes to the national discourse on health and politics in lectures, publications, and the books she writes.

Brian Kampschroer became ill in 2021 with what was later diagnosed as COVID-19. His recovery took place over a period of weeks, but thereafter, he felt "back to normal." The pandemic has focused the medical community on the vulnerabilities of kidney transplant patients. Susceptible to viral and other uncommon infections as "immunosuppressed hosts," kidney transplant patients were on heightened alert during the pandemic. As the virus raged across the U.S., it became clear that immunosuppressed patients were at high risk for infection and death from COVID-19. While the rapid development of vaccines and deployment of vaccination programs held out a lifeline for the general population, kidney transplant patients realized that they did not develop the same antibody response to vaccines as seen in others without ESRD. A paper in *JASN* in 2021 by French investigators highlighted the relatively poor antibody response in kidney transplant patients, even after three vaccinations.[82] Morbidity and mortality remained elevated for ESRD (including kidney transplant patients) as well as CKD patients.[83] It remains to be seen how the coronavirus infection will affect the kidney transplant population over the next several years.

Novel Federal Policy Initiatives

Alex Azar II wanted to change the statistics regarding the distribution of transplantation within the ESRD population. Azar attended Dartmouth College and graduated from Yale University with a degree in law in 1991. He served as clerk for Supreme Court associate justice Antonin Scalia from 1992 to 1993. Azar was the general counsel of the Department of Health and Human Services from 2001 to 2005. He became the deputy secretary of Health and Human Services in 2005, a position he held until 2007. Azar worked for Eli Lilly and Company from 2007 to 2008 and rejoined the company in 2009. Azar served as the president of Lilly USA from 2012 to 2017. In 2018, after the resignation of Dr. Tom Price (because of a scandal regarding the ethics of his government travel), Azar became the secretary of Health and Human Services (HHS) under President Donald J. Trump.

Azar was forthright about the reasons for his interest in kidney disease. His father, a physician, had developed ESRD and was treated with dialysis for several years before he received a kidney transplant. Azar appreciated the differences in survival and quality of life experienced by patients with treatment of kidney failure with dialysis compared with those who received successful kidney transplantation. Azar wanted to reduce the costs of the ESRD program and increase the availability of transplantation for people with advanced kidney disease. He was able to use the levers of power within the government to change the landscape of care for ESRD patients. Under Azar's aegis, HHS released a position paper entitled "Transforming Kidney Care in America: Innovative Initiatives across the U.S. Department of Health and Human Services Designed to Improve Care Delivery and Treatment Options for Patients with Kidney Disease." Azar spoke of his vision in remarks at the National Kidney Foundation in March 2019. He outlined three objectives with ambitious goals. The government would initiate and strengthen efforts to prevent the development of ESRD in patients. The policies would involve preventing CKD or slowing its progression to end-stage and would enhance "person-centered treatment," meaning increasing the choices available to patients for treatment of ESRD. This goal would increase the use of home treatments, such as home hemodialysis and peritoneal dialysis, as well as advance research on wearable artificial kidneys. Finally, the ESRD program would increase use of kidneys from deceased donors and minimize the number of organs discarded as well as provide incentives to increase the number of living donors. The net result of these efforts, Health and Human Services officials hoped, would be to decrease the growth and size of the ESRD program, incentivize home dialysis treatments, and increase the number of patients receiving kidney transplantation. The number of patients treated by in-center hemodialysis, the overwhelmingly most common treatment modality, would decrease dramatically, in their opinion. The plan was aspirational with lofty, and perhaps unattainable, goals, but the approach would change the whole structure of ESRD care. Organ Procurement Organizations would have to change to meet new benchmarks, and Medicare payments for services would be altered, as might physicians' incomes.

Clinicians and dialysis organizations were skeptical regarding whether these goals could be achieved.

Azar's speech was followed by the release of Executive Order 13879, Advancing American Kidney Health, by the administration of President Trump on July 10, 2019. Arguably the biggest policy advance for people with kidney disease since 1973, the order stated:

> My Administration is dedicated to advancing American kidney health. The state of care for patients with chronic kidney disease and end-stage renal disease (ESRD) is unacceptable: too many at-risk patients progress to late-stage kidney failure; the mortality rate is too high; current treatment options are expensive and do not produce an acceptable quality of life; and there are not enough kidneys donated to meet the current demand for transplants.

The order tasked HHS to support research on preventing, treating, and slowing the progress of kidney disease and to radically increase the number of kidney transplants performed in the U.S. HHS envisioned exceptional growth in home ESRD therapies, by developing new payment models and economic incentives for companies and physicians in order to "improve quality of life and care for Medicare beneficiaries" with CKD. The order supported "breakthrough" technologies, such as wearable artificial kidneys, through efforts like KidneyX, a public-private partnership between HHS and the American Society of Nephrology that offers prizes to innovators. The order outlined changes in Organ Procurement Organizations, including greater oversight and "enforceable objective metrics," which would hopefully increase the supply of deceased donor kidneys, and increased incentives for living donors.

Besides effects on patients, the executive order had potentially profound implications for large dialysis organizations, the OPOs, UNOS, and physicians and health-care providers involved in the care of patients with kidney disease. The ramifications of these revisions in incentives for dialysis and the institution of changes presumably making kidneys more available to patients who desire renal transplantation will necessarily have to be assessed and may only become apparent over the next decade.

Congress passed HR5534—the Comprehensive Immunosuppressive Drug Coverage for Kidney Transplant Patients Act of 2020—and it was subsequently signed by President Trump. The act extended insurance coverage for immunosuppressive drugs to kidney transplant Medicare patients indefinitely. This was a policy that had been advocated by the Levinsky and Rettig IOM report almost thirty years previously.

The National Academies of Science, Engineering, and Medicine held a workshop in March 2021, at the request of the Social Security Administration, bringing together experts in transplantation, law, and public policy to assess the current state of solid organ transplantation and understand the extent of and ramifications related to disability in patients who were waiting for or who had received transplants.[84] A key element of the workshop was the extent to which transplant patients and their family members and significant others participated in the proceedings.

The workshop included perspectives of different speakers from diverse disciplines and backgrounds culminating in the understanding that while patients may survive and have better quality of life after transplantation, a large proportion of the patients were quite ill before the procedure and continued to have underlying medical problems afterward. The speakers pointed out the chronic conditions that may have led to kidney transplantation, such as high blood pressure and diabetes, were not cured by the gift of a kidney, and those health conditions still posed challenges and obstacles after a successful procedure. Immunosuppressive drugs have clinical side effects that are sometimes unavoidable and can affect the health and quality of life of the patients who take them on a long-term basis. In addition, depression and anxiety, as well as substance use disorders and the effects of the social determinants of health, play key roles in rehabilitation and are often undetected or untreated if physicians concentrate on assessing outcomes by evaluating only S[Cr] levels. Many adult kidney transplant patients, although experiencing good quality of life, are not participating or are not able to participate in the workforce.

The reasons for these discrepancies and relatively low employment rates are unknown, primarily because of lack of data collection regarding these outcomes, especially over longer follow-up periods. The causes underlying low employment rates are presumably multifactorial, including the increasing age of the adult kidney transplant population, the presence of coexisting medical problems (such as diabetes) in this group of patients, as well as possible financial disincentives. Considerations in pediatric kidney transplant recipients are necessarily quite different from those in adults. Unfortunately, many pediatric transplant patients might never be able to put in a forty-hour workweek in the current workplace for a variety of reasons, including the burden of underlying illnesses, educational and social limitations experienced during development, and the effects of drugs used to maintain immunosuppression. Future research is needed to understand the reasons for these challenges to patient outcomes.

The workshop also highlighted that there are not enough publications on transplant outcomes beyond five years of follow-up, for financial as well as logistical reasons, interfering with the ability of policymakers to meaningfully plan for patients with ESKD, especially those who are children. Drs. Segev, Ferris, and Montgomery participated in the workshop. Tellingly, Montgomery was a speaker in the patient experience segment of the workshop and shared the story of his own heart transplant from an HCV-positive donor in the context of thinking about long-term outcomes, recent advances in increasing the donor pool, and consideration of responses of patients who might have been struggling with comorbid illnesses and mental health challenges over the long haul after successful transplantation.

Backward Glances and Current Challenges

Kidney transplantation represents an astounding advance in medicine, improved over the last more than seventy years by the work of numerous clinicians and investigators, including surgeons, nephrologists, immunologists, pharmacologists, sociologists, psychiatrists, psychologists and social workers, biostatisticians, and public health officials as well as the patients who volunteered for experiments and participated in clinical trials. Altruistic donors have played a key role in experimental studies and clinical care continuously over the past seven decades in advancing the field of kidney transplantation. Transplantation provides patients who have irreversibly lost kidney function with life in the face of otherwise certain death—extended in time and enhanced in quality.

The success of kidney transplantation resulted in the development of cardiac and liver transplantation and then lung, intestinal, and other organ transplants, including the provision of two organs simultaneously. These procedures have provided life, improved survival, and better health to hundreds of thousands of patients with a range of chronic debilitating and life-threatening illnesses in the U.S. and across the globe. Over the past sixty years, access to kidney transplantation and survival of recipients have progressively increased. However, the limited availability of deceased and living kidney donors means that not every person with ESRD who desires and qualifies for renal transplantation can receive a kidney. And access to kidney transplantation for African American ESRD patients has lagged and been inadequate. Monica Fox provided a personal viewpoint on these issues from the perspective of a patient in CJASN in 2021.[85] Dr. Vanessa Grubbs told her own story, from the perspective of a nephrologist, about donating a kidney to a loving partner in her memoir, *Hundreds of Interlaced Fingers: A Kidney Doctor's Search for the Perfect Match.*[86]

The Progress Report on Understanding the Long-Term Health Effects of Living Organ Donation to Congress for 2020 noted that revisions had been made to the Living Donor Reimbursement Grant Program to enhance financial support for living donors, in accordance with Executive Order 13879 in 2019. (Such policy changes were also envisioned by the Levinsky and Rettig IOM report in 1991.) Specifically, funds were made available to donors who needed help with reimbursement for childcare and elder-care costs as well as lost wages. The report also described the deleterious effect that COVID infection had had during the first nine months of 2020, resulting in decreased numbers of living donations compared to the previous year. During the first nine months of 2020, kidney paired donations accounted for approximately one in six transplants, a proportion that increased dramatically over the decade, more than doubling over that period. Kidney donation is safe over the relative short term, but in the long term, prospective studies are necessary to establish statistics for donors for more than about ten years. And the vision of Dr. Satel for lifelong medical coverage for living kidney donors has gone unfulfilled, in part because of the legal complexities involved in insurance systems. (It should be noted that Satel's views do not necessarily reflect those of the kidney transplantation establishment.)

Long-term statistics on the outcomes of people who donated kidneys had not been kept by transplant organizations in the past, but a registry to follow donors prospectively has been established. Such registry information must be enhanced by studies that use comparison populations to put individual patients' risk into perspective. Dr. Morgan Grams, a nephrologist now at NYU, and colleagues, including Drs. Kasiske and Segev, suggested in a paper in the *NEJM* in 2016 that based on numbers from administrative databases, the risk of developing ESKD in living donors was quite low (less than 1%) but that there was a statistically significant greater chance for Black donors than there was for White donors.[87] Dr. Kasiske and colleagues have published several papers following living kidney donors,[88] showing kidney function remains relatively stable in donors compared to a reference group, and that relatively few changes in laboratory tests can be shown to occur in the donors over time. Although this group's evaluations are extensive, the follow-up time for the donors is still less than ten years.

Current challenges include attempting to extend the long-term survival of kidneys and transplant recipients as the potential kidney transplant pool becomes larger, older, and sicker or, more precisely perhaps, more "medically complex." Contemporary immunosuppression regimens primarily include tacrolimus and mycophenolate mofetil, with or without steroids. Belatacept, a potentially better drug that does not injure the transplant kidney, is only used in a small minority of patients, primarily because of its cost. In those treated with steroids, long-term minimization of the dose or elimination of its use are constant goals. Wojciechowski and Wiseman, in a paper in 2021, described providing the proper immunosuppression to kidney transplant patients over the long course as "a balancing act" between maintaining a kidney from another person in a host with a different genetic background and the side effects inherent in a complex medication regimen.[89] Complications encountered in patients treated with kidney transplantation, even if successful, include the development and progression of heart and blood vessel disease, susceptibility to common and uncommon infectious diseases, and the emergence of many types of cancer as a result of immunosuppression as well as the onset or progression of bone disease. The long-term course of transplanted kidneys may be affected by immunologic factors related to the response of the recipient or to nonimmunologic factors similar to those present as people age or in patients with the early stages of chronic kidney disease. Disability, even after successful transplantation, remains an issue for many patients, perhaps reflecting their health status before the procedure. Transplant clinicians have turned from using the term chronic allograft nephropathy, or CAN, to IFTA, standing for "interstitial fibrosis and tubular atrophy" to describe the reasons for the slow decline of kidney function in recipients, just as the public, physicians, and patients have changed the nomenclature from "cadaver kidneys" to "gifts from deceased donors." The complexity and expense of doing studies, especially randomized controlled clinical trials, in patients where outcomes are evaluated after more than ten years is immense. Although new monitoring tools and techniques may confer some advantages, these difficult issues pose significant barriers to the possibility of science improving long-term outcomes in patients who receive kidney transplants.

Over the last forty years, the ESRD program has grown in size and expanded to cover older and sicker patients, as well as poorer individuals. While it has accommodated the needs of underrepresented groups, many of whom have markedly increased risk of developing and suffering from kidney disease due to genetic susceptibility, the program still contains inequities in care, specifically related to access to a superior therapy that conveys longer and improved quality of life, for women and members of minority groups. Over the decades, institutional biases and the search for corporate profits have been consistently linked by reputable researchers to these differences in access and care.[90] UNOS has, over the last three decades, worked to make sharing and allocation systems more equitable for the patients who need kidney transplants, but progress has been limited. It is hard to reject the notion that systemic racism and sexism underlie the results of the U.S. ESRD transplant program and have resulted in past and ongoing disparities and inequities that characterize patient demographics and outcomes. Patients with kidney disease awaiting transplantation and those who have received kidneys exist in a complex environment, dealing with their families, friends, and employers as well as physicians, surgeons, transplant coordinators, nurses, insurance companies, medical regulatory entities, and local and national political forces. Policymakers, physicians, and the leaders of large dialysis organizations, in cooperation with advocacy groups and patients, must work together, with the assistance of the government, to rectify the ongoing and substantial inequities in access to and delivery of care for patients with advanced kidney disease.

EPILOGUE

Where are we now, and what does the future hold? There are more than 800,000 ESRD patients in the U.S., and estimates suggest approximately 20 million or more worldwide. In the U.S. approximately 550,000 people are treated with dialysis and almost 250,000 have functioning kidney transplants. Because of the improved survival of kidney transplant patients, the proportion of transplanted patients has steadily increased over the years, even though the number of transplants performed yearly in the U.S. is limited. We are faced with a tragic imbalance. The number of kidneys available for transplantation remains low, and the number of patients on the kidney transplant waitlist continues to be stubbornly high. Currently, approximately a third of U.S. ESRD patients have transplants. These numbers only represent the tip of the iceberg. Various scientific and advocacy groups have suggested that up to one-seventh or one-eighth of the population has CKD. AKI remains an important cause of morbidity and mortality, disproportionally for elderly and African American patients in the U.S. There are still no treatments for the most common underlying causes of AKI.

The COVID pandemic has had a profound effect on patients with kidney disease in the U.S. The USRDS reported in 2022 a dramatic decrease in the number of dialysis patients, because of deaths of ESRD patients between 2020 and 2022 attributed to the viral illness.[1] Despite the best attempts of dialysis personnel, dialysis patients were indoors, in close proximity, and often being transported in small vehicles several days a week during the time when the viral infection raged out of control. ESRD patients did not mount an immune response comparable to that of patients without kidney disease, and vaccinations were less effective in the ESRD population. Kidney transplant patients, because of their immunosuppression, were particularly at high risk. The number of kidney transplants decreased in 2020 as the virus plagued the health-care system.

What is the future of kidney failure and its treatments? Two main prospects come to mind related to dialysis and transplantation. First, how well will the dialysis organizations deal with stresses on their payment models, which can limit their profits? Dr. Frederic Finkelstein, a clinical professor of medicine at the Yale University School of Medicine, observes that dialysis profits are already extremely limited and that the profitability of large dialysis organizations in the U.S. is currently dependent on payments from patients with commercial insurance rather than those provided by Medicare to the vast majority of ESKD patients. In addition, changes instituted by CMS, pursuant to the Executive Order on Advancing American Kidney Health of 2019, could further limit corporate profits. The executive order called for a dramatic decrease in the number of patients treated with in-center hemodialysis and an increase in the use of home therapies, such as peritoneal dialysis and home hemodialysis. Perhaps most importantly, the executive order mandates an improvement in transplantation rates for patients treated with dialysis. The extent of commodification of in-center hemodialysis, rendering it a business rather than a treatment, was highlighted by conferences held by Columbia University in May 2022 and May 2023, focused on "Nephroeconomics," rather than primarily on patient treatment or well-being. The proposed changes in CMS payments elicited anxiety in members of the academic clinical nephrology community regarding the future of their mission and the financial viability of their operations. Mitchell H. Rosner, Charles R. Manley, Edward V. Hickey III, and Jeffrey S. Berns, writing from academic, advocacy, and patient perspectives, however, recently castigated the two largest U.S. dialysis organizations for maximizing corporate profits, shareholder buybacks, and the salaries of chief executive officers, rather than investing more capital toward enhancing patient outcomes. They championed patients as the true stakeholders of large dialysis organizational efforts, and called for greater corporate accountability.[2]

A paper published in June 2023 in the *NEJM* from European investigators reported improved patient survival with hemodialfiltration compared with hemodialysis in a randomized trial.[3] If other studies confirm these findings, and patients and physicians demand changes, large dialysis organizations might face the challenge and costs of providing new technologies for patient care.

In addition, a major concurrent challenge for large dialysis organizations is to improve the referral for and accomplishment of kidney transplantation in their patients, an urgent issue of racial equity. African American patients, who comprise approximately 12% to 13% of the U.S. population, constitute about one-third of dialysis patients, a remarkable threefold overrepresentation. Yet, over the past twenty-five years or more, African American dialysis patients are less likely to be referred for or to receive a kidney transplant. Since the death of George Floyd in May 2020, as part of a broad societal response, tremendous focus has been directed by the federal government toward inequities in the ESKD population, reflected by a resurgence of funding opportunities regarding disparities in kidney disease and its treatment, the publication of research findings on this topic, and the acceptance for publication of proposals for solutions related to kidney disease by high-impact journals. Dr. Ebony Boulware, an internist trained in epidemiology at Johns Hopkins with a special interest in CKD and ESRD patients, currently a professor at Wake Forest University, has led a study of interventions to improve transplant referrals in U.S. African American patients funded by the NIDDK. Concern exists regarding outcomes in other race and ethnic groups with CKD and ESRD. The NIDDK has leapt to the forefront of championing research aimed at combatting the negative influences of structural racism on outcomes of kidney disease in patients of color with ESRD and CKD. The effort is led by Dr. Raquel Greer, an internist with a long-standing interest in equity for patients with kidney disease who was recruited by the NIDDK to conduct research in this space, reflecting an ongoing commitment to bring science to bear with the goal of promoting social justice.[4] These calls for research proposals will bring new investigators to the field to plan trials to address medical aspects of structural racism in U.S. patients with kidney disease.

Finkelstein has been a champion of research focusing on the psychosocial status of patients tethered to a machine thrice weekly to survive for almost half a century. He and his wife, Susan, a social worker, with colleagues performed early studies on marital and family responses to treatment of ESRD, concentrating on how people with kidney disease felt during and after their treatment. Finkelstein believes that the next wave of research studies may focus on how patients successfully adapt to the stresses of kidney disease and its treatment and their perceptions of quality of life. Jennifer S. Scherer, assistant professor of medicine at NYU, also believes that attention to the feelings and emotional and social responses of ESRD patients may be the next step in research in nephrology. Scherer, motivated by the suffering she witnessed in ESKD patients during her training and subsequent career, has devoted her research to the palliative care of patients with CKD. She has recently become interested in the role that CKD patients' spiritual needs and resources have played in determining their outcomes.

Despite its successes, one aspect of the failure of dialysis as a therapy was highlighted almost forty years ago, initially in the *NEJM* in 1986 by Drs. Neu and Kjellstrand,[5] who showed a relatively large proportion of dialysis patients died after making a well-informed decision to withdraw from dialysis. Author James Michener was probably the most prominent person to take this route after a long successful period of treatment with dialysis during which he continued to teach.[6] Withdrawal from dialysis still remains the reason for death in many dialysis patients, representing a challenge for this therapeutic modality.[7] One recent report estimated withdrawal accounted for 13.7% of deaths in hemodialysis patients.[8] But it is still unclear if and how the quality of life of dialysis patients can be improved in the absence of transplantation. A recent prospective study of European patients who began dialysis for ESKD highlighted that the quality of life perceived by patients before the start of dialysis was poor but noted that a year after starting dialysis, although perception of physical status deteriorated after treatment, the Mental Component Score actually improved.[9] This novel finding elicited controversy. Dr. S. Vanita Jassal, a Canadian nephrologist who has long been interested in palliative and conservative care for elderly ESKD patients, argued in an accompanying editorial coauthored by a colleague, Jorge I. Fonseca-Correa from the Instituto Nacional de Ciencias Médicas y Nutrición, Salvador Zubirán, in Mexico City, that the benefits of dialysis were not outweighed by the outcomes, an admittedly pessimistic viewpoint, bolstered by a theoretical trajectory of perception of quality of life in patients.[10] Many nephrologists disagreed. In the glass-half-empty or half-filled world, I would suggest that the maintenance or improvement of people's emotional lives, measured by this crude quality of life measure, represents a remarkable, positive outcome for elderly patients who otherwise would have died. How many of these patients would ask to withdraw from dialysis because their life had no meaning or going on was not worth it?

Prospective studies focusing on more refined aspects of the perception of quality of life of patients treated by dialysis are still urgently needed. Indeed, the onus remains on dialysis physicians to provide clear informed consent regarding the benefits and travails of dialysis treatment and to employ measures to improve the experience of dialysis and the ability of patients to cope with an ongoing, burdensome, time-consuming, but life-saving treatment. The NIDDK held a workshop in May 2023 on the postdialysis fatigue syndrome, highlighting its devastating effects on patient well-being. Dialysis has also been attacked as environmentally deleterious, generating medical waste as well as involving huge quantities of water, electricity, plastic tubing, and other precious resources, especially compared to the smaller carbon footprint of successful kidney transplantation.

Daniel Cukor, Ph.D., a clinical psychologist, became interested in the psychological needs and resources of patients with kidney disease, including those treated with dialysis, more than twenty years ago. After performing studies linking the perception of quality of life of dialysis patients with other factors, such as depression, pain, and attendance at dialysis sessions, he embarked on a study of cognitive behavioral therapy (CBT) to treat depression in dialysis patients. His small study, published in *JASN* in 2014, showed a short course of CBT could markedly ameliorate symptoms of depression and improve perception of quality of life in hemodialysis patients.[11] His work has been instrumental in helping the nephrology and research communities acknowledge that the study of the psychosocial status and well-being of patients with kidney disease is as important as understanding their laboratory tests.

Indeed, NIH and NIDDK have become interested in the psychosocial status of patients with kidney disease. The NIDDK supported a trial of antidepressant therapy in CKD patients initiated by Dr. Susan Hedayati of the University of Texas, Southwestern Medical Center, in Dallas, Texas.[12] Other federally funded studies have evaluated virtual reality therapies, and studies of sleep disorders, insomnia, and depression and the interaction of psychosocial and medical factors in CKD patients. The Patient-Centered Outcomes Research Institute (PCORI) funded the ASCEND study, in which Drs. Cukor and

Hedayati, along with principal investigator Dr. Rajnish Mehrotra of the University of Washington, compared outcomes of hemodialysis patients with depression treated with antidepressant medications or CBT. Remarkably, the study, published in 2019, showed that both therapies resulted in significant improvement in the level of depressive affect.[13]

Since the seminal studies of Yitzchak Binik and colleagues in Canada, first reported in *Kidney International* in 1982,[14] it has become increasingly apparent that pain is an important part of the experience of a large proportion of patients treated with dialysis, which affects their perception of quality of life. Nephrologists increasingly learned this lesson over the subsequent decades.[15] In 2019, the HEAL (Helping to End Addiction Long Term) Program at the NIH, initiated to address the opioid epidemic in the U.S. and to alleviate pain in our general population, included the HOPE (Hemodialysis Opioid Prescription Effort) study, administered by NIDDK. The HOPE study, designed to test whether a cognitive behavioral therapy–like intervention would improve the perception of pain in hemodialysis patients and reduce opioid use over the short and long term, includes eight clinical centers and a scientific and data research center.[16] The study involves up to 643 hemodialysis patients in a randomized controlled trial and will be the most comprehensive repository of information regarding the psychosocial status of contemporary hemodialysis patients. Study results are expected in 2025.

The HOPE study is also pioneering the participation of patients in the research enterprise. The call for research that initiated the HOPE study asked each grant applicant to identify two patients who would serve in a paid, advisory capacity to the study. Patients advised on aspects of the HOPE intervention, helped create the informed consent document that allows entry into the study, created a video used in recruitment of participants (in which some of the advisers starred), and are participating in the oversight of study results on an ongoing basis. Patient participants in the HOPE study have also provided advice to the entire HEAL program. The NIDDK has heralded its efforts to include patients in all aspects of contemporary research in kidney disease.

The second major issue, consistent with Executive Order 13879, is increasing the number of ESRD patients treated by kidney transplantation. The number of patients on kidney transplant waiting lists in the U.S. has remained high and stubbornly relatively static, while the number of deceased and living donors remains inadequate to the demand. As mentioned earlier, over the past fifty years, xenotransplantation has been somewhat of a pipe dream and perhaps a joke among American physicians. This dramatically changed one morning in the autumn of 2021 with the publication of a story in *USA Today* and subsequently in the *New York Times* regarding the implantation of a porcine kidney in a brain-dead patient at New York University Medical Center by Dr. Montgomery and colleagues. The genetically modified pig kidney did not undergo the rapid, hyperacute rejection typically characteristic of interspecies transplants during the very short period of this proof-of-concept study. Suddenly, it was apparent to patients and physicians that the world had changed and that xenotransplantation was a real possibility for the future. In addition, unlimited organs from pigs might alleviate much of the inequity in ESRD treatment in the U.S. Shortly thereafter, another report, from Dr. Jayme Locke and colleagues of the University of Alabama, described anastomosis of a porcine kidney in a brain-dead recipient in January 2022.[17] The results corroborated those generated at New York University. Montgomery and colleagues subsequently reported the clinical details of xenotransplant function in two brain dead patients at NYU in the *NEJM* in 2022.[18] Rivka Galchen, the psychiatrist, novelist, and staff writer at the *New Yorker*, contributed a piece on xenotransplantation for a general audience in the magazine in February 2022. Beecher would have been proud that brain-dead patients were providing important research insights as a model of evaluating the feasibility of xenotransplantation.

On June 30, 2022, the *Wall Street Journal* highlighted a possible change in FDA regulations for research in xenotransplantation. The *Journal* reported the FDA was considering clinical trials of transplantation of porcine organs into humans. The article stemmed from the seventy-third Cellular, Tissue, and Gene Therapies Advisory Committee meeting on June 29 and 30, hosted virtually by the FDA. In addition to standing committee members, temporary voting members were appointed with expertise in veterinary medicine, molecular biology, infectious complications of clinical transplantation, clinical nephrology, cardiology, transplantation surgery, and human immunology. The roster included Paul Conway of the American Association of Kidney Patients as a patient representative and Kathleen O'Sullivan-Fortin of ALD CONNECT Inc.

as a consumer representative. The committee was chaired by Lisa Butterfield, Ph.D., vice president of research and development at the Parker Institute for Cancer Immunotherapy and adjunct professor of microbiology and immunology at the University of California, San Francisco. I participated in the deliberations as a temporary voting member.[19]

Committee members were asked to address six questions regarding research needed if clinical xenotransplantation of porcine organs were to occur in the U.S. Committee members were told by Dr. Wilson W. Bryan, director of the Office of Tissues and Advanced Therapies at the FDA, that the committee would not consider ethical issues involved in xenotransplantation during the meeting. One might have thought that the meeting was galvanized by the electronic publication of a paper in the *NEJM* by Drs. Bartley P. Griffith and Muhammad M. Mohiuddin and colleagues on June 22, the week before the meeting, that described the treatment of a man with advanced heart disease at the University of Maryland with transplantation of a pig heart, beginning with surgery on January 7, 2022.[20] The patient lived for an astounding sixty days after surgery but ultimately succumbed. It was unclear what role porcine cytomegalovirus infection might have played in the patient's demise.

Drs. Joachim Denner of the Institute of Virology of the Free University of Berlin, Richard Pierson III of the Center for Transplant Sciences of the Massachusetts General Hospital in Boston, Eckard Wolf of the Department of Biochemistry Molecular Animal Breeding and Biotechnology of the Ludwig-Maximilians University of Munich, and Kristi Helke of the Department of Comparative Medicine of the Medical University of South Carolina gave presentations to the committee. These talks by outside experts were sobering. Committee members were told that pigs have many viral infections and that attention should be paid to infection of patients by these viruses as well as the consequences that could result if such infections were transmitted beyond organ recipients. These include porcine circovirus 3 (PCV3) and porcine cytomegalovirus (PCMV). In addition, swine genetic material contains several porcine endogenous retroviruses (PERVs), with similarities to human immunodeficiency virus. Some of these viruses were known to infect human cells, and some were thought not to. In some cases, however, the potential for human infection was unclear. It was also unknown whether other viruses infecting pigs might pose threats to patients. It was clear, however, that pigs to be used for xenotransplantation had to be free of viruses as well as other infectious agents that could harm humans. Pigs providing organs for human transplantation would need to be bred under scrupulous conditions in germ-free environments. Several biotech firms had confronted these problems over the last twenty or more years, and their results were reported in the medical literature. In addition to "knocking out" (or removing) PERVs from the porcine genome with a new technology invented relatively recently by Nobel laureate Dr. Jennifer Doudna and colleagues, genetically modified pigs had been created with human genes inserted ("knocked in") to minimize possible immune reaction from hosts and the precipitation of inflammatory and clotting cascades as well as attacks by the human complement system. The pig used in the transplantation of the Baltimore heart patient had a complex genetic design that included four knocked-out genes and several knocked-in human genes. Detecting infection in donor pigs, preventing infection in humans, and preventing the unwanted growth of transplanted porcine organs were all critical issues that needed to be addressed and resolved before human studies could succeed. The purity, identity, and sterility of porcine tissues or organs, as well as their efficacy, function (or potency), and safety all had to be determined before human studies could take place.

The committee was invited to discuss these issues as well as the genetic modifications necessary to limit organ rejection and ensure xenograft survival and research needed in animal models before human xenotransplantation might go forward. A final question focused on the performance of pig kidneys in the complex environment of a sick patient with multiorgan system disease being treated with a variety of medications. There were few definitive answers to the questions posed by the FDA, and several other pertinent clinical and scientific questions were raised during the meeting. A general acknowledgment emerged that many of the questions could only be answered by initial studies in desperately ill patients who agreed to xenotransplantation with unknown consequences. I opined that the clinical and research landscape was similar to the situation before the successful twin transplantation at the Brigham in 1954. The group consensus was that the first patients undergoing xenotransplantation would indeed be heroic pioneers. The committee did not make recommendations.

Research proposals for transplantation of porcine kidneys into patients with ESKD are already being submitted.

A festering concern regarding the integrity of the U.S. system for obtaining and allocating organs for transplantation was publicly raised in February 2022. The National Academies of Science, Engineering, and Medicine (NASEM) had been charged by Congress with evaluating current systems for organ procurement, sharing, and allocation, including focusing on equitable outcomes and information technology capacity. NASEM convened an ad hoc distinguished expert panel to assess the issues and reported its findings to Congress. The public report emphasized inequitable access to organs and variation across U.S. transplant centers, as well as failures of computer systems, and highlighted that one in five kidneys procured for transplantation ended up discarded. Later that year, at the same time the Senate was grappling with the protean issues involved in securing funding for health benefits, initiatives to address climate change, and changes in the tax code under the aegis of reconciliation, its Finance Committee held a hearing on UNOS, whose thirty-six-year-old contract for administering the U.S. Organ Transplant Procurement Network (OPTN) was scheduled for renewal in 2023. The weekend before the hearing, the *Washington Post* highlighted two reports: one to the government about the inadequacy of the computer systems used by the OPTN and an article by Lenny Bernstein and Todd C. Frankel, released just before the hearing, that cited the NASEM workshop and reviewed the complaints leveled against UNOS. The articles commented that the system operated "with seemingly little regulatory oversight" and reported that over a thousand complaints had been filed with UNOS between 2010 and 2020 while acknowledging that these mishaps accounted for only a "tiny fraction" of the 174,338 organs processed from 2008 to 2015. In a rare show of bipartisan unity as well as contempt, on August 3, senators from both sides of the aisle condemned current UNOS practices, including its oversight of the fifty-seven Organ Procurement Organizations (OPOs), citing the transplantation of infected kidneys, and the loss and disposal of viable kidneys after their "harvesting." Brian Shephard, the chief executive officer of UNOS, tried to shift some of the blame onto CMS for its failure to deal with problematic OPOs, but the organization was attacked to various extents by witnesses, including Barry Friedman, R.N., executive director of AdventHealth Transplant Institute of Orlando, Florida, Diane Brockmeier, R.N., president and CEO of Mid-America Transplant of St. Louis, Missouri, and Dr. Jayme Locke of the University of Alabama at Birmingham. The government recently announced that new contracts for organ procurement functions will be divided among several smaller domains.

Some bright lights exist regarding the future. Drs. Shuvo Roy, William Fissell, and Victor Gura were recognized at the American Association of Kidney Patients' Fourth Annual Global Summit in August 2022 as having moved the field of wearable or implantable kidneys forward, although progress has been slow and the end is not yet in sight. The Kidney Health Initiative, a joint effort of the FDA and the American Society of Nephrology that includes a consortium of industry partners, has pushed for the development of new therapies and has meaningfully elevated the patient voice in these efforts. KidneyX, a prize program to foster the development of innovative approaches to ESRD therapy, involves the Department of Health and Human Services and the American Society of Nephrology. After receiving a $1 million grant from Otsuka and Visterra, the ASN in August 2022 announced the KidneyCure Diversity, Equity, Inclusion, and Justice Research Grant, to be awarded every other year to a scholar from an underrepresented minority or specifically proposing such research. The ASN published a statement against racism in June 2020. The NKF published a statement deploring racial violence and disparities in America in June 2020. The American Society of Transplantation has issued several statements on racism since 2020. Dr. Lilia Cervantes has made clear the plight of undocumented immigrants with ESRD who cannot receive dialysis care in the U.S. without going through emergency services, sometimes resulting in untimely death. Her work has had the effect of changing treatment policies. The Renal Physicians Association authored a paper supporting policies to provide payment for the care of such patients. The ASN and the NKF convened a working group of scholars to propose GFR estimating equations that removed race parameters from the algorithm. (The supporting studies were reported in the *NEJM* and elsewhere in 2021.)[21] These joint efforts have generated an enormous amount of commentary as the new equations have been disseminated across the clinical arena.[22] The AAKP issued a statement in August 2022 signaling that it as an organization was going to hold insurers to the fire for failing to support payments for innovative therapies desired by patients with kidney disease. In her presidential address at the ASN Kidney Week meeting in November 2022, Dr. Susan Quaggin called for a world in which kidney disease was eradicated. The world is indeed changing.

Who are the heroes of this long and complex saga regarding treatment of patients with kidney failure? Racism and poverty derail the progress of treatment for those with nephropathy. Drug development and use strategies can put primacy of profit over patient welfare. The global specter of kidney disease, with widespread acute kidney injury, often attributed to poor sanitation and water treatment, and catastrophic endemic illnesses, such as malaria and schistosomiasis, affects the public health of low- and middle-income nations. Poor countries do not have the resources to provide dialysis services to their citizens in need. Western lifestyles put patients at risk for developing kidney failure from the ravages of diabetes and hypertension in the high-income world, while genetic architectures differing between groups, abetted by these factors, put people of recent African descent at tragic susceptibility to nephropathy. The number of not-for-profit dialysis centers in the U.S. has dwindled, and most ESRD dialysis patients are currently treated under the purview of large, for-profit dialysis organizations. Perverse financial disincentives and business interests may have functioned to keep patients on dialysis rather than prioritizing kidney transplantation. Black patients are less likely to go through the steps resulting in successful transplantation compared to White patients. Women are more likely to be donors than recipients of kidney transplants. African American children with ESRD have less access to transplantation and have less success after transplantation than their White counterparts. Much must be accomplished by researchers and clinicians, working with patients, to rectify these problems, hopefully over the next few years but probably necessitating decades.

Of course, in dramatic advances since the middle of the last century, the medical scientists, physicians, and surgeons who performed the experiments on cell lines and organs, in animal studies, and in humans all served to make dialysis and transplantation lifesaving treatments for the many patients who have lost all kidney function. In particular, the place of Drs. Murray, Starzl, and Terasaki in the pantheon of pioneers of kidney transplantation remains secure.

Dr. Merrill was a key influence in the development of modern techniques of transplantation and dialysis who stood on the shoulders of such giants as Drs. Willem Kolff and George Thorn. Drs. Scribner and Schreiner (and others) worked in scientific, medical, and political arenas to make dialysis (and meaningful survival) a reality for people with ESKD while ensuring the provision of payments for dialysis and kidney transplantation. In addition, patients who volunteered for treatments that were largely experimental, such as transplantation in the days before modern immunosuppression, and those involved in early dialysis studies, in Seattle and elsewhere, helped make ESRD treatments the viable therapies they are today. Spouses and family members suffered when patients became ill or died and rejoiced when therapies provided meaningful extensions of life and improvements in the well-being of loved ones. Their agonies and ecstasies were documented by such pioneers in the evaluation of the emotional status of patients by visionaries such as Drs. Fox and Simmons.

Industry scientists have provided major breakthroughs in the treatment of complications of advanced kidney diseases and for the immunosuppression necessary to make transplantation successful. Contemporary medical treatment of ill patients is inconceivable without the participation of a vibrant corporate pharmaceutical and biotechnology infrastructure. The remarkable efficacy of the sodium-glucose cotransporter 2 (SGLT2) inhibitors in improving outcomes for patients with kidney disease is just the most current example of triumphs achieved for patients by the pharmaceutical industry. It is, however, important that the profit motive be tempered by an unflinching regulatory oversight focus on the safety of patients and the efficacy of new and established treatments. This requires the action of forces external to the commercial enterprise, responsive to public health concerns and the body politic.

In addition, I am impressed with the role that federal scientists and regulators have played in the advances in kidney therapies over the last fifty years, since patients have been entitled to treatment for ESRD. Government employees, sometimes termed bureaucrats, who provided early analyses of the characteristics of the patients treated with dialysis under the aegis of the ESRD program and documented disparities in the deployment of these lifesaving therapies, helped patients and researchers confront unknown clinical and research challenges. Federal regulators at the FDA ensured that erythropoietin treatment would be as safe as possible and acted to prevent the deployment and proliferation of therapies that might not be the safest or most efficacious. These government employees have worked tirelessly to safeguard patients with kidney disease in the U.S. In addition, federal scientists and administrators have played important roles in administering the ESRD program and evaluating the pathogenesis and therapy of kidney diseases without the remuneration provided by academic institutions and industry. FDA officials have been in the vanguard of advancing the patient voice in regulatory aspects of drug development in their meetings and through participation in the Kidney Health Initiative. Department of Health and Human Services officials, working in tandem with the American Society of Nephrology, have spearheaded KidneyX, an initiative that aims to revolutionize ESKD treatment in the U.S. and across the globe by reaching out to industry and academic innovators to jump-start technologic research that may have a long horizon until clinically useful products emerge for patients. NIH intramural scientists work on projects to find cures for acute kidney injury, polycystic kidney disease, and focal segmental glomerulosclerosis, while extramural NIDDK scientists provide guidance to major clinical studies affecting patients with kidney disease and promote research in the academic community to dismantle structures that sustain inequitable access to the most promising, and perhaps most expensive, treatments. Executive Order 13879 holds the prospect of changing the landscape of ESKD therapies to meaningfully improve the quality of life of patients with a presently incurable disease in perhaps the greatest governmental advance in kidney disease therapies since the original support of payment for dialysis and transplantation in 1973.

But the real heroes of kidney disease are the patients. Patients with ESKD undergo dialysis treatments three times a week in centers or at home and participate in research through registries. They wait patiently for kidneys that may not arrive in their lifetimes. To the extent allowed by dialysis organizations and encouraged by researchers, patients participate in research that may not help them directly but may help others in the future. Patients participate in randomized controlled trials to provide the only definitive evidence regarding whether specific treatments work, or don't. Patients are beginning to raise their voices as participants in drug development and in oversight of research, including their work on the council of the NIDDK, among other venues. In the Kidney Precision Medicine Project, patients who would not necessarily need a renal biopsy for diagnosis or treatment altruistically put their lives on the line to provide knowledge that may (or may not) identify new effective treatments. Patients suffering from ESKD will be asked to be pioneers in the evaluation of xenotransplantation, a high-risk endeavor that could result in triumph or despair for individuals and society. They will face many challenges, defeats, and roadblocks. Their role will be similar to that of the trailblazers who underwent kidney transplantation before the Herrick brothers changed the clinical landscape and modern immunosuppression became a viable treatment for desperately ill people. The patients are the real heroes of the story, who have participated in the quest to solve the enigma of kidney disease from before the days of Richard Bright to the current era.

ACKNOWLEDGMENTS

First, I would like to thank my friends Kevin Kampschroer and Sally Satel, whose lives inspired and formed the basis for this book, for allowing me to tell their stories. As I labored on the manuscript, they provided me new details about their histories, of which I was previously unaware. They are courageous combatants in the war against kidney disease. I will never forget the trust they placed in me nor the gratitude I feel toward them.

There are many people for me to mention who knowingly or unwittingly were involved in the creation of *The Body's Keepers*. I hope I have acknowledged all (or most) of them below. (Apologies to those whom I may have inadvertently omitted from this list. You presumably know who you are—and know you helped me greatly.)

Steven Peitzman, Il Miglior Fabbro, is an incredible historian of kidney disease—and a friend and mentor, who gave me much good advice as I wrote. I learned an enormous amount from him. I continue to read and reread his beautiful books and papers with pleasure.

I've known Brian Kampschroer since 1968. He revealed the most intimate details of his life to me (and to you, the reader), with the hope of helping others. His story is truly a triumph of humanity over disease. I am especially grateful to him for his generosity of spirit.

I am indebted to Brendan Kildunne—a careful reader, and an outsider to the field who was not afraid to voice his views on the book and its progress with me. (Even if sometimes it was an uphill fight in the chapter on erythropoietin.) He has been my good friend for a long time, and is a good critic. John Brennan, Dan Goessling, and Linda Wetzel, also good friends, read early versions of the chapter on kidney physiology and gave me brutally frank but useful feedback. Thanks so much!

I'd like to thank the many people who talked with me and allowed me to get their perspectives as I prepared *The Body's Keepers*. My friend Paul Eggers, perhaps the most preeminent scholar of the ESRD program, read several chapters and gave me critical feedback. He hates reading multiple drafts but indulged me, as usual. Aliza Thompson provided me with a path toward reviewing and understanding the FDA documents that were critical in reporting the evaluation of roxadustat and daprodustat. Ellis Unger, although he had constraints in discussing the specific details of decisions he was involved in at the FDA, spoke with me regarding many general aspects of FDA reviews. I very much valued our conversation. David Goodkin and Anatole Besarab were generous with their time, sharing their knowledgeable views on the Normal Hematocrit Trial. Allen Nissenson and Fred Finkelstein helped me understand the modern economics of large dialysis organizations.

Richard Formica and Krista Lentine provided me with feedback on contemporary aspects of kidney transplantation. Jeffrey Perlmutter updated me on efforts of the Renal Physicians Association to address aspects of systemic racism, and Robert Blaser of the same organization helped me understand current economic, regulatory, and legislative challenges affecting the ESRD program. Ganesh Bhat, Moro Safilu, and Chaim Charytan graciously shared information with me about the early days of dialysis in New York City, and Fiona Karet advised me on some aspects of nomenclature.

Suzanne Watnick and Stephanie Pitts of the Northwest Kidney Center, Joseph Bonventre and Catherine Pate of the Brigham and Women's Hospital, and Jessica Murphy of the Countway Library graciously made historical images of kidney treatments available to me. Joseph Vassalotti of the National Kidney Foundation, Erin Kahle of the Association of Kidney Patients, and Meghan Kennedy of the American College of Surgeons discussed aspects of their archives with me. I thank Julie Ingelfinger for her kind assistance.

Virginia Postrel made herself available to give me background on her decision to donate a kidney and its aftermath.

Juan Bosch, one of my mentors, reminisced with me about the early days of erythropoietin treatments. Dennis Cotter and Mae Thamer, my friends for a long time, helped me better navigate the complex, fraught relationship between

Ortho and Amgen in the late 1980s and early 1990s. Maria Ferris shared her time and experiences as a physician and mother with me, helping me understand issues related to kidney transplantation in children in a personal way. Daniel Coyne and Jay Wish spoke with me at length about hypoxia-inducible factor prolyl hydroxylase inhibitors, and their views on commercial, regulatory, medical, and pharmacologic issues. Michael Kolber and Jacob Kronenberg gave me valuable editorial advice.

Steve Korbet, an expert in kidney biopsies, talked with me about Dr. Robert Kark, a pioneer of the procedure. James Winchester added to my recollections of the details of the Capri Conference, which we both attended.

David Clive read the final manuscript and helped me decide on the limited number of figures that were used in the book.

Louis Begley and Barbara Paul Robinson gave me background on their mentor Oscar Ruebhausen. I was sorry I was not able to use all their stories in this book.

Marla Levy spent a long time with me outlining her experience of her complicated illness and her heroic journey to regain her health. She was frank and enthusiastic about making her story known to readers. She is another warrior in the fight against kidney disease.

Three pediatric kidney transplant patients who are now adults, Ted Ferris, Michael Mittelman, and Austin Lee, generously told me their stories about growing up with kidney disease. (I think they have provided readers with unique insights into the world of pediatric kidney transplantation and the transition of such patients to adulthood.) I am grateful for their time and candor. I only wish I had more space to tell the stories of more patients.

Robert Montgomery gave unstintingly of his time to enlighten me about the underpinnings of recent advances in kidney transplantation, many of which he pioneered. In addition, he candidly shared his unique perspective as a patient as well as a surgeon and researcher. I am deeply appreciative of his work and his help in crafting *The Body's Keepers*.

Jennifer Scherer described the landscape of patient care from a contemporary viewpoint for me and was open in her opinions regarding future prospects for clinical research and improvements in outcomes for patients with kidney failure.

Cherie Winkler, a key player in the identification of the association of *APOL1* variants and the presence of kidney disease, reviewed the chapter on *APOL1* from personal and historical vantage points. Her insights were invaluable, and I thank her for her assistance.

Rebekah Rasooly helped me by reviewing molecular biologic techniques and keeping the glossary honest. John Hansen-Flaschen, my friend from the first day of medical school, talked with me at length about the Pulmonary, Allergy, and Critical Care Division at the University of Pennsylvania. Robert Alter, in email exchanges, enlarged on biblical conceptions of the kidneys.

Paul Conway and Richard Knight gave their time and expertise to this work, with unique insights into the workings of the systems behind the regulations and rules that affect the lives of patients and the practice and livelihood of physicians who care for those with kidney disease.

Andy Narva, my colleague, spoke in great detail about the structures and economics of contemporary dialytic care, allowing me to use new ideas to assess old problems. I thank Marva Moxey-Mims for her gracious assistance.

Thad Garret and Joanne Pierre of the Cosmos Club helped me finish this long project. Thad Garrett in particular proved adept at finding the right text from the popular literature that could shed light on the early days of kidney transplantation and dialysis. The staff of the Himmelfarb Library at George Washington University were invariably helpful to me as I roamed the literature in search of obscure references.

I thank Erik Koritzinski, who provided beautiful illustrations, which I hope elucidate complex scientific concepts for general readers.

Eric Lupfer took a chance on an author, perhaps a bit long in the tooth, with experience in academic publishing but without a track record of writing for the general public. His grasp of the trajectory of a nonfiction work is, in my opinion, extraordinary. I deeply appreciate all he has done for me and thank him for his assistance.

Daniela Rapp of Mayo Clinic Press expressed confidence in this project from the beginning, which was sincerely appreciated. She supported my work in the community and writes beautifully. She consistently embodied the perspective of the interested outsider, who would need assistance navigating the vocabulary of the medical industrial complex. She is equipped with a finely honed critical sensibility.

I'd like to thank the cover designer, Olya Kirilyuk, Kelly Hahn, Jasmine Souers, Dana Noble, and Alan Bradshaw at Mayo Clinic Press, and Carol McGillivray at Amnet who took a long list of words and turned it into, in my opinion, a beautiful book.

Prudence Kline read so much of the manuscript, so many times, and consistently and honestly provided me with sage advice. She is capable of reducing a three paragraph complicated argument into a one-sentence devastating but understandable quip. I often had to prevent this from occurring. I will forever be in her debt for her gracious, skillful assistance on this book and in life.

I received a great deal of assistance from those mentioned and others as I researched the literature while writing *The Body's Keepers*. Any mistakes in the text are, of course, mine.

GLOSSARY AND SELECTED NORMAL LABORATORY VALUES

acquired immunodeficiency syndrome	AIDS, a late stage of human immunodeficiency virus (HIV) infection.
acute kidney injury	AKI, a sudden diminution in glomerular filtration rate. Many syndromes and diseases may be associated with its presence. May be reversible or irreversible, often complicating the course of CKD.
acute renal failure	ARF, an older term for AKI, delineating three categories: prerenal azotemia (an often reversible diminution of blood flow to the kidneys engendered by diverse causes), intrinsic disease of the kidney tissue, or urinary tract obstruction.
albumin	a common protein circulating in the blood, which supports the blood volume. In people with normal renal function, albumin only appears in very low levels in the urine.
albuminuria	abnormal, excess albumin in the urine, a sensitive sign of glomerular disease.
aldosterone	a hormone produced by the adrenal cortex, released in cases of volume or sodium depletion, which acts on the collecting duct of the distal nephron to produce salt retention by facilitating the reabsorption of sodium ions.
American Association of Kidney Patients	AAKP, founded in 1969. The National Association of Patients on Hemodialysis (NAPH), changed its name to AAKP in 1989.
American Journal of Kidney Diseases	*AJKD*
American Journal of Medicine	*AJM*
American Journal of Transplantation	*AJT*
American Society for Artificial Internal Organs	ASAIO
American Society of Nephrology	ASN

amino acid	the chemical building blocks of proteins, composed of carbon, hydrogen, oxygen, and nitrogen. There are twenty-two amino acids, such as lysine, serine, and arginine, appearing in the DNA code.
anaphylaxis	profound allergic reaction to a foreign protein or other chemical, often characterized by rapid onset of severely decreased blood pressure, skin rash, constriction of the bronchi of the lungs, and potentially death if untreated.
anemia	a decrease in the amount of red blood cells in the blood; laboratory tests show decreased levels of hemoglobin and hematocrit.
anephric	"Without kidneys."
Annals of Internal Medicine	*AIM*
antibody	molecules with a characteristic structure, produced by B-cells, in response to challenge with an antigen. Antibodies engage and help neutralize invaders such as microorganisms as part of the immune response.
anticoagulant	colloquially, a blood thinner; a substance that delays or suppresses the clotting of the blood. Heparin is used intravenously during hemodialysis treatments as an anticoagulant. Warfarin (or Coumadin) is an older oral anticoagulant. Newer oral anticoagulants have been developed over the last twenty years.
antidiuretic hormone	ADH, a hormone produced by the pituitary gland, in response to dehydration or volume loss, which acts on the collecting duct of the distal nephron to produce concentrated urine by facilitating the reabsorption of water.
antigen	a substance, often a protein, capable of eliciting an immune response.
anuria	no urine output.
aorta	the largest artery in the body, emanating directly from the left ventricle of the heart.
apolipoprotein L1	*APOL1*, a gene that codes for this protein, involved in immunity and other cellular functions. People with two variant versions of this gene are at increased risk for developing kidney disease. Not all people with two variants will develop kidney disease during their lifetime.
Aranesp	trade name for darbepoetin, a longer-acting version of Epogen; an acronym for "a novel erythropoiesis-stimulating protein."

azathioprine	derivative of mercaptopurine, a purine antagonist that interferes with DNA synthesis. An immunosuppressant drug, formerly used quite often in kidney transplant recipients. Now largely replaced by mycophenolate mofetil.
B-cell, B-lymphocyte	a type of lymphocyte (a subset of white blood cells). On stimulation by an antigen, they can transform into plasma cells that release antibodies.
bladder	distensible sac located in the pelvis, into which the ureters drain, that retains urine until it is excreted.
blood typing	the ABO system is the major classification system for blood typing. Classification is based on the different proteins associated with red blood cells.
blood urea nitrogen	BUN, a waste product of the breakdown of proteins that attains high levels in the circulation when kidney function is diminished. Urea may be excreted in high levels in normal urine. Normal BUN values are variably up to 20 mg/dL. Higher levels indicate derangement of kidney or circulatory function or, occasionally, gastrointestinal bleeding.
bone marrow	material filling the bone cavity, made up of blood forming cells and supporting tissue.
British Medical Journal	*BMJ*
calcineurin inhibitor	immunosuppressant, often used in transplant medicine. Examples include cyclosporine and tacrolimus. By inhibiting the action of calcineurin, it impairs production of interleukin-2 and other cytokines by T-cells, inhibiting their action. They are used to prevent rejection.
carbohydrate	molecule made up of carbon, oxygen, and hydrogen atoms. Sugars, for example, are carbohydrates.
catecholamines	hormones synthesized primarily by the adrenal glands, often part of the "fight or flight" response, which can affect blood vessels and increase blood pressure.
Centers for Medicare and Medicaid Services	CMS, the agency that currently administers the Medicare and Medicaid programs.
chromosome	a long strand of DNA, comprised of many genes, found in the cell nucleus. Twenty-three pairs of chromosomes form the human genome. One chromosome of the pair is inherited from the mother, the other from the father.
chronic kidney disease	CKD, typically defined by a decrease in kidney function (GFR) and/or abnormal albuminuria, lasting for more than three months.

chronic renal failure	CRF, variously described as the stage of progressive chronic kidney disease in which counterregulatory systems begin to break down—now a relatively obsolete term.
chronic renal insufficiency	CRI, variously described as a decrement of renal function usually in the absence of abnormal laboratory tests or symptoms—now a relatively obsolete term.
Clinical Journal of the American Society of Nephrology	*CJASN*
collecting tubule	a segment of the distal nephron, which contributes to the final volume and concentration of the urine by reabsorbing water, sodium, and other ions, often against concentration gradients, under the influence of hormones such as ADH or aldosterone.
continuous arterio-venous hemofiltration	CAVH, a procedure to treat fluid overload and electrolyte disturbances, often in the presence of acute kidney injury. The procedure involves a dialysis cartridge, linked to catheters connecting the arterial and venous circulations of the patient. The pressure gradient between the artery and the vein drives the filtration of fluid. Now largely superseded by CVVH.
continuous renal replacement therapies	CRRTs, including continuous arterio-venous hemofiltration (CAVH) and continuous venovenous hemofiltration, (CVVH). These treatments are used in patients with fluid overload and electrolyte disturbances, usually in the setting of AKI, often in an intensive care unit.
continuous veno-venous hemofiltration	CVVH, a procedure to treat fluid overload and electrolyte disturbances, often in the presence of acute kidney injury. The procedure involves a dialysis cartridge, linked to catheters connecting the venous circulations of the patient. The pressure gradient is often supplied by a pump.
creatinine	molecule circulating in the bloodstream. A product of muscle metabolism, its circulating levels are inversely related to glomerular filtration rate. Various equations have been used to estimate GFR using the serum creatinine concentration, S[Cr].
cubic centimeter	cc, one-thousandth of a liter, or a milliliter (mL, about 0.0042 cups).
cyclosporine	various spellings and trade names. First developed as an immunosuppressive drug by Borel and colleagues at Sandoz in the 1970s and 1980s. It was the first of the class of calcineurin inhibitors. Used in patients who have received a transplant to prevent rejection.

daprodustat	an ESA, in the class of hypoxia-inducible factor prolyl hydroxylase inhibitors, developed by GlaxoSmithKline. It was approved for use in the treatment of anemia in dialysis-dependent CKD patients in February 2023.
darbepoetin	Aranesp, a modification of erythropoietin with a longer-lasting half-life, developed by Amgen in the 1990s and approved by the FDA in 2001.
deciliter	dL, one-tenth of a liter, about one-fifth of a pint, or 42% of a cup.
Department of Health and Human Services	HHS. The agency contains, among others, the NIH, FDA, and CMS.
diabetes insipidus	a disease resulting from inadequate production or action of antidiuretic hormone, typically characterized by thirst and frequent urination (polyuria and polydipsia), leading to the passage of large amounts of dilute urine throughout the day and night.
diabetes mellitus	DM, a collection of metabolic diseases characterized by inability to maintain circulating blood glucose levels in a narrow reference range. The most common types of DM in the U.S. include type 2, characterized by high circulating insulin levels but resistance to the action of insulin, closely linked to obesity, most commonly seen in adults. The rarer type 1, defined by failure of the pancreas to secrete insulin, is an autoimmune disease frequently affecting children and young adults. There are various forms of DM. DM is commonly complicated, usually after years of the illness, by the development of CKD.
dialysis	first described by the Scottish scientist Thomas Graham (1805–1869), outlining the movement of ions or solutes across a semipermeable membrane according to their concentration gradients. Now most often the treatment of kidney disease using a semipermeable membrane with the patients' circulation on one side and a fluid designed to normalize abnormalities in electrolyte concentrations and facilitate the diffusion of wastes in another compartment. Can include various forms of dialysis using the bloodstream (hemodialysis) or the peritoneal cavity (peritoneal dialysis).
diuretic	Drug that increases urine flow, or phase of acute tubular necrosis during which increased urine flow is apparent.
Division of Kidney, Urologic and Hematologic Diseases	DKUHD, the division of NIDDK concerned with grants and contracts related to kidney disease, nonmalignant urologic disease, and selected blood diseases.

DNA	deoxyribonucleic acid, the building block of the genetic code. Composed of nucleotides made from the bases adenine, cytosine, guanine, and thymine and sugar and phosphate groups.
encephalopathy	dysfunction of the brain.
end-stage kidney disease	ESKD, a new, currently widely accepted term for ESRD. The clinical situation where dialysis or kidney transplantation is required to maintain life, health, or well-being.
end-stage renal disease	ESRD, now referring to the U.S. program to reimburse dialysis and transplantation, after certification of need for treatment for irreversible disease by a physician. Replaced clinically by ESKD.
epigenomic	see omics.
Epogen	Amgen trademark. Erythropoietin to be used in patients treated with dialysis, identical to Procrit, marketed by Ortho Biotech.
erythrocyte	a red blood cell (RBC).
erythropoiesis-stimulating agent	ESA, a drug, usually (although not always) a modification of erythropoietin that has similar effects on red blood cell synthesis and release.
erythropoietin	EPO, a hormone synthesized by the kidney that supports the development, production, and release of red blood cells into the circulation.
estimated glomerular filtration rate	eGFR, a derived measurement of kidney function, calculated from factors such as age and sex, and circulating creatinine or cystatin C concentrations.
expression	the production of proteins from their RNA templates.
extracellular fluid	ECF, a part of the body water that includes the plasma.
ferritin	an iron-containing blood protein. Its circulating levels are used to evaluate patient iron stores and use.
fistula, A-V fistula	AVF, a surgical connection between an artery and a vein that matures to sustain repeated cannulation for access to the bloodstream for hemodialysis.
focal, segmental glomerulosclerosis	FSGS or FGS, a primary kidney disease typically associated with large losses of protein in the urine (proteinuria or nephrotic syndrome). Can also manifest as a secondary kidney disease, the complication of another illness. Defined by histologic characteristics noted on a kidney biopsy.
Food and Drug Administration	FDA

gene	the biologic unit of heredity, as stretches of DNA arranged on chromosomes in the cell nucleus, composed of a discrete set of purine or pyrimidine base pairs—including adenine, cytosine, guanine, and thymine—and sugars and phosphates.
genomics	see omics.
glomerular filtration rate	GFR, a fundamental measurement of kidney function, defined as the amount of a substance not acted on by the tubules and removed from the bloodstream each minute through the glomeruli.
glomerulonephritis	GN, inflammation of the filtering portion of the nephron (the glomerulus), often resulting in proteinuria and hematuria and decrease in kidney function (as measured by GFR).
glomerulus (pl., glomeruli)	the filtering component of the nephron, composed of a ramification of blood vessels emerging from the afferent arteriole and culminating in the efferent arteriole, situated within Bowman's capsule.
glycoprotein	a molecule composed of a chain of amino acids linked to carbohydrates.
graft, A-V graft	an artificial vessel, surgically implanted, to provide access for hemodialysis.
gram	variably g, gm, a unit of mass (weight).
Health Care Financing Administration	HCFA, previously provided oversight and payment for the ESRD program; now superseded by CMS.
Health Care Financing Review	HCFR
hematocrit	the percentage (by volume) of red blood cells in the blood. Often determined using automated laboratory testing. Can be determined at bedside by a clinician as the level of red cells in a centrifuged specimen of blood. Normal values vary between men and women and across laboratories. Typical normal values range between 37.5 and 51.0%.
hematuria	red blood cells appearing abnormally in the urine.
hemochromatosis	a set of illnesses characterized by iron overload. Several mechanisms may lead to inability to properly use iron stored in the body.
hemodiafiltration	a technique of renal replacement therapy combining aspects of hemodialysis and hemofiltration, used in continuous therapies. For in-center treatment, hemodiafiltration techniques were far more commonly used in Europe than in the U.S.
hemodialysis	see dialysis.

hemofiltration	a technique of renal replacement therapy using a dialysis semipermeable membrane. The technique primarily employs ultrafiltration (no dialysis fluid) with replacement of the fluid removed with intravenous fluid approximating the chemical composition of normal plasma. Not often used in the U.S.
hemoglobin	Hb, a protein containing iron that binds oxygen and transports it from the lungs to all the tissues of the body. Found primarily in red blood cells. Normal values vary between men and women and across laboratories. Typical normal values range between 12.6 and 17.7 g/dL.
hemolysis	destruction of red blood cells within the circulation, releasing hemoglobin.
heparin	a substance (mucopolysaccharide) with potent anticoagulant properties, used clinically to prevent clotting in various renal replacement therapies.
hepatitis B virus	HBV, a DNA virus causing acute and chronic liver injury.
hepatitis C virus	HCV, a RNA virus causing acute and chronic liver injury.
hirudin	a peptide produced by leeches with anticoagulant properties, used in early dialysis experiments.
histology	the study of tissues, generally using microscopic techniques.
hormone	a substance, usually but not exclusively a protein, secreted by a gland that has an action on another organ. Typical examples include insulin, corticosteroids, estrogen, and testosterone.
human immunodeficiency virus	HIV
Human Leukocyte Antigen	HLA, a type of molecule making up the tissue type, found on most cells of the body. The "flags" that signal the tissue type to surveillance immune cells.
hydrocephalus	excessive fluid in the ventricular system of the brain resulting in an increase in the pressure inside the cranium.
hyperkalemia	increased level of circulating potassium concentration.
hypernatremia	increased level of circulating sodium concentration.
hypertension	high blood pressure.
hypokalemia	decreased level of circulating potassium concentration.
hyponatremia	decreased level of circulating sodium concentration.
hypoxia	low levels of blood oxygen.
Institute of Medicine	IOM, now renamed the National Academy of Medicine, a part of NASEM.

insulin	a hormone made by the pancreas that facilitates the transfer of glucose from the bloodstream into the tissues of the body.
interstitial nephritis	IN, inflammation of the interstitium of the kidney, typified by infiltration of white blood cells in kidney tissue, detected by light microscopy. May result in decrease in GFR and detection of white blood cells in the urine.
intracellular fluid	ICF, the largest component of the total body water.
iothalamate	radiocontrast agent containing iodine, often used to determine glomerular filtration rate.
Journal of Biological Chemistry	JBC
Journal of Clinical Investigation	JCI
Journal of the American Medical Association	JAMA
Journal of the American Society of Nephrology	JASN
kidney	a Middle English term with unknown antecedents that describes the two organs that filter blood, modify and excrete drugs, and create urine as well as various hormones and chemicals.
kilogram	kg, one thousand grams, a measure of mass (weight) in the metric system, equal to about 2.2 pounds (the weight of a liter of water).
laparoscope	a fiberoptic instrument that can be inserted into the abdomen, used in many different medical procedures.
laparoscopy	procedure using the laparoscope.
"library"	in molecular biology, a collection of molecules or genes, that is present in specific tissues and can be screened to link amino acids, proteins, and genetic material.
liter	L, a kilogram of water, about a quart.
loop of Henle	a portion of the nephron connecting the proximal tubule and more distal portions of the nephron, first described by Friedrich G. J. Henle in 1862. It is composed of the thin descending limb, the thin ascending limb, and the thick ascending limb. Loop of Henle function is involved in the concentration and dilution of the urine and in electrolyte transport.
lymphocyte	a white blood cell involved in immune responses, often categorized as B- or T-cells, among other subtypes.
major histocompatibility complex	MHC, a set of genes on chromosome 6 coding proteins involved in presenting antigens to T-cells.

messenger RNA	mRNA, the RNA type that transcribes information from DNA, ultimately for synthesizing proteins.
metabolomics	see omics.
milliequivalent	mEq, a measure related to the amount of mass and chemical activity of an ion dissolved in a solution, such as serum or plasma. A measure of concentration.
milligram	mg, one-thousandth of a gram.
milliliter	mL, one-thousandth of a liter, also known as a cubic centimeter (cc) of fluid.
molecular biology	the science of DNA, RNA and protein interactions.
molecule	smallest unit of a chemical compound.
National Academies of Science, Engineering, and Medicine	NASEM
National Association of Patients on Hemodialysis	NAPH; see American Association of Kidney Patients.
National Cancer Institute	NCI
National Heart, Lung, and Blood Institute	NHLBI
National Human Genome Research Institute	NHGRI
National Institute of Allergy and Infectious Diseases	NIAID
National Institute of Dental Research	NIDR
National Institute of Diabetes and Digestive and Kidney Diseases	NIDDK
National Institute on Minority Health and Health Disparities	NIMHD
National Institutes of Health	NIH
National Kidney Foundation	NKF
National Nephrosis Foundation	precursor to NKF
nephritic	a syndromic classification of inflammatory kidney diseases, usually involving the glomeruli. To be differentiated from "nephrotic."

nephritis	inflammation of the kidneys, usually a nonspecific term.
nephrolithiasis	having kidney stones, or relating to kidney stone formation.
nephron	the functioning unit of the kidney, composed of the glomerulus and its accompanying tubule.
nephrotic	a syndromic classification of kidney diseases, usually involving the glomeruli, associated with markedly increased urinary protein excretion and signs such as edema (swelling) and high blood pressure. To be differentiated from "nephritic."
neuropathy	a set of medical conditions associated with nerve dysfunction.
New England Journal of Medicine	*NEJM*
nocturia	needing to urinate after falling asleep for the night.
nucleic acid	typically refers to DNA or RNA.
nucleoside	a compound of a purine or pyrimidine base (including adenine, cytosine, guanine, thymine, and uridine) linked to a sugar, typically found in DNA or RNA.
nucleotide	a compound composed of a purine or pyrimidine base (nucleoside) linked to a sugar and phosphate.
oligonucleotide	short synthetic regions of DNA or RNA.
oliguria	low urine output.
omics	shorthand for contemporary techniques for evaluating tissue. Examples include genomics (evaluating gene expression), epigenomics (evaluating change in DNA methylation or packaging), transcriptomics (evaluating RNA), proteomics (evaluating protein production and levels), and metabolomics (evaluating various compounds).
Organ Procurement and Transplantation Network	OPTN
Organ Procurement Organizations	OPOs, U.S. not-for-profit organizations tasked with collecting organs from deceased donors to use in transplantation procedures.
pathology	study of disease, often involves evaluating tissue and laboratory specimens for diagnostic purposes.
peginesatide	a synthetic erythropoietic stimulating agent, no longer on the market.
peptide	short string of amino acids; constituents of proteins.
peritoneal dialysis	several different forms of dialysis accomplished by using fluid instilled into the abdominal cavity, and its lining, the peritoneum, as the semipermeable membrane.
physiology	the science of organ function.

plasmapheresis	a procedure for separating and removing plasma from a patient, involving different therapeutic replacement strategies.
polycystic kidney disease	PKD, a common inherited genetic disorder of the kidneys, characterized by abnormal cyst formation and kidney growth, accompanied by diminution in kidney function, usually, but not exclusively in middle age.
polydipsia	excessive thirst.
polymerase chain reaction	PCR, a molecular biologic method for making many copies of a specific DNA segment; invented by Dr. Kary Mullis, who won the Nobel Prize for his work.
polyuria	excessive or frequent urination.
post-transplant lymphoproliferative disorder	PTLD, a group of diseases, following transplantation and use of immunosuppressive drugs, in which B-lymphocytes (immune cells) multiply, often interfering with the function of the transplanted organ as well as other organs.
potassium	K, the nineteenth element. Potassium is the major ion in the intracellular fluid. Circulating normal levels are typically between 3.5 and 5.5 mEq/L. High and low levels of circulating potassium ions may interfere with heart and nerve functions.
Procrit	Ortho Biotech trademark, this brand of erythropoietin (identical to Epogen, marketed by Amgen) was to be used in patients with CKD not treated with dialysis and for other nondialysis indications.
prostate	gland found below the bladder in men that surrounds the urethra. Its growth with aging can result in urinary tract obstruction and the development of AKI or CKD.
proteinuria	abnormal, excess protein in the urine, a sensitive sign of kidney disease.
proteomics	see omics.
proximal tubule	PT, like Gaul, divided into three parts. This portion of the nephron reabsorbs sodium, potassium, amino acids, glucose, and phosphate, generally according to their concentrations in the circulation and the tubular fluid, without much change in the character of the fluid (isosmotically).
purine	aromatic organic compound containing nitrogen consisting of two fused rings. Two purines, adenine and guanine, are components of DNA. Other purines include caffeine and uric acid.
pyrimidine	organic compound containing nitrogen. Two pyrimidines, cytosine and thymine, are components of DNA.

quality of life	QOL, a construct evaluating overall well-being, often divided into physical functioning and emotional or satisfaction domains. Many questionnaires have been used to assess the diverse aspects of QOL.
randomized controlled trial	RCT, a study, typically of an intervention (drug or procedure) in which roughly half of the participants are randomly assigned (by chance) to the intervention and roughly half do not receive the intervention, functioning as a "control" or "comparison" group.
receptor	proteins, often on the surfaces of cells, that interact with biochemicals (such as hormones) to receive signals or cause effects within the cell.
red cell aplasia	a set of diseases in which the production of red cells by the bone marrow is diminished or abrogated, resulting in anemia.
red blood cell	RBC, a cell without a nucleus, filled with hemoglobin, which allows transfer of oxygen from the lungs to the peripheral tissues through the blood circulation.
red blood cell cast	RBC cast, a collection of RBCs in the urine, usually signifying glomerulonephritis.
renal	of or related to the kidneys, from the Latin *renes* and the Old French *reins*.
renal osteodystrophy	bone disease of CKD, now termed CKDMBD, or CKD-related metabolic bone disease. Before the availability of treatment with potent vitamin D analogues, renal osteodystrophy could have profound anatomic consequences for patients.
renal replacement therapies	various forms of dialysis and hemofiltration.
RNA	ribonucleic acid, which serves as the intermediary between DNA and protein synthesis, composed of the bases adenine, guanine, uracil, and thymine.
roxadustat	an ESA, in the class of hypoxia-inducible factor prolyl hydroxylase inhibitors. It was not approved for use in the treatment of anemia in CKD patients in the U.S.
serum calcium concentration	S[Ca], in laboratories normal range is typically 8.6 to 10.2 mg/dL. (Normal values vary among laboratories.)
serum creatinine concentration	S[Cr], in laboratories normal range is typically between 0.6 and 1.3 mg/dL. (Normal values vary among laboratories.) Reference values are often different for men and women. The higher the value, the lower the renal function.
serum phosphate concentration	S[P], in laboratories normal range is typically between 2.5 and 4.6 mg/dL. (Normal values vary among laboratories.)
serum potassium concentration	S[K], in laboratories normal range is typically between 3.5 and 5.5 mEq/L. (Normal values vary among laboratories.)

serum sodium concentration	S[Na], in laboratories normal range is typically between 135 and 145 mEq/L. (Normal values vary among laboratories.)
sirolimus	an immunosuppressant drug (m-Tor inhibitor) used in patients who have received a kidney transplant to prevent rejection.
6-mercaptopurine	6-MCP, a purine antagonist, used as a chemotherapy agent in the treatment of certain hematologic malignancies.
sodium	Na, the eleventh element, the major positive ion in the extracellular fluid. Circulating normal levels are typically between 135 and 145 mEq/L. High and low levels of circulating sodium ions may interfere with heart and nerve functions.
sodium-glucose cotransporter-2 (SGLT2) inhibitors	a class of drugs that inhibits glucose reabsorption by the proximal tubule of the kidney, resulting in loss of glucose in the urine. Used as blood glucose–lowering drugs, many in this class have been demonstrated to improve kidney and heart outcomes in patients with kidney disease.
tacrolimus	an immunosuppressant drug (calcineurin inhibitor) used in patients who have received a kidney transplant to prevent rejection.
T-cell, T-lymphocyte	a type of lymphocyte (a subset of white blood cells). Interacting with B-cells, T-cells can modify antibody production. Certain types of T-cells have actions on tissues, including killing functions, and production of chemicals that modify immune and cellular functions.
tissue plasminogen activator	TPA, a drug used to treat patients with various types of thromboses (or clots). Available for clinical use as a result of biotechnological advances.
transcriptomics	see omics.
transfection	placement of DNA or RNA into cells, typically to allow the production of an associated protein.
United Network for Organ Sharing	UNOS
United States Renal Data System	USRDS, a registry of U.S. ESRD patients (treated by dialysis and kidney transplantation), supported by a NIDDK contract since 1989. The USRDS issues an Annual Data Report (ADR) and has expanded to consider national statistics regarding CKD and AKI.
uremia	a constellation of signs and symptoms associated with (acutely or chronically) diminished kidney function, including lack of appetite, nausea and vomiting, skin changes, chest or abdominal pain, swelling, seizures, disordered consciousness and somnolence, or coma, as well as anemia, high blood pressure, clotting disorders, and disorders of mineral and electrolyte handling and metabolism.

uremic	of or pertaining to having uremia.
ureter	the tubes connecting each kidney to the bladder, through which urine flows.
ureterostomy	surgery to establish a urinary diversion, often by making an opening in the ureter, and creating a conduit for passage of urine.
urinary tract obstruction	a cause of AKI or CKD, usually occurring as a result of prostatic hypertrophy, or gynecologic tumors.
white blood cell	WBC, circulating cells of a variety of types, which often ingest bacteria as a line of defense and contribute to the inflammatory response to infectious and other stimuli.
white blood cell cast	WBC cast, a collection of WBCs in the urine, often signifying interstitial nephritis.
xenotransplantation	The use of organs from other species, such as swine, for transplantation into humans. Such organs may be genetically altered to improve outcomes.

NOTES

Prologue

1 Personal communication, Robert Alter, March 19, 2022.

1. Two Roommates and Four Kidneys

1 Eric A. Engels, Gary E. Fraser, Bertram L. Kasiske, Jon J. Snyder, Jason Utt, Charles F. Lynch, Jie Li et al., "Cancer Risk in Living Kidney Donors," *American Journal of Transplantation* 22, no. 8 (2022): 2006–15.

2. What the Kidneys Do and When They Don't

1 Rex L. Jamison and R. H. Maffly, "The Urinary Concentrating Mechanism," *New England Journal of Medicine* 295, no. 19 (1976): 1059–76; William T. Abraham, and Robert W. Schrier, "Body Fluid Volume Regulation in Health and Disease," *Advances in Internal Medicine* 39 (1994): 23–47; Peter Bie and Mads Damkjaer, "Renin Secretion and Total Body Sodium: Pathways of Integrative Control," *Clinical and Experimental Pharmacology and Physiology* 37, no. 2 (2010): e34–e42; Susan D. Crowley and Thomas M. Coffman, "Recent Advances Involving the Renin-Angiotensin System," *Experimental and Cellular Research* 318, no. 9 (2012): 1049–56; John Feehally and Maryam Khosravi, "Effects of Acute and Chronic Hypohydration on Kidney Health and Function," *Nutrition Reviews* 73, no. suppl. 2 (2015): 110–19; Mark A. Knepper, Tae-Hwan Kwon, and Soren Nielsen, "Molecular Physiology of Water Balance," *New England Journal of Medicine* 372, no. 14 (2015): 1349–58; John Danziger and Mark L. Zeidel, "Osmotic Homeostasis," *Clinical Journal of the American Society of Nephrology* 10, no. 5 (2015): 852–62; Eric Feraille, Ali Sassi, Valérie Olivier, Grégoire Arnoux, and Pierre-Yves Martin, "Renal Water Transport in Health and Disease," *Pflügers Archiv-European Journal of Physiology* 474, no. 8 (2022): 841–52.

3. Acute Renal Failure—World War II, the Blitz, and Drs. Kolff and Merrill

1 Jay L. Xue, F. Daniels, Robert A. Star, Paul L. Kimmel, Paul W. Eggers, Bruce A. Molitoris, Jonathan Himmelfarb, and Allan J. Collins, "Incidence and Mortality of

Acute Renal Failure in Medicare Beneficiaries, 1992 to 2001," *Journal of the American Society of Nephrology* 17 no. 4 (2006): 1135–42.

2   F. C. Davies, and R. P. Weldon. "A Contribution to the Study of 'War Nephritis,'" *Lancet* 190, no. 4900 (1917): 118–20.

3   Seigo Minami, "Über Nierenveränderungen nach Verschüttung," *Virchow Archive Pathol Anatomy Physiol* 245 (1923): 47–267.

4   Garabed Eknoyan, "Emergence of the Concept of Acute Renal Failure," *American Journal of Nephrology* 22 (2002): 225–30.

5   D. Beall, Eric G. L. Bywaters, R. H. R. Belsey, and J. A. R. Miles, "Crush Injury with Renal Failure," *British Medical Journal* 1 no. 4185 (1941): 432–34.

6   R. Mayon-White and O. M. Solandt, "A Case of Limb Compression Ending Fatally in Uraemia," *British Medical Journal* 1, no. 4185 (1941): 434–435.

7   Eric G. L. Bywaters and Desmond Beall, "Crush Injuries with Impairment of Renal Function," *British Medical Journal* 1, no. 4185 (1941): 427–32.

8   Ronald G. Henderson, "Recovery from Uraemia Following Crush Injury," *British Medical Journal* 2, no. 4205 (1941): 197.

9   Maurice B. Strauss, "Acute Renal Insufficiency Due to Lower-Nephron Nephrosis," *New England Journal of Medicine* 239, no. 19 (1948): 693–700.

10 B. Lücke, "Lower Nephron Nephrosis (The Renal Lesions of the Crush Syndrome, of Burns, Transfusions, and Other Conditions Affecting the Lower Segments of the Nephrons)," *Military Surgeon* 99, no. 5 (1946): 371–96.

11 G. M. Bull, A. M. Joekes, and K. G. Lowe, "Renal Function Studies in Acute Tubular Necrosis," *Clinical Science* 9, no. 4 (1950): 379–404.

12 K. G. Lowe, "The Late Prognosis in Acute Tubular Necrosis: An Interim Follow-Up Report on 14 Patients," *Lancet* 259, no. 6718 (1952): 1086–88.

13 Nils Alwall, "On the Artificial Kidney I: Apparatus for Dialysis of the Blood In Vivo," *Acta Medica Scandinavica* 128, no. 4 (1947): 317–25; Nils Alwall and L. Norvitt, "On the Artificial Kidney II: Effectivity of Apparatus," *Acta Medica Scandinavica*, supp. 194 (1947): 250–59; Nils Alwall, L. Norvitt, and A. M. Steins, "Clinical Extracorporeal Dialysis of Blood with Artificial Kidney," *Lancet* 1 (1948): 60–62; Willem J. Kolff, "Artificial Kidney," *Journal of the Mount Sinai Hospital* 14 (1947): 71–79.

14 Poul Brandt Rehberg, "Studies on Kidney Function: The Rate of Filtration and Reabsorption in the Human Kidney," *Biochemical Journal* 20, no. 3 (1926): 447–60.

15 Jean Oliver, Muriel MacDowell, and Ann Tracy, "The Pathogenesis of Acute Renal Failure Associated with Traumatic and Toxic Injury: Renal Ischemia, Nephrotoxic Damage and the Ischemuric Episode," *Journal of Clinical Investigation* 30, no. 12 (1951): 1307–1439.

16 Willem J. Kolff. "First Clinical Experience with the Artificial Kidney," *Annals of Internal Medicine* 62, no. 3 (1965): 608–19.

17 John J. Abel, Leonard J. Rowntree, and Bernard Benjamin Turner, "On the Removal of Diffusible Substances from the Circulating Blood of Living Animals by Dialysis II: Some Constituents of the Blood," *Journal of Pharmacology and Experimental Therapeutics* 5, no. 6 (1914): 611–23; John J. Abel, Leonard George Rowntree, and Bernard Benjamin Turner, "On the Removal of Diffusible Substances from the Circulating Blood by Means of Dialysis," *Transactions of the Association of American Physicians* 28 (1913):

51–54; John J. Abel, Leonard G. Rowntree, and Bernard Benjamin Turner, "On the Removal of Diffusible Substances from the Circulating Blood of Living Animals by Dialysis," *Journal of Pharmacology and Experimental Therapeutics* 5, no. 3 (1914): 275–316.

18   Kolff, "First Clinical Experience."

19   Gordon Murray, Edmund Delorme, and Newell Thomas, "Development of an Artificial Kidney: Experimental and Clinical Experiences," *Archives of Surgery* 55, no. 5 (1947): 505–22; Gordon Murray, Edmund Delorme, and Newell Thomas, "Artificial Kidney," *Journal of the American Medical Association* 137, no. 18 (1948): 1596–99; Gordon Murray, Edmund Delorme, and Newell Thomas, "Artificial Kidney," *British Medical Journal* 2, no. 4633 (1949): 887; Leonard T. Skeggs Jr. and Jack R. Leonards, "Studies on an Artificial Kidney: I. Preliminary Results with a New Type of Continuous Dialyzer," *Science* 108, no. 2800 (1948): 212–13; Leonard T. Skeggs Jr., Jack R. Leonards, and Charles R. Heisler, "Artificial Kidney. II. Construction and Operation of an Improved Continuous Dialyzer," *Proceedings of the Society for Experimental Biology and Medicine* 72, no. 3 (1949): 539–43; Leonard T. Skeggs, Jack R. Leonards, Charles Heisler, and Joseph R. Kahn, "Artificial Kidney III: Elimination of Vasodepressor Effects Due to Cellophane," *Journal of Laboratory and Clinical Medicine* 36, no. 2 (1950): 272–75; Alwall, "Apparatus for Dialysis of the Blood In Vivo"; Alwall and Norvitt, "Effectivity of Apparatus"; Alwall, Norvitt, and Steins, "Clinical Extracorporeal Dialysis of Blood with Artificial Kidney"; Nils Alwall, L. Norvitt, and A. M. Steins, "On the Artificial Kidney: Some Experiences during the Study of Dialytic Treatment of Animals with Uremia Caused by Mercuric Chloride Poisoning," *Acta Medica Scandinavica* 132, no. 5: (1949) 477–82; Nils Alwall, "Some Experiences and Problems in Treating Renal Insufficiency I: Extracorporeal Dialysis of the Blood In Vivo in Cases of Uremia; 22 Treatments on 18 Cases II: Fluid Balance Problems in Cases of Acute Oliguria; Anuria Due to Acute Nephritis, Incompatible Blood Transfusions, Lower-Nephron Nephrosis and so on Illustrating the Risks of Excessive Electrolyte-Fluid Supply and Illustrating the Risks of the Modern Electrolyte Fluid Therapy and the Importance of Continual Weight Control," *Acta Medica Scandinavica*, suppl. 239 (1950): 33–34.

20   Kolff, "First Clinical Experience"; Kolff, "Artificial Kidney"; Willem J. Kolff, *New Ways of Treating Uraemia* (London: Churchill, 1947).

21   "Artificial Kidney," *Journal of the American Medical Association* (hereafter, *JAMA*) 128, no. 4 (1945) 288–89.

22   Willem J. Kolff, H. Th. J. Berk, Nurse M. Welle, A. J. W. Van Der Ley, E. C. Van Dijk, and J. Van Noordwijk. "The Artificial Kidney: A Dialyser with a Great Area," *Acta Medica Scandinavica* 117, no. 2 (1944): 121–34.

23   Isadore Snapper, "Treatment of Uremia," *JAMA* 131, no. 3 (1946): 251–52.

24   Alfred P. Fishman, Irving G. Kroop, H. Evans Leiter, and Abraham Hyman, "Experiences with the Kolff Artificial Kidney," *American Journal of Medicine* 7, no. 1 (1949): 15–34.

25   Alfred P. Fishman, "A Physician-Scientist's Tale," in *The Pulmonary Circulation and Gas Exchange* (Armonk, NY: Futura Publishing, 1994), 381–87.

26   George W. Thorn, John P. Merrill, and Stephen Smith, "Clinical Application of the Artificial Kidney," *Transactions of the American Clinical and Climatological Association* 61 (1949): 798–99.

27 John P. Merrill, George W. Thorn, Carl W. Walter, Edmund J. Callahan, and L. Hollingsworth Smith, "The Use of an Artificial Kidney I: Technique," *Journal of Clinical Investigation* 29, no. 4 (1950): 412–24; John P. Merrill, Stephen Smith, Edmund J. Callahan, and George W. Thorn, "The Use of an Artificial Kidney II: Clinical Experience," *Journal of Clinical Investigation* 29, no. 4 (1950): 425–38.

28 John P. Merrill, "Present Role of the Artificial Kidney in Clinical Therapy," *Annals of Internal Medicine* 33, no. 1 (1950): 100–107.

29 John P. Merrill, "The Artificial Kidney," *New England Journal of Medicine* 246, no. 1 (1952): 17–27.

30 Murray Epstein, "John P. Merrill: The Father of Nephrology as a Specialty," *Clinical Journal of the American Society of Nephrology* 4, no. 1 (2009): 2–8.

31 John P. Merrill, "The Legacy of 'Pim' Kolff," *Nephron* 36, no. 3 (1984): 153–55.

32 Robert A. Grossman, Robert W. Hamilton, Bruce M. Morse, Audrey S. Penn, and Martin Goldberg, "Nontraumatic Rhabdomyolysis and Acute Renal Failure," *New England Journal of Medicine* 291, no. 16 (1974): 807–11.

33 Lowe, "Late Prognosis in Acute Tubular Necrosis"; John T. Finkenstaedt and John P. Merrill, "Renal Function after Recovery from Acute Renal Failure," *New England Journal of Medicine* 254, no. 22 (1956): 1023–26.

34 Areef Ishani, Jay L. Xue, Jonathan Himmelfarb, Paul W. Eggers, Paul L. Kimmel, Bruce A. Molitoris, and Allan J. Collins, "Acute Kidney Injury Increases Risk of ESRD among Elderly," *Journal of the American Society of Nephrology* 20, no. 1 (2009): 223–28.

35 Richard L. Amdur, Lakhmir S. Chawla, Susan Amodeo, Paul L. Kimmel, and Carlos E. Palant, "Outcomes Following Diagnosis of Acute Renal Failure in US Veterans: Focus on Acute Tubular Necrosis," *Kidney International* 76, no. 10 (2009): 1089–97.

36 Lakhmir S. Chawla and Paul L. Kimmel, "Acute Kidney Injury and Chronic Kidney Disease: An Integrated Clinical Syndrome," *Kidney International* 82, no. 5 (2012): 516–24; Lakhmir S. Chawla, Paul W. Eggers, Robert A. Star, and Paul L. Kimmel, "Acute Kidney Injury and Chronic Kidney Disease as Interconnected Syndromes," *New England Journal of Medicine* 371, no. 1 (2014): 58–66.

37 Talat Alp Ikizler, Chirag R. Parikh, Jonathan Himmelfarb, Vernon M. Chinchilli, Kathleen D. Liu, Steven G. Coca, Amit X. Garg et al., "A Prospective Cohort Study of Acute Kidney Injury and Kidney Outcomes, Cardiovascular Events, and Death," *Kidney International* 99, no. 2 (2021): 456–65.

38 Peter W. J. D. F. Kramer, P. W. Wigger, J. Rieger, D. Matthaei, and F. Scheler, "Arteriovenous Haemofiltration: A New and Simple Method for Treatment of Over-Hydrated Patients Resistant to Diuretics," *Klinische Wochenschrift* 55, no. 22 (1977): 1121–22.

39 Allan Lauer, Anna Saccagi, Claudio Ronco, Mario Belledone, Sheldon Glabman, and Juan P. Bosch, "Continuous Arteriovenous Hemofiltration in the Critically Ill Patient: Clinical Use and Operational Characteristics," *Annals of Internal Medicine* 99, no. 4 (1983): 455–60.

40 Ravindra L. Mehta, John A. Kellum, Sudhir V. Shah, Bruce A. Molitoris, Claudio Ronco, David G. Warnock, and Adeera Levin, "Acute Kidney Injury Network: Report of an Initiative to Improve Outcomes in Acute Kidney Injury," *Critical Care* 11, no. 2 (2007): 1–8.

41 Ian H. de Boer, Charles E. Alpers, Evren U. Azeloglu, Ulysses G. J. Balis, Jonathan M. Barasch, Laura Barisoni, Kristina N. Blank et al. "Rationale and Design of the Kidney Precision Medicine Project," *Kidney International* 99, no. 3 (2021): 498–510.

42 Marla Levy and Sarah Krumholz, "'Miracle Patient' Received the Gift of Life," UCSF Adult Cardiothoracic Surgery, Department of Surgery, January 16, 2015, https:// surgery.ucsf.edu/patient-center/patient-story.aspx?id=63234.

43 Edward D. Siew, Kathleen D. Liu, John Bonn, Vernon Chinchilli, Laura M. Dember, Timothy D. Girard, Tom Greene et al. "Improving Care for Patients after Hospitalization with AKI," *Journal of the American Society of Nephrology* 31, no. 10 (2020): 2237–41.

4. The Birth of the ESRD Program

1 National Institute of Diabetes and Digestive Kidney Diseases (NIDDK), *United States Renal Data System Annual Report*, 2022, National Institute of Health, U.S. Department of Health and Human Services, https://usrds-adr.niddk.nih.gov/2022.

2 Richard A. Rettig, "Origins of the Medicare Kidney Disease Entitlement: The Social Security Amendments of 1972," in *Biomedical Politics*, ed. Kathi E. Hanna (Washington, D.C.: National Academy Press, 1991), 176–208.

3 Abel, Rowntree, and Turner, "On the Removal of Diffusible Substances from the Circulating Blood by Means of Dialysis."

4 Alwall, "On the Artificial Kidney I: Apparatus for Dialysis of the Blood In Vivo."

5 Christopher R. Blagg, *From Miracle to Mainstream: Creating the World's First Dialysis Organization: Early Years of Northwest Kidney Centers* (Seattle, WA: Northwest Kidney Centers, 2017).

6 Wayne Quinton, David Dillard, and Belding H. Scribner, "Cannulation of Blood Vessels for Prolonged Hemodialysis," *ASAIO Journal* 6, no. 1 (1960): 104–13; Belding H. Scribner, R. Buri, J. E. Z. Caner, R. Hegstrom, and James M. Burnell, "The Treatment of Chronic Uremia by Means of Intermittent Hemodialysis: A Preliminary Report," *ASAIO Journal* 6, no. 1 (1960): 114–22.

7 Shana Alexander, "They Decide Who Lives, Who Dies: Medical Miracle Puts Moral Burden on Small Committee," *Life* 53 (1962): 102–25.

8 James E. Cimino, Michael J. Brescia, and Reuben Aboody, "Simple Venipuncture for Hemodialysis," *New England Journal of Medicine* 267, no. 12 (1962): 608–9.

9 Michael J. Brescia, James E. Cimino, Kenneth Appel, and Baruch J. Hurwich, "Chronic Hemodialysis Using Venipuncture and a Surgically Created Arteriovenous Fistula," *New England Journal of Medicine* 275, no. 20 (1966): 1089–92.

10 Richard A, Rettig, "The Politics of Health Cost Containment: End-Stage Renal Disease," *Bulletin of the New York Academy of Medicine* 56, no. 1 (1980): 115; Norman G. Levinsky and Richard A. Rettig, eds., *Kidney Failure and the Federal Government* (Washington, DC: National Academies Press, 1991); Norman G. Levinsky and Richard A. Rettig, "The Medicare End-Stage Renal Disease Program: A Report from the Institute of Medicine," *New England Journal of Medicine* 324, no. 16 (1991): 1143–48.

11 Committee members included Dr. Lewis Bluemle, who acquired one of the first artificial kidneys in the United States and later worked with a young nephrologist at the University of Pennsylvania, interested in techniques, Dr. Lee Henderson, to spearhead work in the hemofiltration component of dialysis, which they suggested might increase the efficiency of the procedure, perhaps shortening the necessary lengthy treatment times for improved patient care and acceptance. Bluemle advanced academically to become an associate dean at the University of Pennsylvania School of Medicine but left Penn in 1969 to become the president of the State University of New York Upstate Medical Center in Syracuse, New York. He went on to become the president of the Oregon Health Center (from 1974 to 1977). In 1977, Bluemle returned to Philadelphia to become the second president of the Thomas Jefferson University. Dr. Donald W. Seldin, widely acknowledged as a genius and an exacting but masterful teacher, became the youngest chair of a department of medicine in the country, founding the University of Texas Southwest Branch. His work included performing seminal research on the function of nephron segments using the response to diuretics as a clinical and research tool. George Schreiner, the preeminent nephrologist at Georgetown University in Washington, D.C., brought academic, technical, and political experience to the committee. Dr. John S. Najarian had been a forceful advocate for the role of transplantation, pushing research into improving immunosuppressive regimens for patients and advocating for this modality of therapy for children and to improve the quality of life of ESRD patients. Dr. Bernard Amos, a tumor immunogeneticist, was chief of the Division of Immunology in the Department of Microbiology at Duke University. Dr. William A. Greene had trained in both medicine and psychiatry and served as the president of the American Psychosomatic Society in 1968. He was interested in the relationship between psychologic function and heart disease, particularly regarding the relatively new technique of cardiac catheterization. Herbert E. Klarman of Johns Hopkins University was a health economist who was interested in costs. Gerald D. Rosenthal served on a federal panel on wages in the health industry and studied cost effectiveness in chronic kidney disease with Klarman. Oscar M. Ruebhausen, a distinguished lawyer and partner in Debvoise, Plimpton, Lyons, and Gates, was a Dartmouth classmate of Nelson Rockefeller. Ruebhausen was interested in the intricacies of policy, and served as an informal advisor to Rockefeller, the governor of New York, a leader of the Republican Party and candidate for his party's nomination for the presidency. Ruebhausen served as the general counsel to the Vannevar Bush Committee in the Office of Scientific Research and Development in 1944, which supported the development of the federal scientific research infrastructure. Dr. Robert S. Berliner was one of the most respected renal physiologists in the country, working at NIH and Yale, who had advanced the understanding of the mechanisms involved in kidney function and diseases and had trained numerous students who went on to become respected research pioneers and teachers. Dr. Arnold S. Nash, born in England, had done graduate work in chemistry, philosophy, and sociology. He was a professor of religion at the University of North Carolina (UNC) as well as an Anglican minister. Dr. Bernard Greenberg, active in his religious community, was the founder and chair of the Department of Biostatistics, dean of the School of Public Health, and organizer of the Division of Community Health Service at UNC. His research interests primarily pertained to survey and analytic techniques related to health and disease.

12 Christopher S. Wilcox, "In Memory of George E. Schreiner, MD," *Kidney International* 82, no. 4 (2012): 369–70.

13 Rettig, "Origins of the Medicare Kidney Disease Entitlement."

14 Hearings, Reports, and Prints of the House Committee on Interstate and Foreign Commerce (Washington, D.C.: U.S. Government Printing Office, 1970), 121–29.

15 Rettig, "Origins of the Medicare Kidney Disease Entitlement."

16 Rettig, "Origins of the Medicare Kidney Disease Entitlement," 187.

17 Rettig, "Origins of the Medicare Kidney Disease Entitlement," 190.

18 Rettig, "Origins of the Medicare Kidney Disease Entitlement," 191.

19 Rettig, "Origins of the Medicare Kidney Disease Entitlement," 192.

20 NIDDK, *United States Renal Data System Annual Report*, 2022.

21 Belding H. Scribner and Willem J. Kolff, "2002 Albert Lasker Award for Clinical Medical Research," *Journal of the American Society of Nephrology* 13 (2002): 3027–30.

22 Paul L. Kimmel and Juan P. Bosch, "Effectiveness of Renal Fellowship Training for Subsequent Clinical Practice," *American Journal of Kidney Diseases* 18, no. 2 (1991): 249–56.

5. Kidney Transplant Donors, Recipients, and Nobel Prize Laureates

1 Thomas E. Starzl, "History of Clinical Transplantation," *World Journal of Surgery* 24 (2000): 759–82.

2 Gordon D. W. Murray, "Heparin in Thrombosis and Embolism," *Journal of British Surgery* 27, no. 107 (1940): 567–98.

3 Vivian C. McAlister, "Clinical Kidney Transplantation: A 50th Anniversary Review of the First Reported Series," *American Journal of Surgery* 190, no. 3 (2005): 485–88.

4 Gordon Murray, Edmund Delorme, and Newell Thomas. "Development of an Artificial Kidney: Experimental and Clinical Experiences," *Archives of Surgery* 55, no. 5 (1947): 505–22.

5 Gordon Murray and Richard Holden, "Transplantation of Kidneys, Experimentally and in Human Cases," *American Journal of Surgery* 87, no. 4 (1954): 508–15.

6 Vivian McAlister, "Surgical Limits: The Life of Gordon Murray," *Journal of the Canadian Medical Association* 47, no. 5 (2004): 388–89.

7 William J. Dempster, "Observations on the Behaviour of the Transplanted Kidney in Dogs," *Annals of the Royal College of Surgeons of England* 7, no. 4 (1950): 275–302.

8 Richard H. Lawler, J. W. West, P. H. McNulty, E. J. Clancy, and R. P. Murphy, "Homotransplantation of the Kidney in the Human," *Journal of the American Medical Association* 144, no. 10 (1950): 844–45.

9 Richard H. Lawler, James W. West, Patrick H. McNulty, Edward J. Clancy, and Raymond P. Murphy, "Homotransplantation of the Kidney in the Human: Supplemental Report of a Case," *Journal of the American Medical Association* 147, no. 1 (1951): 45–46.

10 Thomas E. Starzl, "The French Heritage in Clinical Kidney Transplantation," *Transplantation Reviews* 7, no. 2 (1993): 65–71.

11 Nicholas L. Tilney, *Transplant: From Myth to Reality* (New Haven, CT: Yale University Press, 2003).

12 David M. Hume, John P. Merrill, Benjamin F. Miller, and George W. Thorn, "Experiences with Renal Homotransplantation in the Human: Report of Nine Cases," *Journal of Clinical Investigation* 34, no. 2 (1955): 327–82.

13 Joseph E. Murray, C. B. Favour, Courtney T. Wemyss Jr., and Benjamin F. Miller, "A Preliminary Study of Renal Homotransplants in Dogs," *Plastic and Reconstructive Surgery* 11, no. 5 (1953): 353; C. B. Favour, Joseph E. Murray, C. T. Wemyss Jr., A. Colodny, and Benjamin F. Miller, "Serum Complement Levels in Dogs Undergoing Kidney Homotransplantation," *Proceedings of the Society for Experimental Biology and Medicine* 83, no. 2 (1953): 352–56; Joseph E. Murray and Benjamin F. Miller, "Observations on the Natural History of Renal Homotransplants in Dogs," *Surgical Forum* 5 (1955): 241–44.

14 Joseph E. Murray, "The Fight for Life," *Harvard Medicine*, Summer 2011, accessed March 27, 2022, https://hms.harvard.edu/magazine/science-emotion/fight-life.

15 John P. Merrill, Joseph E. Murray, J. Hartwell Harrison, and Warren R. Guild, "Successful Homotransplantation of the Human Kidney between Identical Twins," *Journal of the American Medical Association* 160, no. 4 (1956): 277–82.

16 Joseph E. Murray, "Ronald Lee Herrick Memorial: June 15, 1931–December 27, 2010," *American Journal of Transplantation* 11, no. 3 (2011): 419.

17 Joseph E. Murray, John P. Merrill, Gustave J. Dammin, J. Hartwell Harrison, Edward B. Hager, and Richard E. Wilson, "Current Evaluation of Human Kidney Transplantation," *Annals of the New York Academy of Sciences* 120, no. 2 (1965): 545–57; Joseph E. Murray, John P. Merrill, Gustave J. Dammin, James B. Dealy, Carl W. Walter, Marcus S. Brooke, and Richard E. Wilson, "Study on Transplantation Immunity after Total Body Irradiation: Clinical and Experimental Investigation," *Surgery* 48, no. 1 (1960): 272–84; Joseph E. Murray, John P. Merrill, Gustave J. Dammin, James B. Dealy Jr, Guy W. Alexandre, and J. Hartwell Harrison, "Kidney Transplantation in Modified Recipients," *Annals of Surgery* 156, no. 3 (1962): 337–55; Joseph E. Murray, John P. Merrill, J. Hartwell Harrison, Richard E. Wilson, and Gustave J. Dammin, "Prolonged Survival of Human-Kidney Homografts by Immunosuppressive Drug Therapy," *New England Journal of Medicine* 268, no. 24 (1963): 1315–23.

18 John P. Merrill, Joseph E. Murray, J. Hartwell Harrison, Eli A. Friedman, James B. Dealy Jr., and Gustave J. Dammin, "Successful Homotransplantation of the Kidney between Nonidentical Twins," *New England Journal of Medicine* 262, no. 25 (1960): 1251–60.

19 Michael F. A. Woodruff, J. S. Robson, J. A. Ross, B. Nolan, and Anne T. Lambie, "Transplantation of a Kidney from an Identical Twin," *Lancet* 277, no. 7189 (1961): 1245–49.

20 Roy Y. Calne, "The Inhibition of Renal Homograft Rejection in Dogs by 6-Mercaptopurine," *Lancet* 1 (1960): 417.

21 Roy Y. Calne and Joseph E. Murray, "Inhibition of the Rejection of Renal Homografts in Dogs by Burroughs Wellcome 57–322," *Surgical Forum*, no. 12: (1961) 118–20; Roy Y. Calne, G. P. J. Alexandre, and J. E. Murray, "A Study of the Effects of Drugs in Prolonging Survival of Homologous Renal Transplants in Dogs," *Annals of the New York Academy of Sciences* 99, no. 3 (1962): 743–61.

22 J. E. Murray et al., "Prolonged Survival of Human-Kidney Homografts by Immunosuppressive Drug Therapy."

23 C. F. Zukoski, H. M. Lee, and D. M. Hume, "The Effect of 6-Mercaptopurine on Renal Homograft Survival in the Dog," *Plastic and Reconstructive Surgery* 30, no. 1 (1962): 208–9; C. F. Zukoski, H. M. Lee, and D. M. Hume, "The Effect of Antimetabolites on Prolonging Functional Survival of Canine Renal Homografts," *Journal of Surgical Research* 2, no. 1 (1962): 44–48.

24 Michael F. A. Woodruff, B. Nolan, J. S. Robson, Anne T. Lambie, T. I. Wilson, and J. G. Clark, "Homotransplantation of Kidney in Patients Treated by Preoperative Local Irradiation and Postoperative Administration of an Antimetabolite (Imuran): Report of Six Cases," *Lancet* 282, no. 7309 (1963): 675–82.

25 Thomas E. Starzl, Thomas L. Marchioro, and William R. Waddell, "The Reversal of Rejection in Human Renal Homografts with Subsequent Development of Homograft Tolerance," *Surgery, Gynecology & Obstetrics* 117 (1963): 385–95.

26 Clyde F. Barker and James F. Markmann, "Historical Overview of Transplantation," *Cold Spring Harbor Perspectives in Medicine* 3, no. 4 (2013): a014977.

27 Francis D. Moore, "Common Patterns of Water and Electrolyte Change in Injury, Surgery and Disease," *New England Journal of Medicine* 258, no. 9 (1958): 427–32.

28 Nathan P. Couch, William J. Curran, and Francis D. Moore, "The Use of Cadaver Tissues in Transplantation," *New England Journal of Medicine* 271, no. 14 (1964): 691–95.

29 Henry K. Beecher, "The Powerful Placebo," *Journal of the American Medical Association* 159, no. 17 (1955): 1602–6.

30 Henry K. Beecher, "Experimentation in Man," *Journal of the American Medical Association* 169, no. 5 (1959): 461–78.

31 Henry K. Beecher, "Surgery as Placebo: A Quantitative Study of Bias," *Journal of the American Medical Association* 176, no. 13 (1961): 1102–7.

32 Joshua Mezrich, *How Death Becomes Life: Notes from a Transplant Surgeon* (New York: Harper, 2019).

33 Henry K. Beecher, "Ethics and Clinical Research," *New England Journal of Medicine* 244, no. 59 (1966): 1354–60.

34 Eelco F. M. Wijdicks, "The Neurologist and Harvard Criteria for Brain Death," *Neurology* 61, no. 7 (2003): 970–76.

35 Henry K. Beecher, "Ethical Problems Created by the Hopelessly Unconscious Patient," *New England Journal of Medicine* 278, no. 26 (1968): 1425–30.

36 Henry K. Beecher, "A Definition of Irreversible Coma: Report of the Ad Hoc Committee of the Harvard Medical School to Examine the Definition of Brain Death," *Journal of the American Medical Association* 205, no. 6 (1968): 337–60.

37 The only citation in Beecher's report is from Pope Pius XII's writing "The Prolongation of Life," published in 1958 in *Osservatore Romano*.

38 Francis D. Moore, "Changing Minds about Brains," *New England Journal of Medicine* 282, no. 1 (1970): 47–48; John Shillito Jr., "The Organ's Donor's Doctor: A New Role for the Neurosurgeon," *New England Journal of Medicine* 281, no. 19 (1969): 1071–72.

39 Robert D. Truog, Thaddeus Mason Pope, and David S. Jones. "The 50-Year Legacy of the Harvard Report on Brain Death," *Journal of the American Medical Association* 320, no. 4 (2018): 335–36.

40 Robert D. Truog, "The Uncertain Future of the Determination of Brain Death," *JAMA* 329, no. 12 (2023): 971–72.

41 Benjamin A. Barnes, "Survival Data of Renal Transplantations in Patients," *New England Journal of Medicine* 272, no. 15 (1965): 776–79.

42 Jean Dausset, "Iso-leuco-anticorps," *Acta Haematologica* 20, no. 1–4 (1958): 156–66.

43 Paul I. Terasaki, D. L. Vredevoe, M. R. Mickey, K. A. Porter, T. L. Marchioro, T. D. Faris, and Thomas E. Starzl, "Serotyping for Homotransplanation VII: Selection of Kidney Donors for Thirty-Two Recipients," *Annals of the New York Academy of Sciences* 129, no. 1 (1966): 500–520.

44 Ramon Patel and Paul I. Terasaki, "Significance of the Positive Crossmatch Test in Kidney Transplantation," *New England Journal of Medicine* 280, no. 14 (1969): 735–39.

45 Henry Krakauer, J. S. Grauman, M. R. McMullan, and C. C. Creede, "The Recent U.S. Experience in the Treatment of End-Stage Renal Disease by Dialysis and Transplantation," *New England Journal of Medicine* 308, no. 26 (1983): 1558–63.

46 Robert G. Luke, "Renal Replacement Therapy," *New England Journal of Medicine* 308, no. 26 (1983): 1593–95.

47 Francis D. Moore, Mitchell Goldman, and Christopher Gates, review of *The Courage to Fail: A Social View of Organ Transplantation and Dialysis*, by Renée C. Fox and Judith P. Swazey, *New England Journal of Medicine* 292, no. 12 (1975): 654.

48 Robert McCabe, review of *The Courage to Fail: A Social View of Organ Transplantation and Dialysis*, by Renée C. Fox and Judith P. Swazey, *JAMA* 230, no. 6 (1974): 906.

49 Erdman Palmore, review of *The Courage to Fail: A Social View of Organ Transplantation and Dialysis*, by Renée C. Fox and Judith P. Swazey, *Annals of Internal Medicine*, 81, (1974): 863.

50 Richard L. Simmons and Roberta G. Simmons, review of *The Courage to Fail: A Social View of Organ Transplantation and Dialysis*, by Renée C. Fox and Judith P. Swazey, *Journal of the History of Medicine and Allied Sciences* 30, no. 3 (1975): 286–87.

6. Hemodialysis Matures: It's All About the Money

1 Edmund G. Lowrie, J. Michael Lazarus, Altair J. Mocelin, George L. Bailey, Constantine L. Hampers, Richard E. Wilson, and John P. Merrill, "Survival of Patients Undergoing Chronic Hemodialysis and Renal Transplantation," *New England Journal of Medicine* 288, no. 17 (1973): 863–67.

2 Daniel S. Greenberg, "Washington Report," *New England Journal of Medicine* 298, no. 25 (1973): 1427–28.

3 John K. Iglehart, "Funding the End-Stage Renal-Disease Program," *New England Journal of Medicine* 306, no. 8 (1982): 492–96.

4 Arnold S. Relman, "Academic Medicine and the Public," *Journal of Clinical Investigation* 48, no. 6 (1969): 1169–71.

5 Arnold S. Relman, "The New Medical-Industrial Complex," *New England Journal of Medicine* 303, no. 17 (1980): 963–70.

6 Gina B. Kolata, "NMC Thrives Selling Dialysis," *Science* 208, no. 444225 (1980): 379–82; Gina B. Kolata, "Dialysis after Nearly a Decade," *Science* 208, no. 444302 (1980): 473–47.

7 Edmund G. Lowrie and C. L. Hampers, "The Success of Medicare's End-Stage Renal-Disease Program: The Case for Profits and the Private Marketplace," *New England Journal of Medicine* 305, no. 8 (1981): 434–38.

8 Tim McFeeley, *The Price of Access: The Story of Life and Death and Money and the First National Health Care Program and the Three Doctors Who Changed Medicine in America Forever* (Nashua, NH: MDL Press, 2001).

9 Levinsky and Rettig, *Kidney Failure and the Federal Government*.

10 Prakash Keshaviah and Fred L. Shapiro, "A Critical Examination of Dialysis-Induced Hypotension," *American Journal of Kidney Diseases* 2, no. 2 (1982): 290–301.

11 Juan P. Bosch, Robert Geronemus, Sheldon Glabman, Michael Lysaght, Thomas Kahn, and Beat von Albertini, "High Flux Hemofiltration," *Artificial Organs* 2, no. 4 (1978): 339–42.

12 Beat von Albertini, J. H. Miller, P. W. Gardner, and John H. Shinaberger, "High-Flux Hemodiafiltration: Under Six Hours/Week Treatment," *Transactions of the American Society for Artificial Internal Organs* 30 (1984): 227–31; J. H. Miller, Beat von Albertini, P. W. Gardner, and John H. Shinaberger, "Technical Aspects of High-Flux Hemodiafiltration for Adequate Short (under 2 Hours) Treatment," *Transactions of the American Society for Artificial Internal Organs* 30, no. 1 (1984): 377–81.

13 Edmund G. Lowrie, N. M. Laird, Thomas F. Parker, and John A. Sargent, "Effect of the Hemodialysis Prescription on Patient Morbidity: Report from the National Cooperative Dialysis Study," *New England Journal of Medicine* 305, no. 20 (1981): 1176–81.

14 Frank A. Gotch and John A. Sargent, "A Mechanistic Analysis of the National Cooperative Dialysis Study (NCDS)," *Kidney International* 28, no. 3 (1985): 526–34.

15 Henry Krakauer, J. S. Grauman, M. R. McMullan, and C. C. Creede, "The Recent U.S. Experience in the Treatment of End-Stage Renal Disease by Dialysis and Transplantation," *New England Journal of Medicine* 308, no. 26 (1983): 1558–63.

16 Thomas Parker, "Introduction and Summary: Proceedings from the Morbidity, Mortality and Prescription of Dialysis Symposium, Dallas, TX, September 15 to 17, 1989," *American Journal of Kidney Diseases* 15, no. 5 (1990): 375–83.

17 Other committee members included Drs. Roger W. Evans and Philip J. Held, respectively a sociologist and health economist and data scientist (who had a leadership role in the United States Renal Data System), with expertise in ESRD and quality of life. Internists with expertise in geriatrics, bioethics, health-care research and disparities, and epidemiology also participated. Two transplant surgeons were also committee members: Clive O. Callender, M.D., from the Howard University College of Medicine in Washington, D.C., renowned for his outspoken championship of access to transplantation for members of underrepresented minority groups, and Ronald M. Ferguson, M.D., Ph.D., who subsequently served as a president of the American Society of Transplant Surgeons.

18 Levinsky and Rettig, *Kidney Failure and the Federal Government*.

19 M. James Scherbenske, Ph.D., a renal physiologist at NIDDK, was chair of the planning committee for the Consensus Conference. The director of the Division of Kidney, Urologic, and Hematologic Diseases (DKUHD), Gary E. Striker, M.D., a distinguished renal pathologist; Lawrence Y. Agodoa, M.D., of DKUHD, a clinical nephrologist who had directed the Modification of Diet in Renal Disease (MDRD) and African American Study of Kidney Disease and Hypertension (AASK) studies for the NIDDK; and Gladys H. Hirschman, M.D., a pediatric nephrologist, of DKUHD also participated. Benjamin T. Burton, Ph.D., and Willis R. Foster, M.D., represented

the Disease Prevention and Technology Transfer group of the NIDDK. John H. Ferguson, M.D., and William Hall and Elsa Bray of OMAR served on the planning committee as well.

20 Jose A. Diaz-Buxo, M.D., of Metrolina Nephrology Associates, PA, in Charlotte, North Carolina; Raymond M. Hakim, M.D., Ph.D., of Vanderbilt University; Nathan W. Levin, M.D., originally from South Africa, from the Division of Nephrology at Beth Israel Medical Center, a part of the Mount Sinai system in New York, who had worked with Greenfield Systems, associated with the Henry Ford Hospital; and Thomas F. Parker III, M.D., of Dallas Nephrology Associates, who had hosted the Morbidity, Mortality, and Prescription of Dialysis Symposium, participated on the planning committee.

21 Edmund G. Lowrie and Nancy L. Lew, "Death Risk in Hemodialysis Patients: The Predictive Value of Commonly Measured Variables and an Evaluation of Death Rate Differences between Facilities," *American Journal of Kidney Diseases* 15, no. 5 (1990): 458–82.

22 William F. Owen Jr., Nancy L. Lew, Yan Liu, Edmund G. Lowrie, and J. Michael Lazarus, "The Urea Reduction Ratio and Serum Albumin Concentration as Predictors of Mortality in Patients Undergoing Hemodialysis," *New England Journal of Medicine* 329, no. 14 (1993): 1001–6.

23 Consensus Development Conference Panel, "Morbidity and Mortality of Renal Dialysis: An NIH Consensus Conference Statement," *Annals of Internal Medicine* 121, no. 1 (1994): 62–70.

24 External Advisory Committee members included Dr. Roland Blantz, a nephrologist and expert in kidney physiology; Dr. William Harmon, a pediatric nephrologist; Dr. Lawrence Hunsicker, a nephrologist and clinical trialist; Drs. Joel Kopple and William Mitch, nephrologists and leaders in studies of nutrition in patients with kidney disease; Dr. Allen Nissenson, a nephrologist with expertise in the treatment of hemodialysis patients and clinical trials; Dr. John Stokes, a nephrologist and expert in kidney physiology; and Drs. William Volmer and Robert Wolfe, biostatisticians with expertise in ESRD outcomes and clinical trials science.

25 Garabed Eknoyan, Gerald J. Beck, Alfred K. Cheung, John T. Daugirdas, Tom Greene, John W. Kusek, Michael Allon et al., "Effect of Dialysis Dose and Membrane Flux in Maintenance Hemodialysis," *New England Journal of Medicine* 347, no. 25 (2002): 2010–19.

7. A Triumph of Molecular Biology and the Excesses of Corporate Greed

1 John W. Adamson, Joseph W. Eschbach, and Melvin B. Dennis, "Physiologic Studies in Normal and Uremic Sheep I: The Experimental Model," *Kidney International* 18, no. 6 (1980): 725–31.

2 John W. Adamson, Joseph W. Eschbach, and Clement A. Finch, "The Kidney and Erythropoiesis," *American Journal of Medicine* 44, no. 5 (1968): 725–33.

3 Joseph W. Eschbach Jr., D. Funk, John Adamson, I. Kuhn, Belding H. Scribner, and Clement A. Finch, "Erythropoiesis in Patients with Renal Failure Undergoing Chronic Dialysis," *New England Journal of Medicine* 276, no. 12 (1967): 653–58.

4   L. O. Jacobson, Eugene Goldwasser, W. Fried, and L. Plzak, "Role of the Kidney in Erythropoiesis," *Nature* 179 (1957): 633–34.

5   Paul Carnot and C. Deflandre, "Sur l'activité cytopoietique du sang et des organs regeneres au cours des regeneration du sang," *Comptes rendus de l'Académie des Sciences (Paris)* 143 (1906): 432–35.

6   E. V. A. Bonsdorff and E. Jalavisto, "A Humoral Mechanism in Anoxic Erythrocytosis," *Acta Physiologica Scandinavica* 16, no. 2–3 (1948): 150–70.

7   Joseph W. Eschbach and John W. Adamson, "Anemia of End-Stage Renal Disease (ESRD)," *Kidney International* 28, no. 1 (1985): 1–5.

8   Axel Ullrich, John Shine, John Chirgwin, Raymond Pictet, Edmund Tischer, William J. Rutter, and Howard M. Goodman, "Rat Insulin Genes: Construction of Plasmids Containing the Coding Sequences," *Science* 196, no. 4296 (1977): 1313–19.

9   Lydia Villa-Komaroff, Argiris Efstratiadis, Stephanie Broome, Peter Lomedico, Richard Tizard, Stephen P. Naber, William L. Chick, and Walter Gilbert, "A Bacterial Clone Synthesizing Proinsulin," *Proceedings of the National Academy of Sciences* 75, no. 8 (1978): 3727–31.

10 David V. Goeddel, Dennis G. Kleid, Francisco Bolivar, Herbert L. Heyneker, Daniel G. Yansura, Roberto Crea, Tadaaki Hirose, Adam Kraszewski, Keiichi Itakura, and Arthur D. Riggs, "Expression in *Escherichia Coli* of Chemically Synthesized Genes for Human Insulin," *Proceedings of the National Academy of Sciences* 76, no. 1 (1979): 106–10.

11 John R. Richardson and Morton B. Weinstein, "Erythropoietic Response of Dialyzed Patients to Testosterone Administration," *Annals of Internal Medicine* 73, no. 3 (1970): 403–7.

12 Walter Fried, Olga Jonasson, Gordon Lang, and Franklin Schwartz, "The Hematologic Effect of Androgen in Uremic Patients: Study of Packed Cell Volume and Erythropoietin Responses," *Annals of Internal Medicine* 79, no. 6 (1973): 823–27.

13 Joseph W. Eschbach and John W. Adamson, "Improvement in the Anemia of Chronic Renal Failure with Fluoxymesterone," *Annals of Internal Medicine* 78, no. 4 (1973): 527–32.

14 Takaji Miyake, Charles K. Kung, and Eugene Goldwasser, "Purification of Human Erythropoietin," *Journal of Biological Chemistry* 252, no. 15 (1977): 5558–64.

15 Sylvia Lee-Huang, "Cloning and Expression of Human Erythropoietin cDNA in Escherichia Coli," *Proceedings of the National Academy of Sciences* 81, no. 9 (1984): 2708–12.

16 Kenneth Jacobs, Charles Shoemaker, Richard Rudersdorf, Suzanne D. Neill, Randal J. Kaufman, Allan Mufson, Jasbir Seehra et al., "Isolation and Characterization of Genomic and cDNA Clones of Human Erythropoietin," *Nature* 313, no. 6005 (1985): 806–10.

17 Fu-Kuen Lin, Sidney Suggs, Chi-Hwei Lin, Jeffrey K. Browne, Ralph Smalling, Joan C. Egrie, Kenneth K. Chen, Gary M. Fox, Frank Martin, and Zippora Stabinsky, "Cloning and Expression of the Human Erythropoietin Gene," *Proceedings of the National Academy of Sciences* 82, no. 22 (1985): 7580–84.

18 P. H. Lai, Richard Everett, Fung-Fung Wang, Tsutomu Arakawa, and Eugene Goldwasser, "Structural Characterization of Human Erythropoietin," *Journal of Biological Chemistry* 261, no. 7 (1986): 3116–21.

19 Christopher G. Winearls, D. O. Oliver, M. J. Pippard, C. Reid, M. R. Downing, and P. M. Cotes, "Effect of Human Erythropoietin Derived from Recombinant DNA on the Anaemia of Patients Maintained by Chronic Haemodialysis," *Lancet* 2, no. 8517 (1986): 1175–78.

20 Joseph W. Eschbach, Joan C. Egrie, Michael R. Downing, Jeffrey K. Browne, and John W. Adamson, "Correction of the Anemia of End-Stage Renal Disease with Recombinant Human Erythropoietin," *New England Journal of Medicine* 316, no. 2 (1987): 73–78.

21 Joseph W. Eschbach, Michael R. Kelly, N. Rebecca Haley, Robert I. Abels, and John W. Adamson. "Treatment of the Anemia of Progressive Renal Failure with Recombinant Human Erythropoietin," *New England Journal of Medicine* 321, no. 3 (1989): 158–63.

22 Joseph W. Eschbach, Mohamed H. Abdulhadi, Jeffrey K. Browne, Barbara G. Delano, Michael R. Downing, Joan C. Egrie, Roger W. Evans et al., "Recombinant Human Erythropoietin in Anemic Patients with End-Stage Renal Disease: Results of a Phase III Multicenter Clinical Trial," *Annals of Internal Medicine* 111, no. 12 (1989): 992–1000.

23 Roger W. Evans, Diane L. Manninen, Louis P. Garrison Jr., L. Gary Hart, Christopher R. Blagg, Robert A. Gutman, Alan R. Hull, and Edmund G. Lowrie, "The Quality of Life of Patients with End-Stage Renal Disease," *New England Journal of Medicine* 312, no. 9 (1985): 553–59.

24 Kathleen Sharp, *Blood Feud: The Man Who Blew the Whistle on One of the Deadliest Prescription Drugs Ever*, Center of Medical Consumers (New York: Dutton, 2011).

25 *Ortho Pharmaceutical Corporation v. Amgen, Inc.*, Appellant, 882 F.2d 806 [3d Cir. 1989].

26 R. W. Evans et al, "Quality of Life of Patients with End-Stage Renal Disease."

27 Robert A. Gutman, William W. Stead, and Roscoe R. Robinson, "Physical Activity and Employment Status of Patients on Maintenance Dialysis," *New England Journal of Medicine* 304, no. 6 (1981): 309–13.

28 Roger W. Evans, Barbara Rader, and Diane L. Manninen, "The Quality of Life of Hemodialysis Recipients Treated with Recombinant Human Erythropoietin," *JAMA* 263, no. 6 (1990): 825–30.

29 Allan J. Erslev, "Erythropoietin," *New England Journal of Medicine* 324, no. 19 (1991): 1339–44.

30 Juan P. Bosch, Anna Saccaggi, Allan Lauer, Claudio Ronco, Mario Belledonne, and Sheldon Glabman, "Renal Functional Reserve in Humans: Effect of Protein Intake on Glomerular Filtration Rate," *American Journal of Medicine* 75, no. 6 (1983): 943–50.

31 Allan Lauer, Anna Saccaggi, Claudio Ronco, Mario Belledonne, Sheldon Glabman, and Juan P. Bosch, "Continuous Arteriovenous Hemofiltration in the Critically Ill Patient: Clinical Use and Operational Characteristics," *Annals of Internal Medicine* 99, no. 4 (1983): 455–60.

32 Neil R. Powe, Robert I. Griffiths, Gregory de Lissovoy, Gerard F. Anderson, Alan J. Watson, Joel W. Greer, Robert J. Herbert, Paul W. Eggers, Roger A. Milam, and Paul K. Whelton, "Access to Recombinant Erythropoietin by Medicare-Entitled Dialysis Patients in the First Year after FDA Approval," *JAMA* 268, no. 11 (1992): 1434–40.

33 Anatole Besarab, W. Kline Bolton, Jeffrey K. Browne, Joan C. Egrie, Allen R. Nissenson, Douglas M. Okamoto, Steve J. Schwab, and David A. Goodkin, "The Effects of Normal as Compared with Low Hematocrit Values in Patients with Cardiac

Disease Who Are Receiving Hemodialysis and Epoetin," *New England Journal of Medicine* 339, no. 9 (1998): 584–90.

34 David A. Goodkin, "The Normal Hematocrit Cardiac Trial Revisited," *Seminars in Dialysis* 22, no. 5 (2009): 495–502.

35 John W. Adamson and Joseph W. Eschbach, "Erythropoietin for End-Stage Renal Disease," *New England Journal of Medicine* 339, no. 9 (1998): 625–27.

36 Dennis J. Cotter, Mae Thamer, Paul L. Kimmel, and John H. Sadler, "Secular Trends in Recombinant Erythropoietin Therapy among the US Hemodialysis Population: 1990–1996," *Kidney International* 54, no. 6 (1998): 2129–39.

37 Nicole Casadevall, Joelle Nataf, Beatrice Viron, Amir Kolta, Jean-Jacques Kiladjian, Philippe Martin-Dupont, Patrick Michaud et al., "Pure Red-Cell Aplasia and Antierythropoietin Antibodies in Patients Treated with Recombinant Erythropoietin," *New England Journal of Medicine* 346, no. 7 (2002): 469–75.

38 William F. Owen Jr., Nancy L. Lew, Yan Liu, Edmund G. Lowrie, and J. Michael Lazarus, "The Urea Reduction Ratio and Serum Albumin Concentration as Predictors of Mortality in Patients Undergoing Hemodialysis," *New England Journal of Medicine* 329, no. 14 (1993): 1001–6.

39 Ajay K. Singh, Lynda Szczech, Kezhen L. Tang, Huiman Barnhart, Shelly Sapp, Marsha Wolfson, and Donal Reddan, "Correction of Anemia with Epoetin Alfa in Chronic Kidney Disease," *New England Journal of Medicine* 355, no. 20 (2006): 2085–98.

40 Tilman B. Drüeke, Francesco Locatelli, Naomi Clyne, Kai-Uwe Eckardt, Iain C. Macdougall, Dimitrios Tsakiris, Hans-Ulrich Burger, and Armin Scherhag, "Normalization of Hemoglobin Level in Patients with Chronic Kidney Disease and Anemia," *New England Journal of Medicine* 355, no. 20 (2006): 2071–84.

41 Giuseppe Remuzzi and Julie R. Ingelfinger, "Correction of Anemia—Payoffs and Problems," *New England Journal of Medicine* 355, no. 20 (2006): 2144–46.

42 Robert Steinbrook, "Medicare and Erythropoietin," *New England Journal of Medicine* 356, no. 1 (2007): 4–6.

43 Mae Thamer, Yi Zhang, James Kaufman, Dennis Cotter, Fan Dong, and Miguel A. Hernan, "Dialysis Facility Ownership and Epoetin Dosing in Patients Receiving Hemodialysis," *JAMA* 297, no. 15 (2007): 1667–74.

44 Daniel W. Coyne, "Use of Epoetin in Chronic Renal Failure," *JAMA* 297, no. 15 (2007): 1713–16.

45 Fadlo R. Khuri, "Weighing the Hazards of Erythropoiesis Stimulation in Patients with Cancer," *New England Journal of Medicine* 356, no. 24 (2007): 2445–48.

46 Robert Steinbrook, "Erythropoietin, the FDA, and Oncology," *New England Journal of Medicine* 356, no. 24 (2007): 2448–51.

47 Marc A. Pfeffer, Emmanuel A. Burdmann, Chao-Yin Chen, Mark E. Cooper, Dick De Zeeuw, Kai-Uwe Eckardt, Jan M. Feyzi et al., "A Trial of Darbepoetin Alfa in Type 2 Diabetes and Chronic Kidney Disease," *New England Journal of Medicine* 361, no. 21 (2009): 2019–32.

48 Erslev, "Erythropoietin."

49 Scott D. Solomon, Hajime Uno, Eldrin F. Lewis, Kai-Uwe Eckardt, Julie Lin, Emmanuel A. Burdmann, Dick De Zeeuw et al., "Erythropoietic Response and

Outcomes in Kidney Disease and Type 2 Diabetes," *New England Journal of Medicine* 363, no. 12 (2010): 1146–55.

50 Ellis F. Unger, Aliza M. Thompson, Melanie J. Blank, and Robert Temple. "Erythropoiesis-Stimulating Agents—Time for a Reevaluation," *New England Journal of Medicine* 362, no. 3 (2010): 189–92.

51 Steven Fishbane, Brigitte Schiller, Francesco Locatelli, Adrian C. Covic, Robert Provenzano, Andrzej Wiecek, Nathan W. Levin et al., "Peginesatide in Patients with Anemia Undergoing Hemodialysis," *New England Journal of Medicine* 368, no. 4 (2013): 307–19.

52 Tilman B. Drüeke, "Anemia Treatment in Patients with Chronic Kidney Disease," *New England Journal of Medicine* 368, no. 4 (2013): 387–89.

53 Charles L. Bennett, Sony Jacob, Jeffrey Hymes, Len A. Usvyat, and Franklin W. Maddux, "Anaphylaxis and Hypotension after Administration of Peginesatide," *New England Journal of Medicine* 370, no. 21 (2014): 2055–56.

54 Gregg L. Semenza, "Hypoxia-Inducible Factors in Physiology and Medicine," *Cell* 148, no. 3 (2012): 399–408; Jay B. Wish, "Treatment of Anemia in Kidney Disease: Beyond Erythropoietin," *Kidney International Reports* 6, no. 10 (2021): 2540–53; Daniel W. Coyne, David Goldsmith, and Iain C. Macdougall, "New Options for the Anemia of Chronic Kidney Disease," *Kidney International Supplements* 7, no. 3 (2017): 157–63.

55 Nobel Prize in Phsyiology or Medicine 2019, "Nobel Assembly at Karolinska Institutet Has Today Decided to Award the 2019 Nobel Prize in Physiology or Medicine Jointly to William G. Kaelin Jr., Sir Peter J. Ratcliffe, and Gregg L. Semenza for Their Discoveries of How Cells Sense and Adapt to Oxygen Availability," press release, October 7, 2019, accessed May 20, 2023, https://www.nobelprize.org/prizes/medicine/2019/press-release.

56 Anatole Besarab, Robert Provenzano, Joachim Hertel, Raja Zabaneh, Stephen J. Klaus, Tyson Lee, Robert Leong, Stefan Hemmerich, Kin-Hung Peony Yu, and Thomas B. Neff, "Randomized Placebo-Controlled Dose-Ranging and Pharmacodynamics Study of Roxadustat (FG-4592) to Treat Anemia in Nondialysis-Dependent Chronic Kidney Disease (NDD-CKD) Patients," *Nephrology Dialysis Transplantation* 30, no. 10 (2015): 1665–73; Robert Provenzano, Anatole Besarab, Chao H. Sun, Susan A. Diamond, John H. Durham, Jose L. Cangiano, Joseph R. Aiello et al., "Oral Hypoxia–Inducible Factor Prolyl Hydroxylase Inhibitor Roxadustat (FG-4592) for the Treatment of Anemia in Patients with CKD," *Clinical Journal of the American Society of Nephrology* 11, no. 6 (2016): 982–91; Robert Provenzano, Anatole Besarab, Steven Wright, Sohan Dua, Steven Zeig, Peter Nguyen, Lona Poole et al., "Roxadustat (FG-4592) versus Epoetin Alfa for Anemia in Patients Receiving Maintenance Hemodialysis: A Phase 2, Randomized, 6- to 19-Week, Open-Label, Active-Comparator, Dose-Ranging, Safety and Exploratory Efficacy Study," *American Journal of Kidney Diseases* 67, no. 6 (2016): 912–24.

57 Nan Chen, Chuanming Hao, Bi-Cheng Liu, Hongli Lin, Caili Wang, Changying Xing, Xinling Liang et al., "Roxadustat Treatment for Anemia in Patients Undergoing Long-Term Dialysis," *New England Journal of Medicine* 381, no. 11 (2019): 1011–22.

58 Nan Chen, Chuanming Hao, Xiaomei Peng, Hongli Lin, Aiping Yin, Li Hao, Ye Tao et al., "Roxadustat for Anemia in Patients with Kidney Disease Not Receiving Dialysis," *New England Journal of Medicine* 381, no. 11 (2019): 1001–10.

59 Nonvoting FDA participants included Ellis F. Unger, M.D., the director of the Office of Cardiology, Hematology, Endocrinology, and Nephrology (OCHEN) in the Office of New Drugs (OND) in CDER, who was an author of the FDA paper on ESAs in the *NEJM*. Ann T. Farrell, M.D., a hematologist and medical oncologist and the director of the Division of Non-Malignant Hematology (DNH), OCHEN, OND, CDER; Saleh Ayache, M.D., clinical reviewer, DNH, OCHEN, OND, CDER; and Jae Joon Song, Ph.D., statistical reviewer, Division of Biometrics, Office of Biostatistics, Office of Translational Sciences, CDER, also participated in the meeting. The designated federal officer was Joyce Yu, Pharm.D., of the Division of Advisory Committee and Consultant Management, Office of Executive Programs, at CDER. Ms. Jacqueline D. Alikhaani, of Los Angeles, California, served as the consumer representative, for the American Heart Association. Jerome Rossert, M.D., Ph.D., vice president and head of Clinical Renal at AstraZeneca in Gaithersburg, Maryland, was on the roster as a nonvoting representative of industry. David G. Soergel, M.D., a pediatric cardiologist and the global head of Cardiovascular, Renal, and Metabolism Development of Novartis Pharma, based in East Hanover, New Jersey, was the actual attendee in that capacity at the meeting. Voting members of the committee included Thomas D. Cook, Ph.D., M.S., M.A., a professor in the Department of Biostatistics and Medical Informatics at the University of Wisconsin, Madison; Christopher M. O'Connor, M.D., M.A.C.C., F.E.S.C., F.H.F.A., F.H.F.S.A., professor of medicine at Duke University and president and executive director of the Inova Heart and Vascular Institute, in Falls Church, Virginia; C. Noel Bairey Merz, M.D., F.A.C.C., F.A.H.A., F.E.S.C., the director of the Barbra Streisand Women's Health Center at Cedars-Sinai Medical Center in Los Angeles, California; Edward K. Kasper, M.D., F.A.C.C., F.A.H.A., the director of the Outpatient Cardiology Program at the Johns Hopkins School of Medicine in Baltimore, Maryland; David J. Moliterno, M.D., professor and chairman of the Department of Internal Medicine at the University of Kentucky Medical Center; and Ravi I. Thadhani, M.D., M.P.H., professor of medicine and dean for Academic Programs at Harvard Medical School in Boston, Massachusetts.

Temporary voting members included Leslie S. Cho, M.D., F.A.C.C., F.S.C.A.I., F.E.S.C., the section head of Preventive Cardiology and Rehabilitation and professor of medicine at the Cleveland Clinic Lerner College of Medicine, Case Western Reserve Medical School in Cleveland Ohio; Susan T. Crowley, M.D., M.B.A., F.A.S.N., professor of medicine at Yale University and director of the National Kidney Disease and Dialysis Program at the Veterans Health Administration; Milton Packer, M.D., distinguished scholar in cardiovascular medicine at Baylor Heart and Vascular Institute in Dallas, Texas; Afshin Parsa, M.D., M.P.H., from the NIDDK; and Thomas J. Wang, M.D., professor and chair of the Department of Internal Medicine at the University of Texas Southwestern Medical Center, in Dallas, Texas.

60 The transcript of the meeting can be accessed at https://www.fda.gov/advisory -committees/advisory-committee-calendar/updated-time-information-july-15-2021 -meeting-cardiovascular-and-renal-drugs-advisory-committee#event-materials.

61 Ajay K. Singh, Kevin Carroll, Vlado Perkovic, Scott Solomon, Vivekanand Jha, Kirsten L. Johansen, Renato D. Lopes et al., "Daprodustat for the Treatment of Anemia in Patients Undergoing Dialysis," *New England Journal of Medicine* 385, no. 25

(2021): 2325–35; Ajay K. Singh, Kevin Carroll, John J. V. McMurray, Scott Solomon, Vivekanand Jha, Kirsten L. Johansen, Renato D. Lopes et al., "Daprodustat for the Treatment of Anemia in Patients Not Undergoing Dialysis," *New England Journal of Medicine* 385, no. 25 (2021): 2313–24.

62 Jessica Seo, Pharm.D., was the designated federal officer. FDA staff at the meeting included Tanya Wroblewski, M.D.; Justin Penzenstadler, Pharm.D.; Hylton V. Joffe, M.D., M.M.Sc.; and Van Tran, Ph.D., as well as others. Committee members who had not participated in the roxadustat meeting included Javid Butler, M.D., M.P.H., M.B.A., a cardiologist and distinguished professor of medicine and chairman of the Department of Medicine at the University of Mississippi, who attended the meeting. Kevin C. Abbott, M.D., M.P.H., a nephrologist at NIDDK; Patrick Nachman, M.D., F.A.S.N., a nephrologist and professor of medicine at the University of Minnesota; and Emilia Bagiella, Ph.D., professor of biostatistics at the Icahn School of Medicine at Mount Sinai had joined the committee. The transcript of the meeting can be accessed at Food and Drug Administration Center for Drug Evaluation and Research, Cardiovascular and Renal Drugs Advisory Committee (CRDAC) Meeting, October 26, 2022, https://www.fda.gov/media/164052/download.

63 Janet K. Freburger, Leslie J. Ng, Brian D. Bradbury, Abhijit V. Kshirsagar, and M. Alan Brookhart, "Changing Patterns of Anemia Management in US Hemodialysis Patients," *American Journal of Medicine* 125, no. 9 (2012): 906–14.

64 Marc N. Turenne, Elizabeth L. Cope, Shannon Porenta, Purna Mukhopadhyay, Douglas S. Fuller, Jeffrey M. Pearson, Claudia Dahlerus, Brett Lantz, Francesca Tentori, and Bruce M. Robinson, "Has Dialysis Payment Reform Led to Initial Racial Disparities in Anemia and Mineral Metabolism Management?," *Journal of the American Society of Nephrology* 26, no. 3 (2015): 754–64.

65 John Danziger, Kenneth J. Mukamal, and Eric Weinhandl, "Associations of Community Water Lead Concentrations with Hemoglobin Concentrations and Erythropoietin-Stimulating Agent Use among Patients with Advanced CKD," *Journal of the American Society of Nephrology* 32, no. 10 (2021): 2425–34.

66 Rudolph A. Rodriguez, Saunak Sen, Kala Mehta, Sandra Moody-Ayers, Peter Bacchetti, and Ann M. O'Hare. "Geography Matters: Relationships among Urban Residential Segregation, Dialysis Facilities, and Patient Outcomes," *Annals of Internal Medicine* 146, no. 7 (2007): 493–501.

67 Arnold S. Relman, "The New Medical-Industrial Complex," *New England Journal of Medicine* 303, no. 17 (1980): 963–70.

68 John Geyman, "The Business Ethic vs. Service Ethic in US Health Care: Which Will Prevail?," *Pharos*, Winter 2022: 41.

8. APOL1: Genetics of Kidney Disease, Race, and Equity

1 Michael Harington, Priscilla Kincaid-Smith, and J. McMichael, "Results of Treatment in Malignant Hypertension," *British Medical Journal* 2, no. 5158 (1959): 969–80; W. Grobin, "Malignant Hypertension and Its Treatment," *Canadian Medical Association Journal* 82, no. 11 (1960): 600–601; James W. Woods and William B. Blythe,

"Management of Malignant Hypertension Complicated by Renal Insufficiency," *New England Journal of Medicine* 277, no. 2 (1967): 57–61; E. Z. Rabin, "Malignant Hypertension," *Canadian Medical Association Journal* 118, no. 8 (1978): 941–43; C. H. Gold, C. Isaacson, and J. Levin, "The Pathological Basis of End-Stage Renal Disease in Blacks," *South African Medical Journal* 61, no. 8 (1982): 263–65.

2 Henry Krakauer, J. S. Grauman, M. R. McMullan, and C. C. Creede, "The Recent US Experience in the Treatment of End-Stage Renal Disease by Dialysis and Transplantation," *New England Journal of Medicine* 308, no. 26 (1983): 1558–63.

3 Elizabeth R. Seaquist, Frederick C. Goetz, Stephen Rich, and José Barbosa, "Familial Clustering of Diabetic Kidney Disease," *New England Journal of Medicine* 320, no. 18 (1989): 1161–65.

4 Donna M. Brown, Abraham P. Provoost, Mark J. Daly, Eric S. Lander, and Howard J. Jacob, "Renal Disease Susceptibility and Hypertension Are under Independent Genetic Control in the Fawn-Hooded Rat," *Nature Genetics* 12, no. 1 (1996): 44–51.

5 Louise M. McKenzie, Sher L. Hendrickson, William A. Briggs, Richard A. Dart, Stephen M. Korbet, Michelle H. Mokrzycki, Paul L. Kimmel et al., "NPHS2 Variation in Sporadic Focal Segmental Glomerulosclerosis," *Journal of the American Society of Nephrology* 18, no. 11 (2007): 2987–95.

6 Jeffrey B. Kopp, Michael W. Smith, George W. Nelson, Randall C. Johnson, Barry I. Freedman, Donald W. Bowden, Taras Oleksyk et al., "MYH9 Is a Major-Effect Risk Gene for Focal Segmental Glomerulosclerosis," *Nature Genetics* 40, no. 10 (2008): 1175–84; W. H. Linda Kao, Michael J. Klag, Lucy A. Meoni, David Reich, Yvette Berthier-Schaad, Man Li, Josef Coresh et al., "MYH9 Is Associated with Nondiabetic End-Stage Renal Disease in African Americans," *Nature Genetics* 40, no. 10 (2008): 1185–92.

7 Giulio Genovese, David J. Friedman, Michael D. Ross, Laurence Lecordier, Pierrick Uzureau, Barry I. Freedman, Donald W. Bowden, et al., "Association of Trypanolytic ApoL1 Variants with Kidney Disease in African Americans," *Science* 329, no. 5993 (2010): 841–45.

8 Afshin Parsa, W. H. Linda Kao, Dawei Xie, Brad C. Astor, Man Li, Chi-yuan Hsu, Harold I. Feldman et al., "APOL1 Risk Variants, Race, and Progression of Chronic Kidney Disease," *New England Journal of Medicine* 369, no. 23 (2013): 2183–96.

9 Emily E. Groopman, Gundula Povysil, David B. Goldstein, and Ali G. Gharavi, "Rare Genetic Causes of Complex Kidney and Urological Diseases," *Nature Reviews Nephrology* 16, no. 11 (2020): 641–56; Dervia M. Connaughton, Claire Kennedy, Shirlee Shril, Nina Mann, Susan L. Murray, Patrick A. Williams, Eoin Conlon et al., "Monogenic Causes of Chronic Kidney Disease in Adults," *Kidney International* 95, no. 4 (2019): 914–28.

10 Clinical Centers in the consortium include Wake Forest University, Columbia University (with the University of Pennsylvania), Mount Sinai Medical School (with Cornell University) in New York City, the University of California at San Francisco, Washington University in Saint Louis, the Cleveland Clinic, the University of Wisconsin, Johns Hopkins University, the University of Maryland, Vanderbilt University, Emory University, the University of Alabama, the University of Miami, and the Joslin Clinic and collaborators.

11 Ogo Egbuna, Brandon Zimmerman, George Manos, Anne Fortier, Madalina C. Chirieac, Leslie A. Dakin, David J. Friedman et al., "Inaxaplin for Proteinuric Kidney Disease in Persons with Two APOL1 Variants," *New England Journal of Medicine* 388, no. 11 (2023): 969–79.

12 Winfred W. Williams and Julie R. Ingelfinger, "Inhibiting APOL1 to Treat Kidney Disease," *New England Journal of Medicine* 388, no. 11 (2023): 1045–49.

13 Neil R. Powe, "A Step Forward for Precision Equity in Kidney Disease," *New England Journal of Medicine* 388, no. 11 (2023): 1043–44.

9. Maturity of Kidney Transplantation: Clinical Success and Lingering Inequities

1 Jean P. Borel, A. Vieillard, and A. Randoux, "Effect of Some Purified Plasma Proteins on Collagen Biosynthesis In Vitro," *Agents and Actions* 6 (1976): 207–10.

2 Jean F. Borel, Camille Feurer, C. Magnee, and Hartmann Stähelin, "Effects of the New Anti-Lymphocytic Peptide Cyclosporin A in Animals," *Immunology* 32, no. 6 (1977): 1017–25.

3 Jean F. Borel, and Dorothee Wiesinger," Studies on the Mechanism of Action of Cyclosporin A [Proceedings]," *British Journal of Pharmacology* 66, no. 1 (1979): 66P–67P.

4 Dorothee Wiesinger and Jean F. Borel, "Studies on the Mechanism of Action of Cyclosporin A." *Immunobiology* 156, no. 4–5 (1980): 454–63.

5 Roy Y. Calne, D. J. G. White, Keith Rolles, D. P. Smith, and B. M. Herbertson. "Prolonged Survival of Pig Orthotopic Heart Grafts Treated with Cyclosporin A," *Lancet* 311, no. 8075 (1978): 1183–85.

6 Roy Y. Calne, Kirk Rolles, Sathia Thiru, P. McMaster, G. N. Craddock, S. Aziz, D. J. G. White et al., "Cyclosporin A Initially as the Only Immunosuppressant in 34 Recipients of Cadaveric Organs: 32 Kidneys, 2 Pancreases, and 2 Livers," *Lancet* 314, no. 8151 (1979): 1033–36.

7 Thomas E. Starzl, Richard Weil III, Shunzaburo Iwatsuki, Goran Klintmalm, Gerhard P. J. Schröter, Lawrence J. Koep, Yuichi Iwaki, Paul I. Terasaki, and Kendrick A. Porter, "The Use of Cyclosporin A and Prednisone in Cadaver Kidney Transplantation," *Surgery, Gynecology & Obstetrics* 151, no. 1 (1980): 17–26.

8 European Multicentre Trial Group, "Cyclosporin A as Sole Immunosuppressive Agent in Recipients of Kidney Allografts from Cadaver Donors," *Lancet* 2 (1982): 57–60.

9 R. M. Ferguson, J. J. Rynasiewicz, D. E. Sutherland, R. L. Simmons, and J. S. Najarian, "Cyclosporin A in Renal Transplantation: A Prospective Randomized Trial," *Surgery* 92, no. 2 (1982): 175–82.

10 F. Harder, R. Loertscher, Roy Y. Calne, D. J. G. White, R. Pichlmayr, J. Klempnauer, R. Margreiter et al., "Steroid-Free Treatment of Renal Transplant Patients with Cyclosporin A: A European Multicentre Study," *Klinische Wochenschrift* 60 (1982): 1137–42.

11 Thomas R. Hakala, Thomas E. Starzl, J. T. Rosenthal, B. Shaw, and S. Iwatsuki, "Cadaveric Renal Transplantation with Cyclosporin-A and Steroids," *Transplantation Proceedings* 15, no. 1, 465–70; J. Thomas Rosenthal, Thomas R. Hakala, Shunzaburo

Iwatsuki, Byers W. Shaw Jr, and Thomas E. Starzl, "Cadaveric Renal Transplantation under Cyclosporine-Steroid Therapy," *Surgery, Gynecology & Obstetrics* 157, no. 4 (1983): 309.

12 Canadian Multicentre Transplant Study Group, "A Randomized Clinical Trial of Cyclosporine in Cadaveric Renal Transplantation," *New England Journal of Medicine* 309, no. 14 (1983): 809–15.

13 Robert M. Merion, David J. G. White, Sathia Thiru, David B. Evans, and Roy Y. Calne, "Cyclosporine: Five Years' Experience in Cadaveric Renal Transplantation," *New England Journal of Medicine* 310, no. 3 (1984): 148–54.

14 Bryan D. Myers, Jon Ross, Lynn Newton, John Luetscher, and Mark Perlroth, "Cyclosporine-Associated Chronic Nephropathy," *New England Journal of Medicine* 311, no. 11 (1984): 699–705.

15 Roger W. Evans, Diane L. Manninen, Louis P. Garrison Jr., L. Gary Hart, Christopher R. Blagg, Robert A. Gutman, Alan R. Hull, and Edmund G. Lowrie, "The Quality of Life of Patients with End-Stage Renal Disease," *New England Journal of Medicine* 312, no. 9 (1985): 553–59.

16 John P. Johnson, Clark R. McCauley, and John B. Copley, "The Quality of Life of Hemodialysis and Transplant Patients," *Kidney International* 22, no. 3 (1982): 286–91.

17 Angus Campbell, Philip E. Converse, and Willard L. Rodgers, *The Quality of American Life: Perceptions, Evaluations, and Satisfactions* (New York: Russell Sage Foundation, 1976).

18 Roberta G. Simmons, Susan D. Klein, and Richard L. Simmons, *Gift of Life: The Social and Psychological Impact of Organ Transplantation* (New York: Wiley, 1977); Renée Claire Fox and Judith P. Swazey, *The Courage to Fail: A Social View of Organ Transplants and Dialysis* (New Brunswick, NJ: Transaction Publishers, 1974).

19 Paul W. Eggers, "Effect of Transplantation on the Medicare End-Stage Renal Disease Program," *New England Journal of Medicine* 318, no. 4 (1988): 223–29.

20 Henry Krakauer, J. S. Grauman, M. R. McMullan, and C. C. Creede, "The Recent US Experience in the Treatment of End-Stage Renal Disease by Dialysis and Transplantation," *New England Journal of Medicine* 308, no. 26 (1983): 1558–63.

21 Gerhard Opelz and Paul I. Terasaki, "Improvement of Kidney-Graft Survival with Increased Numbers of Blood Transfusions," *New England Journal of Medicine* 299, no. 15 (1978): 799–803.

22 Steve Takemoto, Paul I. Terasaki, J. Michael Cecka, Yong W. Cho, and David W. Gjertson. "Survival of Nationally Shared, HLA-matched Kidney Transplants from Cadaveric Donors." *New England Journal of Medicine* 327, no. 12 (1992): 834–839.

23 Steve Takemoto, Paul I. Terasaki, David W. Gjertson, and J. Michael Cecka, "Equitable Allocation of HLA-compatible Kidneys for Local Pools and for Minorities," *New England Journal of Medicine* 331, no. 12 (1994): 760–64.

24 Philip J. Held, Barry D. Kahan, Lawrence G. Hunsicker, David Liska, Robert A. Wolfe, Friedrich K. Port, Daniel S. Gaylin, Jose R. Garcia, Lawrence Agodoa, and Henry Krakauer, "The Impact of HLA Mismatches on the Survival of First Cadaveric Kidney Transplants," *New England Journal of Medicine* 331, no. 12 (1994): 765–70.

25 Fred Sanfilippo, "HLA Matching in Renal Transplantation" *New England Journal of Medicine* 331, no. 12 (1994): 803–805.

26 NIDDK, "Transplantation," chap. 7 in *United States Renal Data System Annual Report*, 2022, figures 7.10b and 7.2, https://usrds-adr.niddk.nih.gov/2022/end-stage-renal-disease/7-transplantation.

27 Sally L. Satel, ed., *When Altruism Isn't Enough: The Case for Compensating Kidney Donors* (Washington, D.C.: AEI Press, 2008).

28 Carl M. Kjellstrand, "Age, Sex, and Race Inequality in Renal Transplantation," *Archives of Internal Medicine* 148, no. 6 (1988): 1305–9.

29 Daisy Reyes, Susie Q. Lew, and Paul L. Kimmel, "Gender Differences in Hypertension and Kidney Disease," *Medical Clinics* 89, no. 3 (2005): 613–30.

30 Phyllis August and Manikkam Suthanthiran, "Sex and Kidney Transplantation: Why Can't a Woman Be More Like a Man?" *Journal of the American Society of Nephrology: JASN* 28, no. 10 (2017): 2829–31.

31 Anette Melk, Birgit Babitsch, Bianca Borchert-Mörlins, Frans Claas, Anne I. Dipchand, Sandra Eifert, Britta Eiz-Vesper et al., "Equally Interchangeable? How Sex and Gender Affect Transplantation," *Transplantation* 103, no. 6 (2019): 1094–110.

32 Paul W. Eggers, "Racial Differences in Access to Kidney Transplantation," *Health Care Financing Review* 17, no. 2 (1995): 89–103.

33 John M. Weller, Shu-Chen Wu, C. William Ferguson, and Friedrich K. Port, "Influence of Race of Cadaveric Kidney Donor and Recipient on Graft Survival: A Multifactorial Analysis," *American Journal of Kidney Diseases* 9, no. 3 (1987): 191–99.

34 S. John Swanson, Iman O. Hypolite, Lawrence Y. C. Agodoa, D. Scott Batty Jr., Paul B. Hshieh, David Cruess, Allan D. Kirk, Thomas G. Peters, and Kevin C. Abbott, "Effect of Donor Factors on Early Graft Survival in Adult Cadaveric Renal Transplantation," *American Journal of Transplantation* 2, no. 1 (2002): 68–75.

35 Bertram L. Kasiske, John F. Neylan III, Robert R. Riggio, Gabriel M. Danovitch, Lawrence Kahana, Steven R. Alexander, and Martin G. White, "The Effect of Race on Access and Outcome in Transplantation," *New England Journal of Medicine* 324, no. 5 (1991): 302–7.

36 G. Caleb Alexander and Ashwini R. Sehgal, "Barriers to Cadaveric Renal Transplantation among Blacks, Women, and the Poor," *JAMA* 280, no. 13 (1998): 1148–52.

37 Pushkal P. Garg, Kevin D. Frick, Marie Diener-West, and Neil R. Powe, "Effect of the Ownership of Dialysis Facilities on Patients' Survival and Referral for Transplantation," *New England Journal of Medicine* 341, no. 22 (1999): 1653–60.

38 Levinsky and Rettig, *Kidney Failure and the Federal Government*.

39 John Z. Ayanian, Paul D. Cleary, Joel S. Weissman, and Arnold M. Epstein, "The Effect of Patients' Preferences on Racial Differences in Access to Renal Transplantation," *New England Journal of Medicine* 341, no. 22 (1999): 1661–69.

40 Norman G. Levinsky, "Quality and Equity in Dialysis and Renal Transplantation," *New England Journal of Medicine* 341, no. 22 (1999): 1691–93.

41 Robert A. Wolfe, Valarie B. Ashby, Edgar L. Milford, Akinlolu O. Ojo, Robert E. Ettenger, Lawrence Y. C. Agodoa, Philip J. Held, and Friedrich K. Port, "Comparison of Mortality in All Patients on Dialysis, Patients on Dialysis Awaiting Transplantation, and Recipients of a First Cadaveric Transplant," *New England Journal of Medicine* 341, no. 23 (1999): 1725–30.

42 Jesse D. Schold, Sumit Mohan, Anne Huml, Laura D. Buccini, John R. Sedor, Joshua J. Augustine, and Emilio D. Poggio, "Failure to Advance Access to Kidney Transplantation over Two Decades in the United States," *Journal of the American Society of Nephrology* 32, no. 4 (2021): 913–26.

43 Vikas R. Dharnidharka, Paolo Fiorina, and William E. Harmon, "Kidney Transplantation in Children," *New England Journal of Medicine* 371, no. 6 (2014): 549–58.

44 Maria E. Ferris, Debbie S. Gipson, Paul L. Kimmel, and Paul W. Eggers, "Trends in Treatment and Outcomes of Survival of Adolescents Initiating End-Stage Renal Disease Care in the United States of America," *Pediatric Nephrology* 21 (2006): 1020–26.

45 Adan Z. Becerra, Kevin E. Chan, Paul W. Eggers, Jenna Norton, Paul L. Kimmel, Ivonne H. Schulman, and Susan R. Mendley, "Transplantation Mediates Much of the Racial Disparity in Survival from Childhood-Onset Kidney Failure," *Journal of the American Society of Nephrology* 33, no. 7 (2022): 1265–75.

46 Krista L. Lentine, Jodi M. Smith, Jonathan M. Miller, Keighly Bradbrook, Lindsay Larkin, Samantha Weiss, Dzhuliyana K. Handarova et al., "OPTN/SRTR 2021 Annual Data Report: Kidney," Health and Resources Administration, U.S. Department of Health & Human Resources, accessed April 2023, https://srtr.transplant.hrsa.gov/annual_reports/2021/Kidney.aspx.

47 Sharon M. Bartosh, Glen Leverson, Delores Robillard, and Hans W. Sollinger, "Long-Term Outcomes in Pediatric Renal Transplant Recipients Who Survive into Adulthood," *Transplantation* 76, no. 8 (2003): 1195–1200.

48 Philip F. Halloran, Konrad S. Famulski, and Jeff Reeve, "Molecular Assessment of Disease States in Kidney Transplant Biopsy Samples," *Nature Reviews Nephrology* 12, no. 9 (2016): 534–48.

49 Mannikam Suthanthiran and Terry B. Strom, "Renal Transplantation," *New England Journal of Medicine* 331, no. 6 (1994): 365–76.

50 Baogui Li, Choli Hartono, Ruchuang Ding, Vijay K. Sharma, Ravi Ramaswamy, Biao Qian, David Serur, Janet Mouradian, Joseph E. Schwartz, and Manikkam Suthanthiran, "Noninvasive Diagnosis of Renal-Allograft Rejection by Measurement of Messenger RNA for Perforin and Granzyme B in Urine," *New England Journal of Medicine* 344, no. 13 (2001): 947–54.

51 Thangamani Muthukumar, Darshana Dadhania, Ruchuang Ding, Catherine Snopkowski, Rubina Naqvi, Jun B. Lee, Choli Hartono et al., "Messenger RNA for FOXP3 in the Urine of Renal-Allograft Recipients," *New England Journal of Medicine* 353, no. 22 (2005): 2342–51.

52 Mannikam Suthanthiran, Joseph E. Schwartz, Ruchuang Ding, Michael Abecassis, Darshana Dadhania, Benjamin Samstein, Stuart J. Knechtle et al., "Urinary-Cell mRNA Profile and Acute Cellular Rejection in Kidney Allografts," *New England Journal of Medicine* 369, no. 1 (2013): 20–31.

53 Aude Dorison, Thomas A. Forbes, and Melissa H. Little, "What Can We Learn from Kidney Organoids?" *Kidney International* 102, no. 5 (2022): 1013–29.

54 Peter P. Reese, Peter L. Abt, Emily A. Blumberg, and David S. Goldberg, "Transplanting Hepatitis C-Positive Kidneys," *New England Journal of Medicine* 373, no. 4 (2015): 303–5.

55 David S. Goldberg, Peter L. Abt, Emily A. Blumberg, Vivianna M. Van Deerlin, Matthew Levine, K. Rajender Reddy, Roy D. Bloom et al., "Trial of Transplantation of HCV-Infected Kidneys into Uninfected Recipients," *New England Journal of Medicine* 376, no. 24 (2017): 2394–95.

56 Prem Kumar, James E. Pearson, David H. Martin, Stephen H. Leech, Paul D. Buisseret, Helen C. Bezbak, Francisco M. Gonzalez, John R. Royer, H. Z. Streicher, and W. Carl Saxinger, "Transmission of Human Immunodeficiency Virus by Transplantation of a Renal Allograft, with Development of the Acquired Immunodeficiency Syndrome," *Annals of Internal Medicine* 106, no. 2 (1987): 244–45.

57 Aaron Spital, "Should All Human Immunodeficiency Virus-Infected Patients with End-Stage Renal Disease Be Excluded from Transplantation?: The Views of US Transplant Centers," *Transplantation* 65, no. 9 (1998): 1187–91.

58 Paul C. Kuo and Peter G. Stock, "Transplantation in the HIV+ Patient," *American Journal of Transplantation* 1, no. 1 (2001): 13–17.

59 Paul J. Gow, Deenan Pillay, and David Mutimer, "Solid Organ Transplantation in Patients with HIV Infection," *Transplantation* 72, no. 2 (2001): 177–81.

60 Peter G. Stock, Michelle E. Roland, Laurie Carlson, Chris E. Freise, John P. Roberts, Ryutaro Hirose, Norah A. Terrault et al., "Kidney and Liver Transplantation in Human Immunodeficiency Virus-Infected Patients: A Pilot Safety and Efficacy Study," *Transplantation* 76, no. 2 (2003): 370–75.

61 M. E. Roland, B. Barin, L. Carlson, L. A. Frassetto, N. A. Terrault, R. Hirose, C. E. Freise et al., "HIV-infected Liver and Kidney Transplant Recipients: 1-and 3-year Outcomes," *American Journal of Transplantation* 8, no. 2 (2008): 355–65.

62 Peter G. Stock, Burc Barin, Barbara Murphy, Douglas Hanto, Jorge M. Diego, Jimmy Light, Charles Davis et al., "Outcomes of Kidney Transplantation in HIV-Infected Recipients," *New England Journal of Medicine* 363, no. 21 (2010): 2004–14.

63 Elmi Muller, Delawir Kahn, and Marc Mendelson, "Renal Transplantation between HIV-Positive Donors and Recipients," *New England Journal of Medicine* 362, no. 24 (2010): 2336–37.

64 Elmi Muller, Zunaid Barday, Marc Mendelson, and Delawir Kahn, "HIV-Positive–to–HIV-Positive Kidney Transplantation—Results at 3 to 5 Years," *New England Journal of Medicine* 372, no. 7 (2015): 613–20.

65 Phillipe Selhorst, Catharina E. Combrinck, Kathryn Manning, Francois C. J. Botha, Jan P. L. Labuschagne, Colin Anthony, David L. Matten et al., "Longer-Term Outcomes of HIV-Positive–to–HIV-Positive Renal Transplantation," *New England Journal of Medicine* 381, no. 14 (2019): 1387–89.

66 Jayme E. Locke, Robert A. Montgomery, Daniel S. Warren, Aruna Subramanian, and Dorry L. Segev, "Renal Transplant in HIV-Positive Patients: Long-Term Outcomes and Risk Factors for Graft Loss," *Archives of Surgery* 144, no. 1 (2009): 83–86.

67 Brian J. Boyarsky, Erin C. Hall, Andrew L. Singer, Robert A. Montgomery, Kelly A. Gebo, and Dorry L. Segev, "Estimating the Potential Pool of HIV-Infected Deceased Organ Donors in the United States," *American Journal of Transplantation* 11, no. 6 (2011): 1209–17.

68 Brian J. Boyarsky, C. M. Durand, F. J. Palella Jr., and D. L. Segev, "Challenges and Clinical Decision-Making in HIV-to-HIV Transplantation: Insights from the HIV Literature," *American Journal of Transplantation* 15, no. 8 (2015): 2023–30.

69 Brian J. Boyarsky and Dorry L. Segev, "From Bench to Bill: How a Transplant Nuance Became 1 of Only 57 Laws Passed in 2013," *Annals of Surgery* 263, no. 3 (2016): 430–33.

70 Christine M. Durand, Dorry Segev, and Jeremy Sugarman, "Realizing HOPE: The Ethics of Organ Transplantation from HIV-Positive Donors," *Annals of Internal Medicine* 165, no. 2 (2016): 138–42.

71 Brianna Doby, Aaron A. R. Tobian, Dorry L. Segev, and Christine M. Durand, "Moving from the HOPE Act to HOPE in Action: Changing Practice and Challenging Stigma," *Current Opinion in Organ Transplantation* 23, no. 2 (2018): 271–78.

72 Michael A. Kolber, "HIV Solid Organ Transplantation: Looking beyond HOPE," *AIDS* 32, no. 13 (2018): 1733–36.

73 Brian J. Boyarsky, Mary Grace Bowring, Ashton A. Shaffer, Dorry L. Segev, and Christine M. Durand, "The Future of HOPE Is Now: The State of HIV+ to HIV+ Kidney Transplantation in the United States," *Current Opinion in Organ Transplantation* 24, no. 4 (2019): 434–40.

74 Christine M. Durand, Wanying Zhang, Diane M. Brown, Sile Yu, Niraj Desai, Andrew D. Redd, Serena M. Bagnasco et al., "A Prospective Multicenter Pilot Study of HIV-Positive Deceased Donor to HIV-Positive Recipient Kidney Transplantation: HOPE in Action," *American Journal of Transplantation* 21, no. 5 (2021): 1754–64.

75 Michael A. Rees, Jonathan E. Kopke, Ronald P. Pelletier, Dorry L. Segev, Matthew E. Rutter, Alfredo J. Fabrega, Jeffrey Rogers et al., "A Nonsimultaneous, Extended, Altruistic-Donor Chain," *New England Journal of Medicine* 360, no. 11 (2009): 1096–101.

76 Robert A. Montgomery, Robert A., Bonnie E. Lonze, Karen E. King, Edward S. Kraus, Lauren M. Kucirka, Jayme E. Locke, Daniel S. Warren et al., "Desensitization in HLA-Incompatible Kidney Recipients and Survival," *New England Journal of Medicine* 365, no. 4 (2011): 318–26.

77 Robert A. Montgomery, "Renal Transplantation across HLA and ABO Antibody Barriers: Integrating Paired Donation into Desensitization Protocols," *American Journal of Transplantation* 10, no. 3 (2010): 449–57.

78 Amber M. Reeves-Daniel, John A. DePalma, Anthony J. Bleyer, Michael V. Rocco, Mariana Murea, Patricia L. Adams, Carl D. Langefeld et al., "The APOL1 Gene and Allograft Survival after Kidney Transplantation," *American Journal of Transplantation* 11, no. 5 (2011): 1025–30.

79 Barry I. Freedman, Marva M. Moxey-Mims, Amir A. Alexander, Brad C. Astor, Kelly A. Birdwell, Donald W. Bowden, Gordon Bowen et al., "APOL1 Long-Term Kidney Transplantation Outcomes Network (APOLLO): Design and Rationale," *Kidney International Reports* 5, no. 3 (2020): 278–88.

80 Flavio Vincenti, Lionel Rostaing, Joseph Grinyo, Kim Rice, Steven Steinberg, Luis Gaite, Marie-Christine Moal et al., "Belatacept and Long-Term Outcomes in Kidney Transplantation," *New England Journal of Medicine* 374, no. 4 (2016): 333–43.

81 NIDDK, *United States Renal Data System Annual Report*, 2022.

82 Dominique Bertrand, Mouad Hamzaoui, Veronique Lemée, Julie Lamulle, Mélanie Hanoy, Charlotte Laurent, Ludivine Lebourg et al., "Antibody and T Cell Response to SARS-CoV-2 Messenger RNA BNT162b2 Vaccine in Kidney Transplant Recipients and Hemodialysis Patients," *Journal of the American Society of Nephrology* 32, no. 9 (2021): 2147–52.

83 J. H. Ng, J. S. Hirsch, R. Wanchoo, M. Sachdeva, V. Sakhiya, S. Hong, K. D. Jhaveri, S. Fishbane, and Northwell COVID-19 Research Consortium and the Northwell Nephrology COVID-19 Research Consortium, "Outcomes of Patients with End-Stage Kidney Disease Hospitalized with COVID-19," *Kidney International* 98, no. 1530–1539 (2020): 10–1016; Debasish Banerjee, Joyce Popoola, Sapna Shah, Irina Chis Ster, Virginia Quan, and Mysore Phanish, "COVID-19 Infection in Kidney Transplant Recipients," *Kidney International* 97, no. 6 (2020): 1076–82; Kubra Aydin Bahat, Ergun Parmaksiz, and Serap Sert, "The Clinical Characteristics and Course of COVID-19 in Hemodialysis Patients," *Hemodialysis International* 24, no. 4 (2020): 534–40; Jennifer E. Flythe, Magdalene M. Assimon, Matthew J. Tugman, Emily H. Chang, Shruti Gupta, Jatan Shah, Marie Anne Sosa et al., "Characteristics and Outcomes of Individuals with Pre-existing Kidney Disease and COVID-19 Admitted to Intensive Care Units in the United States," *American Journal of Kidney Diseases* 77, no. 2 (2021): 190–203.

84 Ruth Cooper, Megan Snair, and Laura Aiuppa Denning, *Exploring the State of the Science of Solid Organ Transplantation and Disability: Proceedings of a Workshop* (Washington, D.C.: National Academies Press, 2021).

85 Monica Fox, "Barriers to Kidney Transplantation in Racial/Ethnic Minorities," *Clinical Journal of the American Society of Nephrology* 16, no. 2 (2021): 177–78.

86 Vanessa Grubbs, *Hundreds of Interlaced Fingers: A Kidney Doctor's Search for the Perfect Match* (New York: HarperCollins, 2017).

87 Morgan E. Grams, Yingying Sang, Andrew S. Levey, Kunihiro Matsushita, Shoshana Ballew, Alex R. Chang, Eric K. H. Chow et al., "Kidney-Failure Risk Projection for the Living Kidney-Donor Candidate," *New England Journal of Medicine* 374, no. 5 (2016): 411–21.

88 Bertram L. Kasiske, Tracy L. Anderson-Haag, Daniel A. Duprez, Roberto S. Kalil, Paul L. Kimmel, Todd E. Pesavento, Jon J. Snyder, and Matthew R. Weir, "A Prospective Controlled Study of Metabolic and Physiologic Effects of Kidney Donation Suggests That Donors Retain Stable Kidney Function over the First Nine Years," *Kidney International* 98, no. 1 (2020): 168–75.

89 David Wojciechowski and Alexander Wiseman, "Long-Term Immunosuppression Management: Opportunities and Uncertainties," *Clinical Journal of the American Society of Nephrology* 16, no. 8 (2021): 1264–71.

90 Clive O. Callender, Patrice V. Miles, Margruetta B. Hall, and Sherilyn Gordon, "Blacks and Whites and Kidney Transplantation: A Disparity! But Why and Why Won't It Go Away?," *Transplantation Reviews* 16, no. 3 (2002): 163–76; Aaron Spital, Clive O. Callender, and Patrice V. Miles, "Ethical Issues in Dialysis: Institutionalized Racism and End-Stage Renal Disease; Is Its Impact Real or Illusionary?," *Seminars in Dialysis* 17, no. 3 (2004): 177–80; Paul L. Kimmel, Chyng-Wen Fwu, and Paul W. Eggers, "Segregation, Income Disparities, and Survival in Hemodialysis Patients," *Journal of the American Society of Nephrology* 24, no. 2 (2013): 293–301; Jenna M. Norton, Marva M. Moxey-Mims, Paul W. Eggers, Andrew S. Narva, Robert A. Star, Paul L. Kimmel, and Griffin P. Rodgers, "Social Determinants of Racial Disparities in CKD," *Journal of the American Society of Nephrology* 27, no. 9 (2016): 2576–95; Deidra C. Crews and Tanjala S. Purnell, "COVID-19, Racism, and Racial Disparities in Kidney Disease: Galvanizing the Kidney Community Response," *Journal of the*

American Society of Nephrology 31, no. 8 (2020): 1–3; Neil R. Powe, "The Pathogenesis of Race and Ethnic Disparities: Targets for Achieving Health Equity," *Clinical Journal of the American Society of Nephrology* 1, no. 5 (2021): 806–8; Ebony L. Boulware and Dinushika Mohottige, "The Seen and the Unseen: Race and Social Inequities Affecting Kidney Care," *Clinical Journal of the American Society of Nephrology* 16, no. 5 (2021): 815–17; Jessica P. Cerdeña, Jennifer Tsai, and Vanessa Grubbs, "APOL1, Black Race, and Kidney Disease: Turning Attention to Structural Racism," *American Journal of Kidney Diseases* 77, no. 6 (2021): 857–60; Dinushika Mohottige, Clarissa J. Diamantidis, Keith C. Norris, and L. Ebony Boulware, "Racism and Kidney Health: Turning Equity into a Reality," *American Journal of Kidney Diseases* 77, no. 6 (2021): 951–62; Jesse D. Schold, Sumit Mohan, Anne Huml, Laura D. Buccini, John R. Sedor, Joshua J. Augustine, and Emilio D. Poggio, "Failure to Advance Access to Kidney Transplantation over Two Decades in the United States," *Journal of the American Society of Nephrology* 32, no. 4 (2021): 913–26; John S. Gill, Burnett Kelly, and Marcello Tonelli. "Time to Abolish Metrics That Sustain Systemic Racism in Kidney Allocation," *JAMA* 329, no. 11 (2023): 879–80; Deidra C. Crews, Rachel E. Patzer, Lilia Cervantes, Richard Knight, Tanjala S. Purnell, Neil R. Powe, Dawn P. Edwards, and Keith C. Norris, "Designing Interventions Addressing Structural Racism to Reduce Kidney Health Disparities: A Report from a National Institute of Diabetes and Digestive and Kidney Diseases Workshop," *Journal of the American Society of Nephrology* 33, no. 12 (2022): 2141–52.

Epilogue

1 Eric D. Weinhandl, David T. Gilbertson, James B. Wetmore, and Kirsten L. Johansen, "COVID-19–Associated Decline in the Size of the End-Stage Kidney Disease Population in the United States," *Kidney International Reports* 6, no. 10 (2021): 2698.

2 Mitchell H. Rosner, Charles R. Manley, Edward V. Hickey III, and Jeffrey S. Berns, "Stakeholder Theory and For-Profit Dialysis: A Call for Greater Accountability," *Clinical Journal of the American Society of Nephrology* 18 (2023): 1225–27.

3 Peter J. Blankestijn, Robin W. M. Vernooij, Carinna Hockham, Giovanni F. M. Strippoli, Bernard Canaud, Jörgen Hegbrant, Claudia Barth et al., "Effect of Hemodiafiltration or Hemodialysis on Mortality in Kidney Failure," *New England Journal of Medicine* (2023): 700–709.

4 RFAs DK 22–014 and DK 22–015.

5 Steven Neu and Carl M. Kjellstrand, "Stopping Long-Term Dialysis," *New England Journal of Medicine* 314, no. 1 (1986): 14–20.

6 Mark E. Neumann, "Novelist Michener Dies after Withdrawing from Dialysis," *Nephrology News & Issues* 11, no. 12 (1997): 60–62.

7 Jenny H. C. Chen, Wai H. Lim, and Prue Howson, "Changing Landscape of Dialysis Withdrawal in Patients with Kidney Failure: Implications for Clinical Practice," *Nephrology* 27, no. 7 (2022): 551–65.

8 James B. Wetmore, Nicholas S. Roetker, David T. Gilbertson, and Jiannong Liu. "Early Withdrawal and Non-withdrawal Death in the Months Following Hemodialysis

Initiation: A Retrospective Cohort Analysis," *Hemodialysis International* 23, no. 2 (2019): 261–72.

9   Esther N. M. de Roijj, Yvette Meuleman, Johan W. de Fijter, Saskia Le Cessie, Kitty J. Jager, Nicholas C. Chesnaye, Marie Evans et al., "Quality of Life before and after the Start of Dialysis in Older Patients," *Clinical Journal of the American Society of Nephrology* 17, no. 8 (2022): 1159–67.

10 Jorge I. Fonseca-Correa and S. Vanita Jassal, "Health Care for Older Adults with Kidney Failure," *Clinical Journal of the American Society of Nephrology* 17, no. 8 (2022): 1110–12.

11 Daniel Cukor, Nisha Ver Halen, Deborah Rosenthal Asher, Jeremy D. Coplan, Jeremy Weedon, Katarzyna E. Wyka, Subodh J. Saggi, and Paul L. Kimmel, "Psychosocial Intervention Improves Depression, Quality of Life, and Fluid Adherence in Hemodialysis," *Journal of the American Society of Nephrology* 25, no. 1 (2014): 196–206.

12 S. Susan Hedayati, L. Parker Gregg, Thomas Carmody, Nishank Jain, Marisa Toups, A. John Rush, Robert D. Toto, and Madhukar H. Trivedi, "Effect of Sertraline on Depressive Symptoms in Patients with Chronic Kidney Disease without Dialysis Dependence: The CAST Randomized Clinical Trial," *JAMA* 318, no. 19 (2017): 1876–90.

13 Rajnish Mehrotra, Daniel Cukor, Mark Unruh, Tessa Rue, Patrick Heagerty, Scott D. Cohen, Laura M. Dember et al., "Comparative Efficacy of Therapies for Treatment of Depression for Patients Undergoing Maintenance Hemodialysis: A Randomized Clinical Trial," *Annals of Internal Medicine* 170, no. 6 (2019): 369–79.

14 Yitzchak M. Binik, Andrew G. Baker, Dennis Kalogeropoulos, Gerald M. Devins, Ronald D. Guttmann, David J. Hollomby, Paul E. Barré, Tom Hutchison, Michel Prud'Homme, and Lise McMullen, "Pain, Control over Treatment, and Compliance in Dialysis and Transplant Patients," *Kidney International* 21, no. 6 (1982): 840–48.

15 Paul L. Kimmel, Chyng-Wen Fwu, Kevin C. Abbott, Anne W. Eggers, Prudence P. Kline, and Paul W. Eggers, "Opioid Prescription, Morbidity, and Mortality in United States Dialysis Patients," *Journal of the American Society of Nephrology* 28, no. 12 (2017): 3658–70.

16 Daniel G. Tobin, Mark B. Lockwood, Paul L. Kimmel, Laura M. Dember, Nwamaka D. Eneanya, Manisha Jhamb, Thomas D. Nolin, William C. Becker, Michael J. Fischer, and HOPE Consortium, "Opioids for Chronic Pain Management in Patients with Dialysis-Dependent Kidney Failure," *Nature Reviews Nephrology* 18, no. 2 (2022): 113–28; Carrie E. Brintz, Martin D. Cheatle, Laura M. Dember, Alicia A. Heapy, Manisha Jhamb, Amanda J. Shallcross, Jennifer L. Steel, Paul L. Kimmel, Daniel Cukor, and HOPE Consortium, "Nonpharmacologic Treatments for Opioid Reduction in Patients with Advanced Chronic Kidney Disease," *Seminars in Nephrology* 41, no. 1 (2021): 68–81.

17 Paige M. Porrett, Babak J. Orandi, Vineeta Kumar, Julie Houp, Douglas Anderson, A. Cozette Killian, Vera Hauptfeld-Dolejsek et al., "First Clinical-Grade Porcine Kidney Xenotransplant Using a Human Decedent Model," *American Journal of Transplantation* 22, no. 4 (2022): 1037–53.

18 Robert A. Montgomery, Jeffrey M. Stern, Bonnie E. Lonze, Vasishta S. Tatapudi, Massimo Mangiola, Ming Wu, Elaina Weldon et al., "Results of Two Cases of

Pig-to-Human Kidney Xenotransplantation," *New England Journal of Medicine* 386, no. 20 (2022): 1889–98.

19 Event materials for the meeting can be accessed at https://www.fda.gov/advisory -committees/advisory-committee-calendar/updated-contact-information-october -26-2022-meeting-cardiovascular-and-renal-drugs-advisory#event-materials.

20 Bartley P. Griffith, Corbin E. Goerlich, Avneesh K. Singh, Martine Rothblatt, Christine L. Lau, Aakash Shah, Marc Lorber et al., "Genetically Modified Porcine-to-Human Cardiac Xenotransplantation," *New England Journal of Medicine* 387, no. 1 (2022): 35–44.

21 Lesley A. Inker, Nwamaka D. Eneanya, Josef Coresh, Hocine Tighiouart, Dan Wang, Yingying Sang, Deidra C. Crews et al., "New Creatinine- and Cystatin C–Based Equations to Estimate GFR without Race," *New England Journal of Medicine* 385, no. 19 (2021): 1737–49.

22 Akinlolu Ojo, "Eliminating Racial Inequities in Kidney Health: Much More Than Revising Estimating Equations," *Annals of Internal Medicine* 175, no. 3 (2022): 446–47; Jennifer Bragg-Gresham, Xiaosong Zhang, Dao Le, Michael Heung, Vahakn Shahinian, Hal Morgenstern, and Rajiv Saran, "Prevalence of Chronic Kidney Disease among Black Individuals in the US after Removal of the Black Race Coefficient from a Glomerular Filtration Rate Estimating Equation," *JAMA Network Open* 4, no. 1 (2021): e2035636–e2035636; Pierre Delanaye, Hans Pottel, and Richard J. Glassock, "Americentrism in Estimation of Glomerular Filtration Rate Equations," *Kidney International* 101, no. 5 (2022): 856–58; Chi-yuan Hsu and Alan S. Go, "The Race Coefficient in Glomerular Filtration Rate-Estimating Equations and Its Removal," *Current Opinion in Nephrology and Hypertension* 31, no. 6 (2022): 527–33.

INDEX